Sacred Science

HISTORY AND PHILOSOPHY OF SCIENCE

Heresy, Crossroads, and Intersections

Paolo Palmieri
General Editor

Vol. 6

The History and Philosophy of Science series is part of the Peter Lang Humanities list.
Every volume is peer reviewed and meets
the highest quality standards for content and production.

PETER LANG
New York • Bern • Frankfurt • Berlin
Brussels • Vienna • Oxford • Warsaw

Gregory V. Loewen

Sacred Science

Ritual and Miracle in Modern Medicine

PETER LANG
New York • Bern • Frankfurt • Berlin
Brussels • Vienna • Oxford • Warsaw

Library of Congress Cataloging-in-Publication Data

Names: Loewen, Gregory V., author.
Title: Sacred science: ritual and miracle in modern medicine / Gregory V. Loewen.
Description: New York: Peter Lang, 2017.
Series: History and philosophy of science: heresy, crossroads, and intersections; vol. 6
ISSN 2376-6336 (print) | ISSN 2376-6344 (online)
Includes bibliographical references.
Identifiers: LCCN 2017030387 | ISBN 978-1-4331-4328-1 (hardback: alk. paper)
ISBN 978-1-4331-43298- (ebook pdf) | ISBN 978-1-4331-4330-4 (epub)
ISBN 978-1-4331-4331-1 (mobi)
Subjects: LCSH: Medicine—Religious aspects. | Health—Religious aspects. | Miracles.
Classification: LCC BL65.M4 L64 2017 | DDC 201/.7621—dc23
LC record available at https://lccn.loc.gov/2017030387
DOI 10.3726/b11638

Bibliographic information published by **Die Deutsche Nationalbibliothek**.
Die Deutsche Nationalbibliothek lists this publication in the "Deutsche Nationalbibliografie"; detailed bibliographic data are available on the Internet at http://dnb.d-nb.de/.

29 Broadway, 18th floor, New York, NY 10006
www.peterlang.com

To Dr. G. M. Loewen, M.D., who has spent his life in the service of overcoming human suffering

The highest blessing possible for a human to possess is the health of his body. (Plato, *Gorgias*, 452).

Table of Contents

INTRODUCTION

The Séance of Science

Introduction

In our time, science has assumed the mantle of religion. It is a discursive Napoleon, taking from the metaphysical Pope the vaunted crown of empire and placing it upon its own brow. Its practitioners are not so much appointed, but anointed. This applies especially to those who practice the applied sciences, engineering and medicine. But while the former occupies itself with the world as it is and eschews most extrapolation from the mundane circumstance of utility, the latter aspires to far more. Science may have supplanted religion, but its ultimate purpose and meaning for humankind remains the same: immortality. And medicine constitutes the vanguard of our collective aspiration to become immortal. As the gods had been, so we will be.

That other hit machine of modernity, engineering, certainly elicits both applause and admiration, even awe. But if this or that particular building or bridge, or even if close proximity fly-by images of the Pluto system of planetoids or some such other panorama did not exist, few would lose sleep about it. No, it is medicine that makes us tremble with anticipation and shake with resentful rage. For while engineering constructs the externality of being, medicine reconstructs ontology itself. Engineering makes our mortality more bearable, but medicine holds out the promise of its obsolescence.

And medicine is distinctly personal. Far from the building blocks of infancy and the Legos of youth, the body of most young human beings is in itself both a time capsule and a time-bomb. Genetic proclivities may both aid and sabotage its long term viability. Things can come up at the most unexpected of times, offering to ourselves the most obscene circumstances. Oftentimes it makes the news: an adolescent dying of a rare genetic cancer or heart defect. In countries without universal health care systems a call goes out the community for help. It might be better said that a call *goeth* out, given the link between the idea of godhead still prevalent in such regions and the sense that human beings have much less right to intervene in 'fate'. One is destined to suffer on this earth.

But such places are now becoming almost as rare as the afflictions that so animate them, the United States being the most obvious and blatant example of this general link between religion and health. To secularize health, however, means to make the science of it sacred, and how that has been done over the previous decades, as well as how that transition has been analyzed, is the subject of this book.

In order to chart the dual career of sacralization and secularization, each representing the obverse of the same coin—the coin itself an amalgam of both objective health and how one feels about being 'healthy'; what is health as a scientific construct and what does it mean to be healthy as a person, both physically and mentally etc.—we must look in turn to the boundaries that mark the limits of health and healthiness respectively, as well as the both the dividends and the deficits that accrue to those who dwell within or without these limits. What is it to be the same thing as the ideal type of objectified fully functional living body, or living being? How does the concept of saneness derive from sameness, and then in its own turn exhort its maintenance? What can and cannot be within the boundedness of sacral science in its methods and epistemologies, or again, within the less-blessed half-acre of secular subjectivity, the arc of how one 'feels' today? The much-vaunted dualism between body and mind aside, contemporary discourse is littered with the most exacting references to the sanctions separating what the patient thinks he or she is experiencing and what they are actually undergoing, or what they must do to undergo it and what the doctor is undertaking as a procedure or a treatment. They rarely, if ever, fully identify with each other. Yet one can certainly suggest that the subjectivity of health has also become its own object. Psychoanalysis is merely the most famous example of this. The introduction of homeopathic medicine, or should we rather say, its reintroduction, is a case in point. Allopathic medicine, the medicine of the object, is still dominant. But given the placebo effect and related social facts, alternative health regimes from all over the world have been slowly let in the back door of the applied science edifice, gradually taking more and more a part in the drama of immortality without being shunned as mere melodrama.

This history, perhaps more than any other, demonstrates both the link between fetish and cult, between ideal and real, between end and means. Immortality, whether through artificial intelligence surrogates, cyber-organic prosthesis or some other hitherto unthought of experiment, is merely a reflection of the apparent and presumed general *failure* of modern medicine to make good on its design. No doubt mortal beings become impatient with their mortality over time, both as an individual life course and within a contemporary history that often seems to be a combination of three steps forward and two back, and sometimes even two steps forward and three back. We cannot be entirely faulted for such an attitude. Children already are immortal, and when we, as adults, lose this magical world, we long to return to it. All myths of expulsion have this origin at the subjective level, though they may, more objectively and mytho-poetically reference actual historical events such as the transition to the agrarian mode of production and what have you. Long lost to mortal memory, such changes pale in their thrall compared to the just recollected and just mourned apocalypse of sudden adulthood, legally and morally. At seventeen, for instance, it is illegal to manufacture, possess, view or distribute sexually explicit imagery of whatever sort. But at eighteen it is not. How many young loves occur between seventeen and eighteen year olds in this or that legal region each month? There is no need to belabor such an issue. It is clear that in order to leave childhood behind we must also forsake youthfulness, and it is *this* that gives the expulsion narratives their staying power, even amongst unbelievers, and, perhaps more tellingly, most contemporary believers who take such stories as mere metaphors and do not take seriously the idea of their reference to some historically real event or place.

Indeed, like the legal difference between the child and the adult, the difference between literality and metaphor is seen as a mark of mature being. Ambiguity is real, certitude unreal. Yet in the sacralization of medical science, certitude is a goal, even as the uncertainty that flows forth from any subjective source, the patient's feelings, for example, is rendered as marginal to the process. Subjectivity is a form of childhood in these discourses. It is our own auto-ethnography, our body-double. It can be taken with the utmost seriousness only in its own world, that of the patients and their experiences, or that of the children and their phantasms. Yes, it is also a mark of maturity to repossess, as Nietzsche famously exhorted, the 'seriousness one had as a child at play'. Precisely so, but not for the *purpose* of child's play. Rather, such focus and organization, persistence and dedication must be turned outward into the world-envelope. It no longer dwelleth within, but goes into the world as on a mission. And in this world one finds that others have taken on the mantle of similar missions. Once transparently religious, the auspice has become the hospice, the temple the hospital, the monastery the medical school. What occurs to the individual as one's fate must now navigate a newly minted parallax of currencies, from stem cells to acupuncture, medical marijuana to cybernetic implants. Certainly, the smorgasbord of potential treatments has never been so varied and vast. This alone might be enough to at least give us hope for the future, both collectively and personally.

Results are, however, often found to be wanting. At the very least, the certitude of the child can only rarely be replicated. It is a signal mark of the will to life to be anxious about death. That we have personalized this suggests that one aspect of subjectivity is quite willing, even desiring, to be turned into an object. The more of our selves that can be remade into something other than selfhood, the better chance we have at outlasting the mortal coil. So, the bold predictions regarding the ability to upload our very consciousness into a 'cloud-based' version of the internet spark our imaginations. Perhaps we believe we can be rid of ourselves only to find that we can never be rid of ourselves. And this is in fact a good thing, in the end. Better still, let us upload, construct a cybernetic vehicle, bipedal or more, and then download. No need now to be concerned about a definite loss of self. Technologies of this sort are the plainest signs of the loss of the symbolic process of transfiguration, associated with agrarian metaphysics. Signs replacing symbols is, of course, nothing new. But to imagine that we have overcome the need for a sign to point to something beyond itself is naïve at best.

The 'something else' to which signs must point is in fact muted by the idea of sameness. If there is no other, and all are the same, there can be nothing 'else' at which to point thither. Sameness is the paragon of health and indeed, healthy-mindedness. It is no accident that when James famously remarks on the relationship between hygiene and religion that was to be found in those sectarian movements that 'minded' health in this way, he finds that a transition from the metaphysical to the physical has begun. The physical is first embodied in physique. This is the easiest thing to do, and reminds one of how techne first became noticeable in technique. But more importantly, *being* healthy is something to do with the subject as object. The subject aspires to be an object; this in itself is a *sign* of health. If attained, or at least, approximated relative to age and many other factors, one can be said to *be* generally healthy. And all who are healthy are healthy in the same way, according to the dominant discourses of medicine. No differently than religion, and especially religion before Protestantism, one attains the proximate soteriological privilege by 'getting right with god', though this phrase is incumbently associated with the very beliefs that put sameness, for the time being, on hold. Indeed, one can suggest that Protestantism as a social movement born of rebellion and critique resists the category of the object. It must continually differentiate itself from itself, hence the hundreds of known sects that have developed over the past half-millennia. On average, one for every year since the ninety-five theses were nailed upon the doors to heaven. Luther had given notice. The structure had been condemned and could no longer, in all good conscience, be inhabited. It would be *unhealthy* to do so. Being healthy, minding one's health and keeping a healthy mind, quite apart from all of the puritanical baggage associated with such hygienic and, so it also proved, proto-fascist epithets, was about reconstructing the structure of sameness. If all are naked before God, nakedness is the first sign of health, both physical and mental, as well as moral. One cannot hide anything, from a blemish to a pregnancy, from making eyes to making love.

This is not to claim that regimentation first occurred simply due to one's 'natural' state. No, a state had to become a status. It is this, first and foremost, that sameness addresses unilaterally as it presents itself as the goal of objectification. Thus as with saneness, sameness proceeds to evaluate from a specific set of values; those of equal measure and to be measured objectificity. What cannot be, as a mark of physique to be exposed by technique, merges into what must not be, as a sign of the unelect status of an unhygienic state.

Sameness

> Discourses are not once and for all subservient to power or raised up against it, any more than silences are.
>
> —FOUCAULT (1980, 100–101)

Rather, being the same thing speaks volumes. Not only is there the immediacy of solidarity, there is the further promise of a subjective camaraderie, something that speaks itself into the persons involved. The liquid shape of discourse prohibits it from being annulled by its own powers, let alone that against which it may, from time to time, assert itself. Yet sameness also silences the need for difference. One grows accustomed to the comfort of one's peers. Health becomes an arbiter of intimacy, of career, of offspring and of tenure of retirement, of 'doing one's own thing' at last. We have also grown to disdain the unhealthy, in our latter day Nazism, and the more scientifically based evidence we can muster in defense of our more or less aesthetic claims the better. Even fashion has succumbed to the mobile silence of the discourse of health, as we see more and more curves in media. No doubt the baby-boom demographic, aging and increasingly, and ever more hopelessly, unhealthy has much to do with this transition from the waif to the queen. Even so, it is symptomatic of a discursive backdrop that frames an attitude, an outlook. Protecting silence while proclaiming sameness, the sanity of gravity denying cleavage and posterior is something to be debunked, much as Cervantes sought to demythologize his hero's youth as an allegory for the destruction of the previous era. Quixotic visions become chaotic apparitions.

Histories

And so it is for us: it is indeed our very nature to be healthy and sane, and on top of this to think the same way about it. Alternatives are fine within the realm of technique. Yoga, acupuncture, even past-life regression have been assimilated, though in different degrees and with significantly different levels of authority, as techniques or elements of treatment, not as mindsets or worldviews. As technique is itself sacred to our consciousness, it may then be thought of as part of not only our nature, but of the nature of things. Gadamer reminds us that the idea of nature first appears in Plato's *Phaedo*: "The word had long been used but always only as the nature of something, hence not as the concept of nature" (1998, 34). Likewise, and following from this, the sense that a thing has a material form and thus is not being called upon to demonstrate the existence of matter *per se* (ibid, 82). No one of us can *be* health, personified or allegorized. But due to the exacting sameness of the qualifications for being healthy, and no less the ranges of what constitutes reasonable health age-relative and according to gender and ethnicity—distilled and distended averages resting on actuarial tables and incidences of illness and disease; the more years lived the more healthy the one who has or had lived them—one needs no murky metaphors to explicate how one feels; for better or worse. If I feel good, I mostly feel good about something. But feeling good in and of itself is an amorphous representation of general well-being, that is, hygienic and objectifiable health. Each of the goods that a human being can or could feel good about, whether in oneself or in the world of acts and effects, is predicated on a system of value that states that all is related, and a flaw in character can well be seen as a sign of ill-health; hence the clause in most life insurance packages that notes suicide as a symptom of mental illness and thus pays out on it if it occurs. It is a new cause for a very old effect: "This new order of interlocking natures arises to take the place of an order predicated on an ontic logos. [ ] It is fully compatible with the modern conception of the nature of a thing as made up of the forces which operate within it" (Taylor 1989, 276). It was the force of ill-health, and not weakness of moral character or yet its altruistic strength, that effected a suicide. One kills oneself not because one cannot stand oneself or the world, or both, but because one is *sick*. This immediately implies that no healthy person could be so self-critical, or have become such a trenchant culture critic, to give up in this radical manner. It follows, therefore, that critique itself must be at some point silenced, and not with hemlock, but with some other part of the *Pharmakon* that kills us more softly than ever before.

If illness is the reason for unhealthy acts, if no immoralist or amoralist could be imagined without citing the 'Diagnostic and Statistical Manual', now in its fifth edition, then critique itself falls into the oblivion of a hobby. The 'dreaded' hobby, intones Adorno, threatens to overtake any vocation. Luther could then be seen, as he has very much been, as a kind of schizo-affective hobbyist, with a compulsion for contradicting all authorities and courting attention to himself, no matter how negative. Indeed, the behavior of many a 'lunatic' in our own day could be encapsulated in the idea of attention-seeking, a response to neglectful parenting, of which there is so much about these days. But if sameness cultivates saneness, as we will see later on, the evaluation of human behavior must then proceed from a kind of instrumental and technical reason, not at all the kind of reason that evaluates the morality of a person let alone a culture: "Reason becomes 'legislative of experience'—this was the decisive point that Kant's genius perceived as the real revolution of the new science …" (Barrett 1979, 201). Note how one requires 'genius' to understand the authenticity of reason. No mere sanity will suffice. And genius is the very thing that obviates sameness, that pulls saneness well outside its three standard deviation curvature, at least to the right of the diagram. To stand outside both what is alike and what is reasoned is to see it from the vantage point of the third eye, certainly, but it is also, ironically, to evaluate it from a position that it itself cannot understand, cannot hold within itself. To do so is, at length and perhaps surreptitiously, to mock the concepts altogether. For if only those who harbor a kind of insanity and thus ill-health within them can see through the reason of the language at hand, the language of health and healthy-mindedness, then what does this say about the limits of such a language?

This is why the most recent ancestor of our modern discourse has design rather than reason as its *ne plus ultra*. Without suggesting a regression, we can still appreciate the idea that, given the flawed character of human judgement, prosthetized or no, a source of evaluation that humans merely proselytize has a preferentiality about it that still tempts some today: "… we have an ethic based no longer on inherent hierarchy but rather on marked activities. Reason is still important [ ] but it doesn't suffice to determine the good by serving as the benchmark by which activities are ranked" (Taylor, op. cit, 282). Design of course implies designer, an idea that is distasteful in our own time. But we have at least approached the critique of having to have a 'doer for every deed', if not having overcome the presence of source as blame or fault. Medical discourse has seen fit to transfer the morality of cause and effect in the world of humanity into a non-sentient world of life forms and life forces. That it remains there may be a trick of language, an existential rhetoric, but its illocutionary abilities still give us the strong sense that we are sensing something about either ourselves—we have smoked for sixty years, for instance, and now we have lung cancer—or about the world at large—coal mine dust producing a similar disability—or yet about others to self—the veritable neurosis about sexually transmitted diseases testifies to this last. Even so, design, however muted and translocative, still provides the framework for any subjective discussion of symptoms and diagnostics. Even more so, the cures for the causes or sources of illness are themselves sourced in designs, counter-designed to make the impression upon the original source that it is now humanity that controls the universe, and not some other entity, once deified and majuscule and now as often as not, to be found in the vulgar and miniscule: “But this did signify a real transformation of the natural worldview under the causal-mechanistic mode of perception that attained the fundamental power of its expression in the existence of technology” (Gadamer 2003, 84 [1935]). As if to counterbalance and yet still mimic the miniscule workings of the virus or bacteria, high technology as applied to medicine also contains the spectacle of the very small and sophisticated. After having defeated the gods through the engineering of the larger scales, we now have turned to confront the once invisible vectors of mortality, making them first visible through much smaller scale and finely tuned technologies. In other words, any battle that is waged must be fought with sameness, even as the goal of health retains and remains the idea of becoming uniform. Indeed, at base, the disease vectors that most plague us today from without, microorganisms and viruses, those to which we can nod away any subjective responsibility, are themselves characterized by an essential sameness to which they owe their own otherwise insignificant existence; “Molecular movement in turn corresponds to a certain quantum of energy, so that the common denominator of the elements is energy” (Jung 1959, 251). That we ultimately share this with the most base of life-forms—these owe their *moral* existence to the fact that they make us sick or well; we would likely not notice them otherwise than taxonomically and evolutionarily, and certainly they could not have attained any general fame amongst beings such as ourselves—makes our enemies enough like ourselves to incur our jealous wrath. The stigma which the Greeks used to attach to the sick person has been lifted from him and reattached to the source of the sickness. Such life-forms are less *worthy* than us, and this is by no means a scientific judgement (cf. Sigerist 1977, 391).

Once addressed, the problem of the relative virtue of the denizens of the great chain of being can then be relocated a second time; from differences in order and species to those of individuals. In doing so, morality has come home to roost, as it were. No longer can we look in askance at the facticity of subjectivity. It is very much in the way, right in front of us. No sidelong view permits an egress from it, no circumlocution a locomotion around it: “Our task consists rather in studying the largest number of cases and observing the mechanisms of transformation at work in real life and no longer in artificial situations such as surveys or formal interviews” (Peneff 1990, 42). Diagnosis, the conversation with the patient, is hardly enough to rest the case; it is only a bare beginning. Even in the suite of depth psychologies, the metaphoric couch backdrops only the narratives of manifestation, the descriptions of dreams. The real work deals with the living, and neither the past nor the dreamscape of sleep qualifies. Speech gives way, inexorably and then suddenly, to vision. This is supposed to occur both within the realm of the purely elemental and physical, where 'quanta' of energy may be perceived as motive forces and may even be registered on the most sensitive of equipment, such as super-colliders and the like. Speaking into being is one thing, but in our age, seeing is yet more believable: "... where gazes meet, the individual unique nucleus of these collective phenomena" (Foucault 1973, 25). Foucault immediately reminds us that at the height of the enlightenment, the institutionalization of the gaze is occurring. Sight becomes vision, and vision is a naked sword.

This is hardly limited to medical treatment and discourse. It is symptomatic of an entire revolution in thought. Though we view the enlightenment with a more critical gaze today, we nonetheless still gaze at it. Its horizons are still our own, no matter our efforts to either turn otherwise—back into some nostalgic and altogether unreal fantasy of 'the past', a butter churn or yet a better urn; and make no mistake, nostalgia always betrays our bitterness to ourselves—or to run ahead—into a 'postmodern' op art collage of declining expectations. Even so, both such responses are almost entirely subjective. Meanwhile, objects of science pile up faster than do our objections to the methods by which they are catalogued. This must have been so, at least at first, given "... the linked ideas of inevitable progress and the omnicompetence of science. Here certain ways of thinking that proved immensely successful in the early development of the physical sciences have been idealized, stereotyped and treated as the only possible forms for rational thought across the whole range of our knowledge" (Midgely 2004, 13). And though we have attained a measure of critical freedom vis-à-vis *scientism*, we are so reliant on science in our contemporary lifeway that we cannot avoid accepting into our subjective fold its products, even if they are no longer quite seen as gifts. It would be hypocritical to deny that the *same* methods are at work in both evolution and the automobile, and all those who drive and maintain some belief or other in creationism, for instance, are guilty of this sleight of hand. The scientific revolution, accessed in our day through a kind of metempsychosis, approached through the séance of simultaneous use and abuse, manipulation and elation, not to mention an ek-stasis of envy given that it seems to be our only hope of overcoming our mortality, is premised on a similar revolution, not in physics, but in consciousness: "Now this revolution, at once interior and exterior, which makes philosophy, onto-theological metaphysics, pass over the other edge of itself, is also the condition of its translatability" (Derrida 1995, 70). It calls precisely for a 'community that overflows in tongue', and what laps and then floods endlessly over the lip of the glass and thus bypassing our own lips is the gaze, the most easily extended human sense. Thinking no longer has to do with either being or Being, but with the onticity of *beings* in the world. Its new conditions, stated unequivocally, uttered without breath mark, shift the focus of our consciousness from the mouth to the eye. The mouth can betray both other and self, but the eyes, the 'windows of the soul' can testify to the truth of things. Certainly, they must be adumbrated through technology as to bear more of a witness to the exterior than to the interior, but note as well that 'interior' no longer implies an interiority, as in Augustine, for instance. No, what is inside is simply occluded by the layers of the worlds that envelope it, the viscous flesh of man a machine. There is no 'inner' within the modern conception of what is inside. All is a box that can be opened. There is no seventh seal, no Pandoran evil. All that is required is a more powerful adumbration of the gaze. We are almost to the point where we can behold the cosmic creation, or should we rather say, origin. This, once attained, will be the ultimate proof of not merely our technical prowess, but of the moral gravity by which we have made once again accessible *the* sacred moment of all things, the 'brightness of self-ignition', which has, of late, descended to ourselves. This marks the end-point of sight. There is nothing that came before this that anyone can see or even imagine. The beginning also marks the end of consciousness; we awake from an unimagined dreamless slumber of inexistence: "The transitionlessness of this transition from sleep to wakefulness or from life to death ultimately points toward the enigmatic experience of thinking, which suddenly awakens and then sinks again completely into darkness" (Gadamer 2003, 32 [1974]).

Structures

Sameness itself rests on the idea of the immutable. There is neither beginning nor end. So thought finds itself struggling to replicate the imagined circumstances of stasis, of the One. This is one reason why so-called aesthetic or artistic inspiration is so highly venerated and sought after. It appears to be sourced in that which has access to the One, a singlemindedness of purpose and task. One hears of athletes who are 'in the zone'. There is only one zone and not all can inhabit it at the same time. One play gives way to another, and if one finds that within this or that game or match, players from opposing sides are excelling, we might say that with each sparkle of genius the one or the other has replaced his or her forebear in the 'zone' and thereby has been granted with a singular gift of inspiration. In the arts and letters, clearly there is not as direct a competition for genius. Nevertheless, we understand one of the sacrifices of the arts is to work most often alone, or at least, within the company of one's invisible muse. Like the later idea of godhead, omniscient and omnipotent as well as omnilocal, such an aesthetic muse can be many places at once, gifting many mortals with her genius, though never continuously and ultimately, never over the entire length of a mortal existence. Yet these limitations are held to always be already our own, and never that of the sources of inspiration, whatever and whomever they may be imagined being. Immortality has deigned to extend mortality with its infinite grace. All works of art and culture were once said to be gifts from the gods, and indeed almost all of them directly referenced this gift in some way, either by personification and allegory or through the dramatic and profound scope of their production.

Science is no different in this regard:

> Science begins in the study of the forms and properties of extension by studying not the empirical givens but the ideas of these forms. [ ] This deductive format of science—which would veritably contain knowledge of all the possible figures and relationships of its region of objectivity—was fixed as the ideal of all Western, rational sciences developed after Galileo. (Lingis 1989, 14)

The 'science of deduction', proverbially misattributed to the ultimate genius of detective fiction, imagines the world as it might be, a microcosm that reflects the wider ambit of nature as it is. Yet clearly rational science is but one half of science as a whole, and one might say, the half that more fully participates in the séance of theoretical constructions than in the data of material locale. It falls to the empirical aspect of the modern sciences to rest its nascent and truncated claims upon induction, which is also what the famous detective actually did. Like a figure in a heroic melodrama, the scientist may well test her hypotheses but in doing so, she must encounter that which tests through the inductive method. This is the 'self-correcting' part of science more so than its procedures, which are more like rituals. But if any ritual is not performed correctly, we can expect no results. This structure has been directly inherited from the religious life. Science not only has the same ideals as religion, it uses the same process of interaction. What differs is the attitude the human being brings to it. Or is it so different?

One suspects that the rise of science has denigrated the attitude that previous epochs may have brought to their metaphysical beliefs. Surely the Greeks and other cultures who participated in a diversity of classical cults did not know ahead of time what to expect from their seers, priestesses, and temple oracles. They had only the faith that there would be *some* response. This is no different than the researcher who consults his laboratory apparatus and technology, who mixes the materials in a quasi-alchemical manner with the partial knowledge of all that has already occurred in the history of science. The idea that one approaches one's gods prostrate and submissive, with the certain expectation of one and only one answer is surely a modern myth, proselytized by those newer acolytes of the newer mythic narratives which structure science and its applications. Especially today, we have no certain expectations of the cult of either science or technology. We have hopes, to be sure, but also deeply laden anxieties. This too is absolutely no different than the manner of our ancestors with regard to their religions.

In order to attempt to differentiate our contemporary stance from those that have passed before us and lent us both their credibility and their incredulity to expand upon indefinitely, we are constantly testing our results. In medicine, this is a life and death examination. So, the source and procedures for collecting the material necessary to exonerate this or that hypothesis is given the highest value. Yet this is due to the general adherence of the applied sciences to the larger picture. Like faith constructing godhead, method constructs the object. The goal for both is to *know* the construction as a real force, both in nature and in one's personal life. Thus it was that godhead was eventually imagined, especially in the Christian faiths, as being part one's life through the vehicle of the soul. Data was collected by the faithful as well, and none more so than the Calvinists, regarding the soteriological status of one's soul. Since immortality was a given, the destination of it very much mattered. We find this equation in our modern world in the cast of an immortal Nature—if not quite local due to our latter day degradation of the earth's current environment, then certainly in the wider sense of the word—and thus it very much matters to us how we can adapt ourselves to live on within its indefinite ambit. So, the question then becomes something like this: how is it that mortal consciousness can know the forms of its own beingness, its own being in the non-formal world? "Here a self-interpretation regarding their basic tendency made itself known. As science of physical phenomena, they define these beings just as they show themselves in experience, a definite mode of access to them, and they define them only to the extent that they show themselves" (Heidegger 1999, 53–54). Unlike the 'reality of the invisible' that James famously remarks upon as one of the crucial elements of any religious faith, science eschews this imagined aspect of projected consciousness and does not 'speculate' about it (ibid, 54). In itself sensible and sound, this injunction rapidly gave way to an new expression of the human actor and his anxieties and aspirations; the idea that one could make sense of the world as it was by virtue of a formal set of procedures that did in fact have an *a priori* goal. If the key sensibility is to know the object only to the extent that it 'shows itself'—in the hyletic sphere, this can, according to phenomenology, be only partial at best, even inauthentic—to our experience, and thus the further assumption is made that this 'means' that our experience is our experience *of* these objects—aside from the somewhat jaded questions concerning the reality of the real etc.—and not of something else. It is this assumption that was precisely *not* made in religious thinking. In this, science has inverted the methodological relationship between subject and object. In religion, the primacy of the subject was assured, at length, through the participation of the object, God or the Gods, within the very being of each human being. This is why there is an 'interior', as we suggested above, in pre-modern thought that no longer exists for a strict rationalism today. Nowadays, then, it is rather the object that takes precedence because we have become all too aware of the transitory character of our human nature. But it has become transitory for the very reason of its loss of the soul.

This sounds sentimental and nostalgic, but it is merely a way of expressing the difference between the subjectivity of our ancestors and our own. Lamented by liberal thinkers such as Taylor and Nussbaum, apparently critically celebrated by the 'anti-humanists' like Bataille and Foucault, the 'soulless' solace of modernity nevertheless offers to us a liberating kick. And it is a kick that has catapulted the ball of knowing in a number of different directions, not all of them salutary to self-understanding. The social sciences as well as those applied have suffered from a too extreme and over-didactic interpretation of objectivity, for instance: "A sort of operational orgy rapidly spread throughout these disciplines. The expressions 'using operational method', 'operational concept and definition', 'operational theory', and so on, have become magical catchwords monotonously canted for the resolution of all controversies" (Sorokin 1956, 32–33). Perhaps it is not a coincidence that the term 'operation' also connotes a physical intrusion into the body. 'Let's operate!' once appeared as a call to arms. Today, of course, and not least of which due to the rising financial costs of medical care, operations are eschewed or at least viewed warily by doctor and patient alike. But metaphoric operations continue to abound. They have the effect of a renunciation. They are enchanted with a ritual quality, as Sorokin notes, as well as possessing the righteousness of all ritualistic behavior. Outside the circles of operationalism, simply one of many specific codewords for the assumed increase in scientific objectivity in the human sciences and elsewhere, researchers may find themselves marginalized. It is commonplace to overhear quantitative scholars and students alike denounce quite publicly those who engage in qualitative research, for example, while corresponding resistance to this is more clandestine due to lack of relative numbers.

And numbers is the name of the game. It is all too facile to imagine that the more numbers, the more knowledge, especially in the applied human sciences that must partake, of their very nature, of those physical. Medicine has always been at this difficult crossroads, and there is present more than just one devil, ready to trade one's soul for this or that technical virtuosity: "… this unprecedented advance in the knowledge and manipulation of matter is making for a lopsidedness which it is of the greatest urgency to rectify by a corresponding scientific exploration of the immaterial or spiritual aspects of the universe" (Westlake 1973, 156). Such sentiments, and from an accomplished medical doctor no less, could well seem at the very least wrongheaded in our contemporary atmosphere. Where is the evidence that such a 'spiritual' realm even exists? How could the immaterial be 'scientifically' explored? Why is it 'urgent' to foment speculation about the cosmos by linking objectivity with emotion? How would one 'operationalize' such ideas or hypotheses? William James, once again, famously attempted to leave such doors ajar, claiming that such matters as have fallen under the rubric of spirituality and religion occur to human consciousness because of aspects of the brain itself. They are not mere will-o-the-wisps in this sense at least. These remarks came at more or less the precise moment of the advent of psychopathological discourse, and offered a competing thread of investigation to that latter. But contemporary psychology has chosen the route of psychopathology and behaviorism. It was not a coincidence that such a route offered a much more convenient buttress for the rise of the legal bureaucracies of the still nascent nation state, also contemporary with both James and his opponents: "… the judicial institution is increasingly incorporated into a continuum of apparatuses (medical, administrative, and so on), whose functions are for the most part regulatory" (Foucault 1980, 144). The focus here is on the living and breathing denizens of the new society, their labour power, or even more fully, their 'bio-power', as Foucault has famously labeled it, and to suggest that there is more to the human being than meets the eye of either the state or the market is to once again allow the church into the mix through the back door, as it were: "A normalizing society is the historical outcome of a technology of power centered on life" (ibid). And it is to life that we owe, as both citizens and persons, our *way* of life. This new worldview patently does not include the afterlife, for instance, in its definition of life, and hence the idea of the 'soul' or spirit, which presumably is the link between human consciousness and the realm in which Westlake and other homeopathically inclined medical specialists are interested, has no place.

Another important aspect is the declension that occurs between scientific research and science based practice, always a weaker link in the chain of both discourse and command: "Although Western medical practice is based on scientific knowledge, the practitioners themselves are typically not scientists. The scientist's objective is to gather empirical data [ ] By contrast, the practitioner's goal is more pragmatic: to deal with the specific conditions of individual patients or clients" (Freund and McGuire 1999, 189–90). It is assumed that once through the clinic or hospital door, one's personhood must be sloughed off in favor of a more anonymous and objectifiable quantity—the 'body'. This is what is always in question, and the fact that cognitive science is so interested in 'mapping the mind onto the brain' bespeaks of nothing other than this reductionistic sensibility. At the same time, it is much more convenient to attempt to understand health through the physical alone. Indeed, a truly hard-nosed veteran of the history of applied science might go so far as to say that *all* talk of something other than the body—even the mind is herein included, recalling Skinner's infamous comment concerning it—is nothing other than leftover nonsense from the previous non-scientific epoch. This criticism also includes within its eponymous ambit the sense that these previous periods were as well anti-scientific and unscientific, terms that carry much more weight of actual disparagement than does the first. That the person is still believed to exist and function is part of the metaphor of socialization. As such, it is relative not only to culture but also to historical period, and cannot be therefore counted as adding to our objective understanding of things: "The *object* of discourse may equally well be a *subject*, without the figures of objectivity being in any way altered" (Foucault 1973, xiv, italics in the original). Personhood, an artifact of the culture at hand, having been dropped off at the front door, one can now get on with a truly scientific investigation of the problem at hand. No matter that one is a mere 'practitioner', one has all the black boxes of pure science at one's back. Such are the discourses of objectivity; their authority emanates from experiment and that means from the world itself, the world of things and forms of things, and not from the fashionable and ever-changing social world, as do persons. This relationship is mimicked in the object of such discursive knowing: "The order of disease is simply a 'carbon copy' of the world of life; the same structures govern each [ ] The rationality of life is identical with the rationality of that which threatens it" (ibid, 7). Therefore, any investigation proceeds along the tried and true axes of what is already known about life itself. How it functions undeterred by the presence of death, for instance, as the outcome of equally rational forces, those that happen to inhabit, through nothing other than the structure of evolutionary existence, other forms of equally viable life that also happen to be our enemies.

Before this kind of discourse arises, death is either personified or at the very least, is understood as anti-rational. It presented to reason its own end rather than helping to attain its ends. Death also covered over the future with an indecipherable cloak. No gaze could penetrate it, no inductive method descry its form, which is why detective fiction, to use perhaps an obvious analog to medical practice, often uses the metaphor of the veil for the villain. But science allows one to see into the very forces that cause death, and thus to anticipate them: "A new alliance was forged between words and thing, allowing one *to see* and *to say*" (ibid, xii, italics in the original). Of course, this alliance must have a large and capable arsenal with which to wage such a battle, as well as many supernumeraries to brandish the visionary swords, laser scalpels and fiber-optic cameras alike. The once person, having stepped into the space of medical discourse, must now be supervised as never before. Medicine, in this sense of both surveillance and sometimes concernful oversight, is not a mere adumbration of society; it *replaces* society: "One began to conceive of a generalized presence of doctors whose intersecting gazes form a network and exercise at every point in space, and at every moment in time, a constant, mobile, differentiated supervision" (ibid, 31). The whole of the parts, as in any organic solidarity, is greater than the sum of the parts. This gestalt is nothing other than discourse 'itself', which is also its own object contradisposed in its parallactic panorama to the objects found within nature and cosmos. Within it one finds that one has been emplaced. There is not so much a loss of power in patient-hood, as many commenters have suggested, rather than a trade, or ongoing bartering of local empowerments. It does feel good, after all, to know one is being 'looked after' in manners beyond our ken, though it might be slightly disturbing as well. At the same time, the placebo effect of simply being *within* a clinical space cannot be underestimated. It is to the advantage of any hospital or other space of medical supervision to transform its façade, however cosmetically, into one that give the new patient a sense that supervision is in fact authentic concern, and that the weapons of discourse are always on the side of the sufferer. More effective treatment might be predicted given such a transformation, and indeed, we do see more and more of this kind of professional ethic in our contemporary scene. It is also less expensive to train health-care practitioners to model this kind of interaction, rather than simply turn out vehicles of discourse alone, those who can only observe, for instance: "The only normative observer is the totality of observers: the errors produced by their individual points of view are distributed in a totality that possesses its own powers of indication" (ibid, 102). Once again, it is the gestalt, the whole which transcends the data as it comes into view, as it is gazed upon by the myriad of mortal points. This metadata reproduces even as it replaces the older idea of godhead, the third eye or omnipresent and omnilocal vantage point. Like the dialectic being polished at the very same time in modern history, the two points along the x-axis, presence and locality, *Langue et Parole*, form the base of a triangle whose synthesis brackets and uplifts the two oppositions into an archiphonemic entablature, that of omniscience.

The séance of science then produces an 'omni-science'. This reconciles the diversity of both episteme and morality that is found along the grounded horizon of opposition, and indeed of all mortal oppositions. The object can now become not merely knowable, but truly known, as if in a proto-phenomenological circumscription: "It is no longer a question of a difference in the object, or the way in which the object is manifested, but of a difference of level of experience of the knowing subject" (ibid, 81). This subject is neither person nor even specific prosthesis, as even here, such tools are used and also checked by many. The transcendental subjectivity that only godhead once possessed, made manifest by its creation of objects in their naked nature through the forces of the naked forms themselves—nudity, following Clarke, appears as the first veil of culture—has now been repossessed by the gestalt of scientific method, observation, and experiment. This was the goal all along.

Processes and Outcomes

But like the old god of morals, the new one of knowledge neither has nor has maintained a monopoly of judgement. There were always alternative religions, even cults. Today, we find that homeopathy and alternative medicine fulfill the cultic role. *Their* practitioners consider themselves elect in their own way, exhibiting a rather smug soteriological privilege when approached by the skeptic, turning away in sometimes sulky silence when confronted by the dominant medical discourse, either in the examination room or the hospital itself. Many persons, of course, avail themselves of both major forms of health-related dogma, switching with ease between the two depending on whether or not there has been a rapid success or even cure sourced in one or the other forms. Though an outgrowth of the alchemical circumstances of pre-modern transmutational epistemology, perhaps ultimately traceable to Aristotle in the West—but also seen, and for the first time assimilated into Western consciousness in the nascent ethnographic vignettes that were to capture the intellectual and aesthetic imagination of the *fin de siècle*—alternative medicines were also given market cantor simply by the Barnumesque dealings and the hurly-burly barter of all those who could not afford to imbibe in official medicine. And these were by far the majority of early nation state populations, at least until the 1950s. So 'alternative' is not really a relevant term for the description of what for approximately two centuries was the going rate for most people, most of the time. They did not, in fact, have an 'alternative'. Nevertheless, now that heavily socialized medical care is available in almost all developed countries and many which are still 'developing' as well, homeopathic discourses can bill themselves as the insightful outsiders rather than merely the wink and nod after-hours clandestination of dubious entrepreneurs: "We are witnessing the most recent manifestation of what has been happening for at least a century: the questioning of objectivity and the undermining of authority. There has been a loss of faith in expert systems" (Williams et al., 1994, 186). It is interesting that the claims of expertise in non-allopathic discourses often ultimately appear to rest on the immaterial, something that is supposedly beyond scientific knowledge, rather than something that is quite knowable and susceptible to science and simply has not yet been recognized as such. The idea of the 'beyond' no doubt has its charms. It is a way of getting round the authority of any rational organization. Homeopathic pundits act as medical vigilantes, taking the justice of health care into their own hands. At least, this is how it is seen from the dominant vantage point. Both categories of discourse make similar claims, however, as they attempt to convince potential consumers that they, and only they, have a firmer grip on the timeless. Indeed, while homeopathy rests its case on the idea of the antiquity of its knowledge and practice—midwifery, herbal remedies, even astrological talking cures, for instance—allopathy reminds its clients that its version of time out of time is that it is not limited by time at all, and rather uses time to constantly improve itself. The analogue between religion and science more generally should be obvious. The methods of science do not change, but their results get better over time.

The results of religion are the same as their methods; they were discovered long ago in a time out of time, and have descended to us as gifts, not of history, but of a metahistory that verges on myth. Yet this approach to the phantasmagorical can only lend further credence to the claims of alternative medicine, even though some of it at least has found its way, often through some partially occluded entrance, into the dominant discourse, especially over the past thirty years.

But indeed this timelessness, the mantle over which the two competing discourses joust, has *already* been transferred from the religious analog to that scientific: "The privilege of its intemporality, which is no doubt as old as the consciousness of its imminence, is turned for the first time into a technical instrument that provides the grasp on the truth of life and the nature of its illness" (Foucault 1973, 144). What is actually occurring, then, is that the 'alternatives' to 'expert systems' discourses—again, a misnomer given that all acolytes of the para-institutional worlds of homeopathic and cross- cultural health care also surely claim as distinct an expertise as do their rivals—are attempting to regain possession of that which has been taken from them some centuries ago. Timelessness, the archiphonemic synthesis of personal experience and objective becoming, was repossessed from its religious origins, suggesting that it itself had been lent even to metaphysical beliefs in some primordial time soon after the advent of the social contract. The true historical origin of belief 'itself' must likely remain obscure, but suffice to say that the organization of what became religious thinking is equally likely *not* the exact birthplace of human thought in general.

And it is human thought that returns to us, eagerly and avidly, when we are ill. The situation demands not only an objective overcoming, but a self-overcoming that in turn forces us to be attentive to a self-understanding that has somehow misunderstood itself: "When confronted with an illness we attempt, so to speak, to overcome nature itself. What we seek to do is master the illness, to gain control of it" (Gadamer 1996, 105 [1991]). That it appears to have gained control of our very selves, pushing us around, bullying us in an anonymous fashion that *feels* very personal, exacts from us the most trenchant call to arms. Anyone or anything willing to be enlisted into the service of the self in these contexts is immediately to be considered an ally. The dueling categories of pre-modern and modern discourses are in fact given their dialectical synthesis not through taking the structural parts that both hold true to and that have animated them historically as siblings, but through the action of the *subject* This is of vital importance: it is our personal experience of ill health that brings together the history of health care, no matter its source and venue, its traditional markets and its institutional authorities. Gods come and go as their franchises wear away or migrate. If even the Gods are susceptible to the subjectivity of human experience, then certainly medicine must also be. Religious belief reaches its crest not so much through religious behavior—one may attend church for no other reason than either authentic community or the somewhat less than ethically authentic appearance of community—but by virtue of the fullest presence of the *disbelief of the world*. One is forced back onto oneself, just as illness forces us back into ourselves. We must reach away then, and grasp part of the objectificity of factical relations, of the matter at hand: "But the more complex in which it is situated becomes, the more *denatured* it becomes" (Foucault 1973, 16, italics in the original). Indeed, Foucault immediately suggests that the hospital, as one example, is a microcosmic equivalent of, if not culture as the essence of human nature, civilization. Though this calls to mind Freud's famous critique, when applied to the relationship between discourse and disease, one can understand it as part of the process of making what is detrimental to cultural life and as such human life more generally, ill at ease in the world. It is doing to disease what disease has already done to us.

The artificial construction of *Ungeheuer* and its projection on the intrusive and lower form of life that usurps its 'natural' position by invading the inner space of our own is tantamount to acknowledging that our being at home in the world is something that is accorded to our status as moral beings. In this, at least, discourses of modern techne lean heavily on their predecessors. It is offensive to be sickened by this or that disease vector, and not merely an inconvenience. Yet to find death offensive would seem to smack of hubris. So, as is common enough for humankind, we tend to split the difference when it comes to having to confront our own mortality. Death is one thing, disease another. If the first cannot yet be avoided—but do not let us forget the ultimate aim of medicine—then the second should not be assuaged in any way. Though the second can lead to the first in certain cases, it *is not* the first. This is more than a faint echo of the 'while there is life there is hope' shibboleth. There is to be made a qualitative distinction between disease and death, and hospitalization is but one form of drawing that boundary, of reframing the ontological status of disease as a passing form rather than a surpassing one. Quantification is another form (cf. Sorokin 1956, 115 and 122). These newly circumscribed spaces of seeing and saying, thence knowing and practicing, desire to bring to the fore not truth *per se*, but evidence. Making visible the unseen, a more precise definition of truth for the Greeks, is taken literally enough in these new spaces of clinical discourse and discipline to obviate or at least ironically obscure the problem of human life as a mode of being conscious (and) self-understanding. Indeed if the disease is 'denatured', then so, in our own unique way, are we.

We cannot simply 'trust in evidence'. This is both naïve, says Heidegger, and makes critical investigations, phenomenological or otherwise, into some form of criminal exhibitionism: "Perhaps once called the conscience of philosophy, it has wound up as a pimp for the public whoring of the mind" (ibid, 37). Making visible the unseen is somewhat tattered at both ends, as it were. Its past argues for the very existence of that which is invisible, much as did religious thought, and its present has only the mutable remains of what, now brought to light, cannot be exactly what it had been when in fact unseen. It is already on its way to decrepitude, though that is one of the moral goals of medical analysis. There are certain exceptions of course, like cancers which, if partially destroyed within the body can return with a renewed vehemence. Like the wars of antiquity, the cancer wars ideally take no prisoners. One seeks total victory. This also reminds us of that other great analogue to how we perceive ancient conflicts, the policies of the Third Reich in the East. Military success was merely a means to a much larger, and more grotesque, outcome. But health insists that it has its own god on its side. Radiation therapies, chemotherapy, excision and amputation, organ replacement and stem cell treatments all attest, in their various methods and applications, to the necessity of making what once was deemed healthy and whole itself once again. One wishes to go back to the origin of life, which includes the presumption of health. Most recently, the advent of genetic solutions to a weak hand dealt at birth testify to this desire. We have made startling progress, if that is the correct term, in the direction of origins, if not as much in the other direction. But one is a test case for the other, like Poland was for France, and like mental patients were for the great masses of later Holocaust victims. Re-engineering our birthright will allow us to overcome what is most demanding of us that also comes directly out of our birthright, our very deaths.

What Cannot Be

That conscious life finds it difficult to imagine its opposite should not decoy us from an examination of all the methods and modes of existence that offer themselves as salves for this lack of imagination. Non-conscious non-being, the kind of 'state' that elementary Buddhist manuals attempt to get one to meditate upon, appears to be something for life to avoid at all costs. And not truly 'life,' nor even 'that which lives', but 'we the living'. Life in general is said to have no consciousness of its own death. Dying, perhaps, as can be observed in animals that are evolutionarily closer to us, especially the social mammals and birds. But it is not part of animal being to recognize its own inherent mortality. For them, inexistence most literally 'cannot be', whereas for us we use this expression as a desperate action, a rhetorical force that really has no ultimate back-up. What has been in fact has been, even if most of this gets lost in the translation from past to present, both writ smaller and larger than ourselves. Our deaths are pre-ordained by our very beings, and as beings in the world as it is, we come to a kind of ethical maturity in not only recognizing this facticity but also in attempting to understand its meaning for us while still alive. Now conscious non-being is something that has been imagined for ages past. Paleoarchaeological discoveries in Turkey and the Near East suggest that it begins to be imagined around the same time as the first fully human sub-specific siblings of ourselves take the scene, perhaps at least a quarter of a million years ago. This makes sense to us in a manner much deeper than merely evolutionarily, though that 'advance' is not lost on us. Perhaps, we might imagine, organismic life evolves a gestalt of consciousness that really *does* transcend its organic basis?

The Problem

This kind of phantasm is not necessarily fantasy, at least not in the discursive sense of the word. It rather represents the ultimate project of action. What might be imaginable if one's consciousness continued indefinitely? As stated previously, we are witness in our own day to a vast machinery of funding and technological virtuosity and even intrigue that has as its simple goal the immortality of consciousness. Forget about the 'soul'. If we have lost it we will make our own, and remake it in our own image. It will be the penultimate part of the 'projective construction' of human *indefinitude*. This is at least something we can both imagine as well as attempt because of the character of the basis for medical science itself. So it is not surprising that the attempt to 'restore' the balance of health within a body, brain, or lifeway, ultimately shifts itself into the mode of reconstruction. One cannot turn back the time on the existential clock, so one has to make a new clock. The old syntagmatic relation of watch and watchmaker can serve for us a purpose after all. Indefinitude may then be defined as a sacral state of being, it is being-desiring-being-fulfilled, if one wishes to combine a phenomenological ethic with an attitudinal complex. Its enactmentality certainly appears to be a kind of ether, but its at homeness with itself is neither aleatory nor alienated. That it is a process is assumed: "The judgement now turns on properties of the activity of thinking rather than on the substantive beliefs which emerge from it" (Taylor 1989, 156). This 'procedural rationality' as Taylor refers to it, guides our contemporary quest to become more than even the mythic heroes were fated to enjoy. Eternity elsewhere no longer impresses us. Life is too good here. It is not at all surprising that this view is hardly shared on a global scale, but this new attitude has within its enactmental complex the ethic of *also* rescuing the 'rest of us' so that all can enjoy the 'new Man'. All of this sounds eerily familiar.

Health, medicine, hygiene and physis were more or less the same as aesthetics, beauty and goodness for the Reich. This is too well known to be dwelt on here, but given life's apparent and imminent materiality, the most obvious first line of both offense and defense against 'decay' and entropy is by way of the physical situatedness of being in the world. The 'as it is' quality of the lifeworld is thereby reduced to something less, and though, as a turning away from the confrontation of Dasein with its ipsissimous beingness—its 'ownmost' way of being it is not something 'lesser' or vacantly amoral etc.—its inauthenticity renders it as the fullest expression of vain desire nonetheless. Medical science can be seen as but a tool in this 'turning aside': "Medicine as it has developed in these modern times is engaged in an ever-increasing elucidation of all the material factors which contribute to healing on the physical plane" (Westlake, op. cit., 142). Westlake continues, suggesting that almost by way of a kind of consolation rather than due to concernful being, psychology has been 'added reluctantly' given the 'emotional' quality of the caring process (ibid). In his mind, this is clearly a textbook case, quite literally, of adding this or that ingredient and stirring, as has sometimes been said regarding gender and the social sciences. But it is clear that an existential claim is being made. Non-material forces are at work, and however occluded they may be to the tools of current science, nevertheless they do exist. Not only this, but what they introduce into the discourses of health is a challenge at the ontological level, a challenge which cannot be confronted by epistemology alone. The problem that was revealed was one of ambiguity striving to attain certainty, of art mimicking life in order to make life more like art: "An uncertainty that was a sign of complexity concerning the object and of imperfection concerning science: no objective foundation was given to the conjectural character of medicine outside the relation between extreme scantiness and excessive richness" (Foucault 1973, 97). One might hazard even the suggestion that science appears to shine so brightly for us because it has borrowed the hidden light of secret things. Jung speaks here of knowledge concerning the 'dark side of matter', and the fact that the 'very roots of life itself' are a primary object of the scientific endeavor (op. cit, 232). This invisible and unseen light, this movement that hides from the world its own motion, is the source of life, the 'life force', as Westlake and others persist in calling it. A combination of being and motion for the Greeks, that was presumed to originate in the unmoved mover and before: "Already in Plato, *dynamis* opens a new ontological perspective, a concept of what is that does not grasp this as something present—as static and permanent givenness—but as something that is motion and leads to motion" (Gadamer 1998, 85). It is easy enough to understand the idea of in-dwelling as movement already and always creating a presence for itself in the world. Even the sick do not cease to feel its presence, though its force may be on the wane. Only in death does movement appear to cease for human consciousness, though the more basic forces of entropic transformation are obviously still at work. *Life* itself does not cease in the death of the one.

And this sensibility of being the one who lives and thus must die is certainly relatively recent. It coincides, more or less, with the nascent idea that health is of the greatest import not only for life, but to live a *good* life. Industrialization, which just as certainly brought about its own original challenges to the good and healthy life, also brought with it the ideal of health proper, the manner in which one could live not only longer but also better. Not merely the industrial revolution, but the intellectual and political revolutions with which it must be intimately associated. This eighteenth century trinity, our modern three-in-one, wrests from the church the polis and then transforms it by way of the concept of health. This new Man is still sacred, and he is no less of his own making here on earth, but the difference lies in his goals. Heaven *on* earth as indefinitude is now the ultimate purpose of earthly existence: "For the first time in history, no doubt, biological existence was reflected in political existence" (Foucault 1980, 142). The politics of health is not just about institutions and budgets, unions and management, techniques and quality of care. This is what appears as a function of a way of thinking; that to denature personhood is not to reduce it but to expose its *essence*. For it is at the level of being that illness strikes us. Disease is dangerous because it works in the world of the unseen, the very world that used to be shrouded *as well* by the veils of metaphysics. These unnecessary layers have been revoked by science, and what has come to light, what has been made visible in the Greek sense of coming to know the truth of things, by both seeing and saying, the gaze and the discourse that emanates from it, is the essence of what it means to be human in the face of diseased dehumanization. So the critics of modern rationalized health care are missing the point, according to this view. It is not institutionalization that dehumanizes, but disease, and the fact that great masses of fellow humans are working very hard and long hours in these systems of care and concern demonstrate the calling of humanity itself.

Only when a kind of inflated authority cascades out of the interface between depersonalized patient and health care professionals does the sense of concernfulness start to wobble. When this occurs, such critiques may have some humane validity, but they cannot be taken as a piece beforehand. Once again, the so-called 'expertise' of rationalized systems is no more than what human beings, past and present, have brought to the examination table. Such expertise is ambiguous in the extreme, even today, and not merely because one does not know the class rank of one's general practitioner. So the presence of outsiders' discourses in taking the archaic form of 'lay' knowledge leaps into the breaches: "… lay knowledge represents a challenge to the 'objectivity' of expert knowledge. It contests the impartiality of that knowledge *vis-à-vis* other forms of knowledge …" (Williams and Popay 1994, 119–20). Not that these 'other' forms, however 'alchemical' or 'astrological', homeopathic or alternative may be when considered in juxtaposition with the heavily industrialized medical scientific discourse, possess an equally alternative 'objectivity'. The salient point is simply that no human knowledge is without its limits. If allopathic medicine can appear to be authoritarian, we witness a case of an action and equally opposing reaction, where the pundit of herbal remedies zealously defends *his* discourse as objective and evidential. But this is hardly Newtonian. Human systems are never closed. We must rather return to the Greeks, who reminded us that motion is by definition part of being, and as long as life persists, this motion is with us and *is* us. On top of this, the human dynamic bears little resemblance to the object realm *a priori*. We are things in the world of things only by a kind of default sense that we must negotiate the world and cannot simply move through it, as it were, as if we were spirits alone. We are in the world but not as any other thing is in the world. For our world is one of a conscious self-understanding, and any critique that exists that ranges itself against an institutional or rational discourse which also exists as a human thing in the world does so precisely and only because of this possessedness of self-understanding. Yes, it is always both partial to itself and incomplete in itself. It is *partial* knowledge in both senses of the word. So it is well within the limits of human knowledge to question the presupposed 'impartiality' of any kind of historical construct. Insofar as 'lay' knowledge does this, it is on solid ground. But if it attempts to hold itself out as a more objective response to the problem at hand, it fails as miserably as would any other such claim.

This is not a new problem. The mythic figures of pre-agrarian societies had similar vexations. The vicissitudes of human existence were as well known to our ancestors as they are to us: "Thus our hero grapples with a problem that perhaps has its parallel in modern science. Two systems which we know to be inadequate present [ ] a differential validity, from both a logical and empirical perspective From which frame of reference shall we judge them?" (Lévi-Strauss 1977, 450). Is it fact alone that can define them as true or not? Or must we take their results into our own way of thinking, symbolically and even ontologically, and thereby discover some meaningfulness to them that would escape any one particular perspective that may or may not share experience with our own? For our devices, in our own time, we readily acknowledge that there is no 'fact' which stands aloof to human concern, which rests alone in the cosmos. Yet we also are equally ready to recognize the existence of facts rather than beliefs or opinions, and have ways in which they may be made recognizable. The discursive apparatuses of science and history, sometimes investigative law and even biography, expose our culture as the culture of the fact. No other human experiment has been so interested in constructing and venerating 'the facts' as are we. So it is no surprise to find that the dominant mode of self-expression with regard to health, both personal and somewhat more shadily, cultural, concerns the facts of the matter at hand. Needless to say, when facts are revealed or reconstituted as such, there is much that must be left to the ellipsis of discursive silence: "We must reexamine the original distribution of the visible and the invisible insofar as it is linked with the division between what is stated and what remains unsaid: thus the articulation of medical language and its object will appear as a single figure" (Foucault 1973, xi). Discourse not only objectifies a world originally separate from itself, it also makes objective a separate world. We might well doubt, after Nietzsche, whether the first of these effects is really the case. Is it not as likely that the world of facts is simply its own world, having little enough to do with nature 'itself'? This suspicion is of course not new, but within medical discourse it must remain unsaid, since it has the potential for unraveling the tapestry of treatments and cures and remaking them into mere regimen and curatives much more rapidly than does any placebo effect. This latter can at least be chalked up to the body's own reconstitutive powers, that is, the body including its brain, and not even so much to the 'power of belief', much vaunted amongst alternative circles. But this proverbial ellipsis within medical treatment itself is hardly the only effect that occurs when the scientific logos assumes predominance.

Its Effects

The more complete story would have include the very understanding of what we are as human beings: "This shift in scientific theory, as we would call it today, involved a radical change in anthropology as well. Plato's theory of the Ideas involved a very close relation between scientific explanation and moral vision. One has the correct understanding of both together, or of neither" (Taylor 1989, 144). Aside from the gradual and growing disbelief in the 'soul', at first disdained and then degraded by reductionisms of sundry sorts, what is more important for us is the effect of rendering a human being as human, period. That is, without 'being'. A human being no longer is able to be in the older sense of the term, attached to Being through the vehicle of the soul, beholden to the wider moral cosmos due to the possibility of judgment both before and after the fact of his or her existence. It is plausible that because of the unprecedented level of judgment each of us faces on earth that the idea of divine judgement or even Karmic reevaluation in the afterlife was discarded. One can only appear in front of so many contextual tribunals before one ceases to care. However that may be, the sense that we embody another form of being that is not entirely human because it is also more than human is transmuted into the technological quest for earthly immortality. We still seek to *replace* the soul, even if we do not want the old soul back: "Technology embodies physically what science has already done in thought when science sets up its own conditions as a measure of nature. The new science is in its essence technological" (Barrett 1979, 202). Its ontic essence, to be sure, but what about its ontological mode of being in a world increasingly transformed by it itself? Gadamer here speaks of an 'artificial human environment', but is this really any more completely justified than Barrett's assertion? (1996, 2 [1972]). To be human is to construct a non-natural surrounding for oneself, even before the discovery of controlled fires. Humanity is and always has been 'artificial' to this regard, and especially with regard to what is perceived as alien and anonymous nature, the universe of instincts and organismic evolution functioning by itself, for itself. Technology is our version of evolution. Like the strictly Darwinian version, the process of population growth, this world-oriented sophistication—this is not to say that such work always represents the *most* sophisticated ideas of the human species—technological complexity and cultural appetite for self-destructiveness amongst other items, human evolution must be seen most fully in its cultural light. After all, it has been at least forty millennia since our last very human cousins shared a small part of this earth with us. The difference between how people lived then and now is likely replicated only in some very remote areas of the Western Amazon, by a scant few hundred 'souls'. Indeed, one wonders, as with Durkheim, whether that term is also a misnomer, and in no ethnocentric manner.

With this in mind, we can retain some skepticism regarding an all too universal condemnation or even description of the lifeworld as somehow 'unnatural' to us. We are not exactly animals, and indeed many other animals reshape the originally natural environment to suit them, from ants to bees to beavers. But it is true that human beings have selected themselves for far more. *Pace* Latour, Woolgar, and others, Gadamer (ibid) makes the finer point that the very fact of scientific fact has constructed its own specific context that precisely appears to be without context. In other words, no previous cultural context, known or imagined, can be said to sit as arbiter on this new invention. This *is* unique in the history of human thought, and is most mindful of the advent of new religious movement which claim, especially during their earliest messianic period, that they are utterly new and cannot be judged by what has been. Even though all religions attempt to gain leverage by comparing themselves against the previous world—'you gave heard it said, *but* I say unto you'—and science is no different to this regard given its universalist claims to be closest to the truth of things, science does differ by the very fact that its facts speak not of Truth itself but of some approximation hitherto unknown to the lights of the times, or yet unknowable by its spirit. So, while religions speak of Truth in an ultimate and innate sense, science eschews both and thereby has emerged triumphant in a world which is nothing but diversity into its truths and its cultural contexts (cf. Taylor 1989, 164ff. concerning Locke's understanding of this effect).

To be content with an approximation to truth and to understand both truth and our knowledge of it to be ever-moving targets realigns our epistemological ventures with those of the Miletian Greeks, if not with say, Plato. But perhaps here we misjudge ourselves a little as well? Isn't it also plausible that due to our halting and oft reluctant recognition that human beings are quite different from one another in how they think and live, and more salient today, how they *want* to think and live, that we have gradually become accustomed to a relative morality that may even be seen as a higher form of ethical maturity given its suasion towards the 'live and let live'? The diversity of morals was no longer to be thought of as an 'effect' of differing environments, even those bio-geographical, for instance, but rather as depicting an ontologically distinct interpretation of being in the world. After 1945, the idea of ontology as essential humanity also had to be revised, lest it continue to skulk undeterred by the defeat of its Nurembergian forces. Thus a morality that was both realistic and ethical in its treatment of others as other could be viewed as a better response to both the world as it is and the fact that we still have to live in it with those others who, if not exactly our best friends, would still have to be tolerated. World courts aside for the moment, we can remind ourselves that we so far have avoided self-destruction since that same fatal year.

At the same time, whether or not Plato or Augustine *et al.* would be able to appreciate our modern situatedness of being-worldly in a world fraught with many elements of non-being, we have not entirely let the idealists founder on the rocks of their own Rhodian forms: "The new audacity of the mathematically structured thinking that we call modern science was really this kind of departure from appearances" (Gadamer 2003, 136 [1995]). Yes, science *is* relative to its own history and to the history of its discoveries, even if it is also cumulative in both a positive and a negative sense. But science is also distinctly anti-relative once its specifically temporal claims have been made. It really *does* state its case as the best case given that very situatedness of human being for which it itself cannot entirely account. So we are left with a puzzle only if we think we also need to know what everyone else thinks to this or that regard as equal partners in the human conversation. Perhaps there are a few ethnographers out there who actually do think this, but the rest of us manifestly do not. And it is not because we think our culture superior on the face of it. No, we simply observe what is occurring globally: everyone wants what we have already got, very much including technology and thus the science behind it. There is little merit to the moralizing argument that tells us that cultures are destroyed in the meanwhile. This may be true to a certain extent, but it is also true to say that cultures and persons adapt. It is not only the other who adapts, we also must remind ourselves that we the possessors of the history of science have not lived up to its human potential in many ways, and have forced various ill-advised and sometimes brutal 'adaptations' on ourselves. This is no apologia for the dominance of experimental science and its global effects. Rather, it is an accounting for the more fundamental structures that have engendered those effects and continue to do so.

No more decisive effects can be charted than in the applied sciences, the home of technology and its spectacular constructions and misconstructions. In medicine itself: "The clinic was probably the first attempt to order a science on the exercise and decision of the gaze" (Foucault 1973, 89). Seeing really was believing. But not quite in the same sense as the Greeks mistakenly imagined wood, for instance, to have as its existential copula the 'ability' to float simply because one could observe this effect. There were those who dove in the classical period but as in most complex cultures, the gap between the experience of the illiterate and that of the literate could only be magnified in periods where elites were a much smaller sample of the general population than even in our own times. Rather, the modern idea of an enclosed space, a laboratory or a clinical arena, allows both what is seen and what is at first unseen to vouch for themselves in a new way: "Immobile, but always close to things, the clinic gives medicine its true historical movement, it effaces systems, while the experience that contradicts them accumulates its truth" (ibid, 56). The manifest induction of the clinic and its growing attendance of associated labs not only confronts the hypothetico-deductive 'system' of thought alongside it, however well-reasoned, but it also constructs a kind of electric currency, an 'inductivity' so to speak, that is the conductor of all new ideas. It transforms the raw resources of the gaze into a discourse, akin to a power generating plant. Even more closely, the social and political power that medicine has attained over the past three centuries is very much due to the translation of induction into a system of its own.

More than this, inductivity's greatest asset lies in its ability to remain *mobile.* It remains 'close' to the originally imagined essence of beings, just as Foucault suggests that it is the character of the clinic and its 'gaze' to hover round any denigration of those beings. Mobility is truly of the essence to medical discourse in any case: "Professors warn students in health professional programs that half of everything they learn may be obsolete in ten years, but it is impossible to predict which half" (Frankel, Speechley, and Wade 1996, 191). Immediately we are also informed that "It is estimated that the health literature grows by approximately 60,000 articles per year" (ibid, 192). The electric aura that inductivity carries within it is also self-generating. It is a certainly a child of von Frankenstein. Far from merely evidencing the usual run of more or less collegial competition, cliques, and the race for funding, such prodigious production speaks more poignantly, if not necessarily compassionately, to the race against mortality. Only the applied sciences can boast of such publication numbers, and health remains the most salient set of these for any modern human who, bereft of soul, ponders the lack of time in which to ponder his or her existence. A discourse that produces and overproduces is also symptomatic of a culture and economy hell-bent on overproduction in Riesmann's famous sense. But such articles, even if they remain incomprehensible to the cases at hand, the living humans who sometimes find themselves at the mercy of research findings—especially those who are female and have to rely on medical data culled from exclusively male trials—testify most importantly to a discourse which, to borrows Weber's proverbial characterization of capital as a whole, is 'riding high' or 'in the saddle', with no serious challenger attempting to joust it off.

Current Reactions

But this all began in the space where case and gaze could first get to know one another: "The clinic figures, then, as a structure that is essential to the scientific coherence and also to the social utility and political purity of the new medical organization" (Foucault 1973, 70). We are still enthralled to, and by, this self-same discursive trinity; this is research that is very much in the public interest in terms of quality of life, an existential modifier, it is of national interest in terms of 'bio-power' and its manipulations, and it is in the scientific interest with regard to evidencing theory and the testing of hypotheses, as well as the not quite accomplished task of convincing the latter day unbelievers that science really does know the truth of things, and that such claims may be judged by the effects that science produces in the world at large. Certain religious sectarians aside for the moment, the vast majority of us are so convinced. So convinced, indeed, that we generally spend more on health care than in any other area of social life. A rapidly aging population in so-called 'mature' capitalist states can only add to this, or, if one is critical of the kind of spending, exacerbate it. Even so, it is to a more fundamental challenge that we must turn to explicate the 'enthralling' quality of medical discourses, one that specifies its product as truthful simply because they are focused in a new and very technical and probabilistic manner: "… it is a requirement of this precision—its posting of a version that fits with its capacity and with its ambition to speak with utter clarity—represents a remodeling of the world that prejudices human enthrallment with it" (Lilburn 1999, 74). The disambiguation, and perhaps also a kind of demythology, that scientific discourse presents to us as the evaluation of what can and cannot be for humans, is also seen here as a major form of disenchantment. We are immediately also told that the logic of Galileo and Descartes are incapable of 'arousing both awe and tenderness'. (ibid). This is not entirely fair. Surely the cornerstones of empirical sciences do arouse awe in their effects, and often this awe is quite authentic to being and not merely a vain result the efforts to extend human beingness into a technological species. Think of the Hubble ultra-deep-field vistas, or even the first sight of our own lonely and fragile world. This *is* awe, and one could just as rightly protest that the mystical visions of our ancestors were rather delusory in this regard. Who knew what they thought they were beholding? But if Lilburn's first point fails, then his second has somewhat more force. Tenderness and compassion are of entirely different orders of magnitude than is awe. They are subjective, first and foremost, and we should not expect the descriptive and logical tools of objectificity to aid, let alone sanctify them in any way. At the same time, it may also be argued that compassion increases by virtue of the disenchantment so proclaimed by the loss of the mystical vision. Indeed, this vision is not at all lost; it has simply moved its gaze elsewhere. We *also* do not know in any certain way if we are not in fact looking at the same thing as did our ancestors in any case, the face of godhead in the heavens, for instance. In sum, we cannot be declamatory regarding the place of either awe or human tenderness in today's world. Awe is both awesome but also awful. This has not changed since mythical epochs. Tenderness has been tendered to the margins more in our own times than any other, and this 'neighborhood' seeks the face to face even if it often fails or is deliberately sabotaged.

Poetic license aside, it is correct to suggest that though both awe and compassion and its siblings may be by-products of scientific thinking, they do not necessarily animate it from the start. Awe is more ancient than is compassion. All agrarian metaphysics had it as a salient component, from the earliest periods of sedentism. But only the later religions of the agricultural epoch would add compassion, Buddhism, Christianity, and Islam, suggesting that the wealthier and more complex societies became, the more leisure time and variegated the classes and occupations there were, the more possible the idea of charity, forbearance, and duty were of being called into existence. Either way, it may suffice to say that both awe and some version of compassion were near the heart of agrarian religious systems in both West and East. Their relationship with science is less clear: "For the Greeks, the essence of knowledge is the dialogue and not the mastery of objects comprehended as proceeding from an autonomous subjectivity, that victory of modern science that has even in a certain sense led to the end of metaphysics" (Gadamer 1998, 70). If agrarianism developed the metaphysical ideas into true and enduring systems of belief, then it fell to us to at the very least redistribute their ontologies and approximation of the Logos into much more air-tight compartments of being in the world. Not unlike social role theory, where we as singularities must occupy a dazzling diversity of contextual scripts and acts, today's metaphysics does not at all shine with a unified light. Perhaps it need not. Subjectivity can have a light of its own, when taken compassionately, bravely and as in Whitman, as a unifying force in a culture and a community.

But the great social experiment of which Whitman was the first to truly embody is hardly outside of the global human experience. Health was of first importance to this body electric, and the inductivity of medical discourse played a not unimportant role in the development of the enlightenment, if not necessarily enlightened, individual: "The breadth of the experiment seems to be identified with the domain of the careful gaze, and of an empirical vigilance receptive only to the evidence of visible contents" (Foucault 1973, xiii). This kind of observation, so well-placed in the clinical atmosphere that its panopticonic surveillance becomes archetypical for an entire society, from prisons to schools to asylums to nursing homes and the military, from Goffman to Foucault and back again during the analytic years of the 1960s and 1970s, also holds forth in its transpersonal court on crime and detective series, perennially popular. It is almost as if each of us imagines that we can know all there is to know simply by training ourselves to observe. Is *this* really why Sherlock Holmes is the most famous figure of all modern storytelling? The apparent ease of control, selection, and viewing, however voyeuristic, that concerns the interface between the user and the internet also has this quality. Research becomes a thing of the visible, wisdom adheres no longer to vision in the vocational or inspirational senses, but to just how much, how many images and the like, one can muster into one's intimate arsenal. Young people and their daring performances, the so-called 'sexting' of teenagers, the jealous rage of adults past their prime, all speak more to the sense that one can *show* oneself without having to be observed by everyone, yet daring everyone to observe after all. The giant collections of erotica to be found on personal computers, for instance, give their viewers a god-like helm. From homework to virtual sexuality and even sex 'itself', the gaze seems to have become triumphantly omniscient.

But if this is so, we must also explore the techniques that the gaze employs and seeks to control. Adults have long been aware and resentful of their children's abilities, whether it be that of learning a new language or their endless libidinal energies and willingness to flout the staid norms of stale bourgeois convention. We may have once been able to do so ourselves, and it is this corresponding loss of freedom that we mourn and seek to destroy in the youth of our societies. *Ressentiment* is perhaps a more true term for these relations, and the gaze as monitoring helps to restore an artificial youth upon those now grown older and more cautious. Technology and technique are harnessed by both the monitor and the monitored in a true Foucauldian wrestling of power relations. Yet each alliance privileges the vision of the gaze. Adults need to see all of what is 'going on', children need to veil it, exposing it only to the right pair of eyes at the right time. The utter nonsense about sexual and psychological health and the supposed risk of bullying and suicide aside—statistically, the risk to minors is almost nil for any of these things given the sheer weight of numbers of sexting 'events' and cases both known and presumed; there is risk in every human activity, including crossing the street on a rainy night—are weapons the resentful adults and sometimes opportunistic 'experts' employ to make themselves feel like they have maintained control over others simply due to the utter bitterness they harbor within their breasts at being forced to control themselves to in fact *be seen* as an adult. Being and seeing are always therefore rendered the same: "The positivist exists so completely in the era of technology that he must strive to justify himself by imitating the technician" (Barrett 1979, 221). The entirety of metaphysics was imagined banished by the

Vienna Circle, for instance, as being part of an *invisible* ether for which no one could ever vouch. One accepts or rejects based on the knowable qualities of the visible alone. This possesses itself a strong streak of the absolute defender of 'morality': "The language of conjecture and refutation is of course, Popperian. It tends to extreme Puritanism: a single refutation means that a theory should be dropped" (Hall 2005, 10). The fact of two suicides in a county of thirty-five million with hundreds if not thousands of sexting events per day means that teens should be banned from sharing their often sincere affections with one another is a reaction that even Karl Popper would not have supported—it has no scientific or objective basis whatsoever. As with all moral panics, such calls to arms carefully skirt the questions that ask why these behaviors are so popular in the first place, not to mention why our reaction to them is so full of condemnation. Such studies as have been done cannot stress the quantitative *per se*, of course, as they tend to obviate any possible point, but even so, we are unable to 'answer the basic question why.' (Sorokin 1956, 139), or to understand the basis upon which sexuality itself has been alienated by transmissive technologies—also, and ironically stuffed down the throats of children by marketeers and the self-same adults who are *also* paranoid about the incidences of sexually transmitted diseases and youthful pregnancies; all of this complex of instrumental discipline and correction point only to the fact that parents have so little sex themselves, due to work schedules and other familistic obligations, and also due to the fact of loss of intimate interest in one another over the life course—and an economy that requires joint household incomes (cf. Lösch 1967, 185 on the relationship between the subject and the 'incidences of independence'). In a word, the presence of children produces both an effect of necessary dependency and thus inevitable control, at least for some years, and the affectation of responsibility. This latter is thrust down *our* throats by the simple fact that most of us, even as adults, incur very little real responsibility in the work-place. The more so even in our marriages, where we have been taught to hold dependency in intimacy as a mark of mental illness let alone a weakness of mature being. The anxious ability to gaze into our children's lives is a despairing compensation for being unable to exert any lasting and satisfying political power in the public realm, or economic power in the world at large.

This said, the metaphoric clinical experience of work, school and socially sanctioned 'activities' for children and adults alike rests its case on the very success it denies when pointing the moralizing finger at the infinitesimal number of cases which go astray and become dangerous in the very manner that adults warn children about. Foucault famously reminds us of how Weberian, even Orwellian, our society is and just how successful it in fact also is. But because of its birthright in the pathology of the diseased case, it must retain its focus on the holism of what threatens the social structure and not how that structure is virtually impenetrable in any case: For "… it is enclosed upon the didactic totality of ideal experience. Its task is not to indicate the individual cases [though these always serve as the cautionary tales used by experts to exemplify their facile 'whys'], with their dramatic points and their particular characteristics, but to manifest the complete circle of diseases" (Foucault 1973, 59). There is a great irony in all of this: such a manifest is also now to be considered a manifest destiny, as its total truth represents the ultimate human freedom. Immortality means the conquest of death, prosthesis the annulment of disease. The more imprisoned we become within the gaze of medical discourse, the more liberated will be our 'spirits'—perhaps today an amalgam of feelings and phantasms, akin to the subjectitude of either work or play—precisely because the body will no longer exist as such. So it is not only science that benefits from the space of vision, but, just as did religion benefit from the arc of the visionary, our very culture will free itself from the 'cancers' afflicting the subjectivity of spirit.

What Must Not Be

Immoralities

Science only appears to eschew morality. It makes good on this sleight of hand due to both the presence of a 'science' of morality, that is, the human sciences, once indeed called the 'moral sciences', and through the idea of objectivity itself. Morality is proverbially relative to time and place. Ethics, to both of these and the individual besides. But discourse, descending from empirical authority, changes only according to the discovery of new data through the unimpeachable non-morality of scientific method. There are many instances of politics that sees in science a moral high-ground precisely, and ironically, due to that very non-morality of which sciences is said to boast: "[Nehru] meant a whole new ideology, a moral approach that would justify using those facts to change society in a quite particular way. And during much of the twentieth century the word 'scientific' has constantly been used in this value-laden sense" (Midgely 2004, 15). In the neo-colonial era, developing countries were reassured that the West could sell them the rope that would not hang them, but that instead would pull them out of their respective regressions. Positivism, emblazoned on the Brazilian flag to this day, was seen as much more than an epistemology. For after all, was it not the very metaphysics of the West that had subjugated the world? Yes, increasingly, from the start of the Columbian conquest onward, the canon of the missionary and the cannons of the mission itself went hand in hand. Nothing impossible here, but one might venture to say that the technology of the emerging sciences had already and always been slung over the shoulders of the dominant morality of the day.

Not a lot has changed in our own time, though the specific rhetorical content of the missionary has altered from a world-overcoming soteriology to a world-developing and thus affirming one. This alteration has occurred not because Western Man has suddenly declined his superiority. No, we wish to demonstrate it in no uncertain terms. This certainty can only be had, according to the new metaphysics, by exemplifying itself in the world as it is, and not by making claims about some other world to come. An added bonus to this shift includes the fact that it is now the case where science and technology can appear in the world as if they have no moral loyalties with the exception of the general betterment of humanity as a whole. But this whole must be remade in *our* own image: 'Intervention' is another term Gadamer follows up with in his description of this historical movement. The greatest effect of technology in the world is homogenization. The greatest effect of science proper is the overcoming of Babel.

But we can look still more deeply into this murky lens, turned upon ourselves, descrying only the silhouettes of desire and of propriety alike. Even as estranged to our sensibilities as are those of the priests of the city of the sun, the Egyptian magicians to whom Moses himself is said to have been apprenticed, nevertheless they contain the first vestiges of science as we have come to know it today, attesting to the historical intimacy religion and science have shared. Speaking of the Heliopolitan story of Creation, Jung suggests:

> Its drastic naturalism, unpleasantly obtrusive in comparison with the reticence of ecclesiastical language, points back on the one hand to archaic forms of religion long since superseded, but forwards, on the other, to a still crude observation of Nature that was just beginning to assimilate the archetype of man. (1959, 207)

Mythic thought also produces effects in the world, perhaps not precisely by itself, as it were, but by becoming part of human consciousness in a rather unconscious manner. It is part of the Durkheimian ether within which each of us is ensconced through our respective cultural socializations. It resists us if we resist it. It defends itself against our transgressions, and yet nonetheless needs these breaches of the peace to maintain belief in its moral architecture. It is certainly the case that "… the most powerful myths are those which influence what people think and do: which are internalized in their ways of thinking, and which they pass on consciously or subconsciously to their children and kin" (Samuel and Thompson 1990a, 14–15). Even when the homiletics of such narratives gradually fade into phantasms, at least for adults, they still exert a power over us (cf. Foucault 1973, 34). It is arguable that the trope of holism is one such myth, given to a latter day resurgence due to the alienation and anomie of capitalist bureaucracies, and their concurrent *Entzauberungen*. Mythic thought has always sought to transcend the object realm, the 'merely' physical', and in so doing, assert and reassert that morality is of more significance than materiality. Modern medical discourse, it is claimed, "… whatever the technical achievements may be, and they are many, is, for medicine, materialistic nihilism, and contemporary medicine is showing signs of having arrived there. The time is over-ripe for a new integrative philosophy of medicine based on a fundamental conception of health" (Westlake, op. cit., xiii). This same call to arms had been already used, in fact, by those intent in working the revolution of consciousness that had occurred across the board in the eighteenth century. But for them it was precisely science and thus also medical science that could be holistic in this sense, and to do so meant, once again, precisely, the overcoming of what Westlake and his allies state must be included in whatever 'fundamental' conception of health the human future should be graced with. Even so, we can discern a shared stealth here, a fealty to the idea that whatever the whole may be, its operation, if not quite its operationalism, must concede the process of interpretation: "… a whole hermeneutics of the pathological fact, based on modulated, coloured experience, is required… " (Foucault 1973, 14). Any hermeneutics seeks to disclose a form of hermetics. The Greek notion of Truth echoes for us still: a disclosedness, a lighting of the space of Being, a making visible of the occluded. No more fertile a ground for this experiment in the idea of truthhood could be imagined than within our own corpus. If consciousness is said to be 'held' within the organic functioning of the body and its brain, where else could one look to find the ultimate truth of Truth itself? "Thus the question that is posed for us today by the confrontation of modern thinking with this Greek heritage is to what extent this ancient heritage offers a truth that remains concealed from us under the peculiar epistemological conditions of modernity" (Gadamer 2003, 121 [1978]). It is of interest to note that the concealment of truth as well extends to truth itself. Truth then must be considered to be its own holism, distinct from any discursive category that can admit to no empirical limits while not letting go of is absolute value; to fill in all the blanks over time (cf. Foucault 1980, 110 on the incest 'taboo' as an example of this tension). A generation before Kuhn, Lösch offered his own approximation of the end-game of the quest for truth that does not admit to the truth of its own limitations: "… science refines the model with as much as the current state of thought permits, and only with this elaboration does the idea come fully to life. Finally the realistic refinement is lost in the details, understanding of the model as a whole is lost, and the period comes to an end" (op. cit., 1967, 358 [1945]). It is as if we imagine that truth is a palimpsest. Squinting into its mirror, we hope to find the finer print of the ontological contract. As with all such textualities, this is where the rub is, so to speak. If the devil is in the details, then, as the original friend of knowledge, he at least must live up to his part of the bargain. For the holistic health practitioners, our collective soul has already been sold down the crossroads of materialism. The key answer that the quest for truth contains for them is of course the manner in which this very soul can be retrieved.

This kind of allegorical narrative may inspire the researcher or scholar, apart from the world. But it is clearly other human beings with political ambitions or access to certain forms of power and the apparatus to redistribute it amongst the culture who in reality have superseded any devil: "… in fact the haters of truth are still as powerful, if not more so, than they ever were. Truth for them is too disturbing and upsetting, and so they turn and rend anyone who has the unenviable and thankless task of proclaiming it …" (Westlake, op. cit., 61). Here, the physician theosopher is speaking of the fate of Wilhelm Reich, and indeed, this is an extreme case of both the immorality of the state and its apparent anti-science bias. But even if Reich's late work in physics has none of the discursive cachet as did his earlier work in psychology, it would still be far better to prove it right or wrong according to the ontologically inclined arbiters of truth. Given the physicists alive in his own day, this could have easily been accomplished. So it is not so much that the 'haters of truth' are such simply because of an emotional or ideological dogmatism, or a palpable fear of change. They are protecting their interests. In the case of Reich, his claim to have found a cure for radiation poisoning would have obviated one of the lynchpins of the cold war, atomic weaponry and its long term effects on human health, though at the same time, one still glances askance at this counter-claim—that is, the one that was being defended by the state—given that even if Reich was correct nuclear weapons could still be used to utterly annihilate all humanity simply due to their awesome and awful short term effects.

Moral Duties

However this may have been, and we have no way of knowing in any certain fashion what the Pentagon or State Department was worried about regarding Reich's Orgone experiments, it is clear that the contestation for 'truth' is generally both a holistic and an invested affair. These two characteristics alone, apart from doxa, dogma, or ideology, sabotage the efforts from the outset: "A *formal indication* is always misunderstood when it is treated as a fixed universal proposition and used to make deductions from and fantasized with in a constructivist dialectical fashion" (Heidegger 1999, 62). One must always have one's truth and the other's too. In a word, one must rather start from vague 'apprehensions', and perhaps this phenomenological term is not as technical as it first appears. It can make one trepidatious to imagine that one seeks something but knows not exactly how or where. Indeed, the 'why' question of existence is what is brought to the fore in phenomenological induction, a sign of authentic being towards the world. The usual distinction between apprehension and apprehensiveness may not always be a necessary one. Like the novice surgeon with a scalpel in hand, each of us feels strongly that we must tread lightly into the unknown, whether in relationships, a new job, the teacher into the classroom, a scholar with a difficult text. This suite of nerves without sure endings, of accelerations without clear horizon, embodies the kind of thing Heidegger exhorts us to search within. This 'world-envelope' towards which Dasein is already and always turned, demands the fullness of being-attentive, or 'concerned', from each of us each day. And it is precisely in the everyday where the signs of Being may be discovered. This aspect of research into the human condition cannot be overtaken by technical means. Reich appears to have stumbled into a realm where what is usually taken as psychosomatic all of a sudden became objective data, or at least, had the potential to do so. Much more work was necessary to be sure of anything, but the very ambiguity of the Orgone concept and its effects in the world and what the subjects claimed still merits both our caution and our concernfulness alike.

To assume either a nomothetic or constructivist standpoint and imagine that either free us from any value-laden standpoint is at best naïve. Everywhere we feel the push and pull of human projections. These cannot be fully delineated by observational study, nor can they be fully explicated by a theory which is itself constructed of scientific projections. But what then, *is* the 'original character of the world', as Neumann puts it? "Thus, stripped of projection, the world becomes objective, a scientific construction of the mind. In contrast to the original unconsciousness and the illusory world corresponding to it, this objective world is now viewed as the only reality" (1970, 341). This kind of 'reality' is dominated, states Neumann, by the masculine archetype, but it might be more reasonable to suggest 'masculinist'. The sense that realities are gendered is of course hardly a revelation. Girls and boys grow up in sometimes radically different worlds, and continue to have difficulty communicating with one another until the grave. But an archetype is also a metaphor for human relationships, both in the externality of the hyletic realm and within and interiority to which empiricism does not admit. We have already noted the disappearance of the interiority of the psyche, and even phenomenology seeks to discuss this aspect of Being in a different manner than do studies of myth. To understand reality as merely the most alert observational sensate is to misunderstand its nature. And it is this specific misunderstanding that became dominant in medical science: "The 'glance' has simply to exercise its right of origin over truth" (Foucault 1973, 4). Yet even here, where the didacticism and precision of a searching eye brooks no veils and is not to be taken in by their adumbrations, interpretation inevitably follows. In some contrast, where one could not view the body of evidence so directly, the need to extrapolate in a sophisticated way was even more clear: "His was a hermeneutic function. With regard to the confession, his power was not only to demand it before it as made, or decide what was to follow after it, but also to constitute a discourse of truth based on its decipherment" (Foucault 1980, 67). A judge, a psychiatrist, or in another world, a priest, are positions that are ironically exposed in their nakedness. The world gazes into them, much like the proverbial abyss, simply because the power of their gaze is limited. But is the outer world of the body, to be vivisected by the ocular surgeon, any less murky? The need to dissect, expose, and view its contents laid out on the table in front of one's eyes for all to see and judge no doubt was a key moment in the history of medicine as a science. It is no surprise the church forbade this practice for centuries. The idea that it was associated with Paganism was a mere ruse. For what could *not* be found, ever, by looking into the body as deeply as this or that technology might allow, was the soul.

Hence morality 'itself' could not, correspondingly, be found in the world no matter how assiduously one searched. The soul as a construct was never of any real concern. As an investiture of social mores and the order of things, however, it was a fail-safe injunction against anarchy. Until it wasn't. By dissecting both the body of discourse concerning what society was and why it existed, along with exposing the inner workings of 'man a machine' or yet as an insect—it was inevitable that Mandeville be called by his contemporary English commentators 'Man-Devil'—the subjective keystone supporting the moral architecture of the day was found to be missing. At least to the gaze. Those 'dissected', or if still living, diagnosed, most often had no trouble locating it, as it was manifestly expressed in their conscience or lack thereof. But this could not be knowledge: "… the patient's view [ ] was never seen as a form of knowledge in itself, but only as evidence of, or a window upon, pathology" (Williams and Popay 1994, 121). How one 'felt', including any pangs of remorse, could now be turned into the data of the new medical discourse. In fact, it became a moral duty to not let morals get in the way of diagnosis, including the increasingly intrusive manner of 'feeling' out the patient from without. Prudery aside, the assault on 'decency' continued apace within the clinic and hospital. Patients were reassured that what transformed their social context into one of indecency, incivility, lack of privacy and yet a corresponding and somewhat facile anonymity was the disease, and not their caretakers. After all, would they even be present if it weren't for their illness? This illness was also, after all, 'their own'. They brought it into the medical arena just as it had brought them in. Health care professionals are merely coincidental to all of this. In being so, they can retain their objectivity, and evaluate the circumstances according to the discourse at hand, free from the morality of the outside world, and also free from the patient's scruples about it. This situation is not itself new: "The judges do not expect the accused to challenge their theory, much less to refute the facts. Rather, they require him to validate a system of which they possess only a fragment; he must reconstruct it as a whole, in an appropriate way" (Lévi-Strauss 1977, 448). Being accused of sorcery in many ethnographically known cultures could mean the death penalty. But depending upon the necessity of the social and kinship position of the accused, most offences were either explained away using a socially sanctioned reinterpretation that split the difference between the defense and the accuser, the facts of the agent and the weight of the accusation. It was the danger of *going through the process* that made the crime horrifying, and not so much its end result. This is simply due to the fact that we undergo social stigma whilst living as a social being. It is a unique torture that no other animal seems to have invented. That we cannot experience our own deaths annuls the ultimate verdict of any judge in any society. No, it is clearly the process itself that presents the danger, and the process of medical examination is no different. Diagnosis, treatment, surgery, after-care, etc., are what the living must face. These are the 'penalties' of illness, and the reason why no one enjoys a visit to the doctor, from waiting room crowds full of other sick people—the sick make one sickened in a manner not that different from the effect of residing in an asylum—to the effort and cost of procuring medicines and altering one's routines to 'get better'. This injunction is a moral one, whether we read it from colleagues or bosses e-mailing us about a missed day at work, or the unholy fascination that a friend's 'get well' card exerts over us. We want to receive it and yet we do not wish to be received into it.

All of this speaks to the dual problem that the person now become patient has no longer a discourse of her own. She has been denuded of morality and the social duty to uphold it. Being sick is also a social role, as sociology has long recognized, but it is one that expresses a distinctive non-function as its function: "It is not the pathological that functions, in relation to life, as a *counter-nature*, but the patient in relation to the disease itself" (Foucault 1973, 8), italics in the original). This kind of function, shorn of its mores, pushes the patient to always turn inward, away from the social world, with the expectation that all of those around her will shore it up in her absence. What becomes valuable in its immanence is not life *per se*, but one's own life. Though one is forced to reflect upon it, especially in times of a health crisis, this process is worked through as *surrogate sociality*. It is as if one is remaking the social world as a circumference into which one places oneself as one's ancestors placed themselves within a magic circle. The truth of this reevaluation becomes much more personal from the standpoint of others as well as more subjective from the standpoint of medicine and science more generally. Thus such a process, whether a dressed rehearsal for an undressed mourning, or for most of us most of the time, a counting of one's blessings and one's dressings, dovetails well with the prevailing scientific value of propositional logic and rationality as objective claims: "True knowledge is ignorant of values, but it has to be grounded on a value judgement, or rather on an *axiomatic* value …" (Monod, in Midgely 2004, 3, italics in the original). From whence these axioms come remains ambiguated by the equally scientific presumption that the human observer cannot match the precision of the ideal method. Akin to the patient's declination into a narrowed subjectitude, the scientist must always exercise caution about his own pressing subjectivity, the 'human equation', the 'observer effect', or yet the 'ghost in the machine' and what have you. As tired as these expressions are, they demonstrate a kind of fatalism in the face of our own idealizations of science *could* be if it weren't for the fact that we invented it. Like Michael Jordan's hall of fame acceptance speech, in which the great athlete nevertheless bemoaned the possibility that he could have been much greater than he was, the self-denigration of scientists in relation to their method and their object would be laughable if it were not for the problem of maintaining a belief that the 'greater' ideal is yet achievable. Perhaps this is another reason why we long for non-human immortality and consciousness.

The inventor of positivism spoke with caution, but nevertheless enjoined, right from the beginning, the scientist to think along these lines: "We must beware of confounding the degree of precision with the certainty of science itself. The certainty of science and our precision in the knowledge of it, are two very different things" (Comte, in Sorokin 1956, 131). What exactly is science 'itself'? Does it refer to the discourse generated from object research? To the objects themselves and the raw data presented by them? To the method alone? To the probability relations that lay claim on various forms of validity given enough cases or experiments? All of these, perhaps. Even so, this complex whole which is the practice of science, its objects and its languages, never once transcends its human context. Science is something human beings do for and by ourselves. Generally, only an epistemologist would care about such smaller issues. When it comes to the sciences of health and life, however, there is much more at stake. To ask the question regarding 'how one knows what one knows' in this realm is to ask a *moral* question, and not one either of method or the study of knowledge proper: "The most important moral problem raised by the idea of the clinic was the following: by what right can one transform into an object of clinical observation a patient whose poverty has compelled him to seek assistance at the hospital?" (Foucault 1973, 83). Today this is no longer a question at all but a given. It is rationalized, perhaps reasonably, by the sense that once one has made the decision to seek help, one places oneself into a milieu wherein one must accept the responsibility for the processes subtended. The element of 'trust', in modern health care rhetoric, as well as the more technical term 'consent', are of the greatest salience. Patients also now have 'rights', including a right to more or less timely care, but this suite of rights does not at all extend into either method or epistemology. Medicine is still medicine. The doctor is still the doctor. Indeed, the contemporary language of patient and care contains the unobtrusive means to turn away from the world and form the institutional context of medical discourse as glosses on the shying away from death itself: "As death is now an offensively meaningless event, so that disease widely considered a synonym for death is experienced as something to hide" (Sontag 1978, 8). Or hide from. The emplacement of the ill within a quarantined space is not merely a logistical consideration. It aids the healthy to keep up the appearances of the general health and welfare of society as a whole, even the 'social body', if we press closer to the increasingly fascist imagery this kind of discourse leans into. The sick are themselves hidden away from the 'unsick', just as they themselves are allowed to hide from their own sickness. And, as all of us have been sick one time or another, the expression unsick applies equally well to all those who have been moved through this modern rite of passage and come out the other end with a new perspective on living, if not life more generally.

Some of this is no doubt salutary to an ethics, but not all. Health care professionals regularly complain of baby-boom patients who come to the hospital under some absurd delusion that in every case there is a cure for what ails them. They are positively offended in discovering this is not necessarily, or seldom, the case. Can't buy me love, perhaps. But we should also be aware that even if the rhetoric of medical accomplishment and technical 'progress' is ever-venerated, the fact remains that mortality has not yet been overcome. If there are fifty ways to leave one's lover, to continue our demographically inclined pop music metaphors, there must be fifty thousand ways to die. It would be better, then, not to speak of them at all: "But this was not a plain and simple imposition of silence. Rather, it was a new regime of discourses. Not any less was said about it; on the contrary. But things were said in a different way; it was different people who said them ..." (Foucault 1980, 27). Death, like sex, big and little, is something for us moderns that we must talk a lot about so that we never ever speak of it.

Moral Statuses

But all this talk serves an even wider purpose. It gives us the impression that we are *concerned*. In *Being and Time*, Heidegger reminds us that inauthenticity in his phenomenological schema is not something lesser or degraded. We turn away from the confrontation with the lifeworld and with our ipsissimous Dasein with our fullest beings, in this way no differently than do we turn toward it. But our attitude of concernfulness is reproachable on another ground. It harnesses the Dasein which we are in a manner ulterior to that authenticity which presents itself when we engage the world as it is. Concernful being is what we are, and though we do not lose it in inauthenticity, we subvert it. Its goals are lesser, but not its being-towards them. Because of this, Heidegger suggests that we are duped, or rather, that it is convenient to engage in duping ourselves, because we do not concern ourselves with noticing how concernfulness itself can disengage from authenticity. Its existential status remains full, but its moral status is what is degraded, or at least, decoyed.

One clue to this always present potential for decoyed concernfulness might be found in our ability to exercise an apokotastasis regarding our existential condition, which of course includes intimately our sense of healthiness. Talking about disease, death, or some other perceived threat to the social body, such as sex or sexuality, is a way in which a nomenclature can be assigned, a manner of controlling or even possessing the threat, perhaps, as above, to quarantine it: "But actually one has acquired nothing more than its name, despite the age-old prejudice that the name magically represents the thing, and that it is sufficient to pronounce the name in order to posit the thing's existence" (Jung 1959, 32). Jung immediately states that our own age has done nothing to defeat this 'conceit', and has simply traded 'intellectual mastery' for magical thinking. The 'talking cure' can be applied culture-wide. Like market 'forces' in economics, or even the market 'itself', is it surprising that in an age of mass media those who talk the most are often the most successful at being heard? Or perhaps overheard is a more apt description of such a state of affairs? Letting in as many voices as possible might at first seem like good policy. Nietzsche's small-eared animals notwithstanding, or further, Muller's man with no ears at all, who cannot hear the petty plaintiffs of the day as he works his way through the winter of humankind, *we* feel a need to stay 'informed'. There is a basic mistrust of information in our day that has the ironic effect of compelling us to pay attention to its dubious sources. Read any list of comments on any news story on any day and you will find this dynamic at work. The *moral status* of the statement is being evaluated and reevaluated moment by moment. No matter if opinions remain individuated. No matter if beliefs are perverted by ideology or plain lust, either for the other or for general control—and the two are not at all necessarily discrete, parents being the most obvious purveyors of this kind of moralizing tactic—in our day 'the people' must have their say. There may be some self-acknowledgement that media, especially as driven through the internet, provides an outlet for false consciousness given the general lack of representation that can be found in national politics. In this way, we might suggest a model, or even a template, for the emerging applied policy discourses of patient's 'rights' and the like. If the doctor is still the doctor and the politician the politician, where exactly are the rights and the voices of people who interact, and are forced to interact, with these systems and regimes?

The status of our morality is really in question, but such a question can be sidestepped by imagining that one is assured of such a status to begin with, and, in applying it to statements made by journalists or government officials or even health professionals, that we are simply reaffirming the given morality that itself is above reproach.

At stake too is the simple dignity of our human relationships. The patient loses much of hers due to the loss of personhood within the health organization and its discourses. Certainly, the professionals who work in the fields also lose much of their own, as they must become roles and at best, persona. One nurse should not be favored over another by this or that patient or doctor alike, for instance. There should be, ideally, no manner in which to distinguish them relative to bedside care, mannerisms, and even appearance. Yet we might do as well to in fact make such distinctions, or some of them, simply to remind ourselves that these roles are occupied by real human beings who are in fact different, willy-nilly, and not just from one another. The dangers to human dignity—this idea is originally religious one, not that the great world systems have always dignified Man in an unequivocal manner—are clear enough within the medical realm. Even so, the model for reconstructing the dignity associated with our vaunted existential status and the presence of our reason also remain relatively clear: "Religious medicine is something else again. Great religions have always provided the social reinforcement of resignation to misfortune by offering a rationale and a style for dignified suffering" (Illich 1975, 53). Medicine cannot, however, fall back on the magical rituals of religion. It must transmute them in some chemical way. This 'new' order of elements can reference its alchemical ancestors only in the most abstract manner, as it can ill-afford to give yet more purchase to alternative therapies that impinge upon the authority and dominance of allopathic and neuroscientific treatments. At the same time, the religious backdrop cannot be entirely dismissed. Most people still rationalize privately their fates, whether or not they are members of some church-going community or network. Medicine, if not an out and out failure regarding human quality of life—and in this partial success human dignity has been also partially redefined—is neither regarded as a full-blooded substitution for soteriological grace, whatever its cultural stripe. For example: "The special status of the sick has become a privileged status. The diseased person has become a participant in the grace of God. To care for him is a Christian obligation, is positively beneficial to the salvation of the soul" (Sigerist 1977, 392). And not merely the soul of the sick person! The gift is well-known in all social contexts to be one to oneself as well as to the other. This is, in fact, the only manner in which human gifts can be given. One always 'gets something' out of it, usually, if nothing material, then an increase in symbolic or cultural capital. 'Virtue', something that thinkers have struggled over pedagogically for millennia, is certainly 'its own reward' given that it itself is a highly sought after symbolic commodity. It needs no other appurtenance to make it valuable.

Even so, the normative status of a social order cannot fail to be recognized by any who participate in the relations so produced by it. If acts of will in all of their modern human freedom, including the gift or individuated versions of grace modeled on the once divine setting, can be cited as the primary source for care of the other and of the self, as well as being the most immanent manifestation of concernful being in the world, then external structures, anonymous and non-human, must be consigned to having only an non-moral status: "In the end, a mechanistic universe was the only one compatible with a God whose sovereignty was defined in terms of the endless freedom of fiat" (Taylor 1989, 161). Health can then be seen as a straightforward confrontation with non-moral forces, biological or otherwise, that threaten a socially defined and constructed order of being, conscious, possessing reason, able to imagine a future for itself that is different from the manner in which the present is lived. That alone assured human beings of their self-styled moral superiority, but it cannot be denied that the ideas of interest, the future as progress, and the hierarchy of existence are all directly inherited from the major religious world systems.

This being so, the problem that remains for medical discourse as a moralizing agent in an anonymous world picture is mostly educative. Its 'mission' is received far and wide, but its message is always lensed through the locale of this or that cultural mix. Bio-power is also a major factor. Populations are left to degrade just in case they are needed by their respective geographic entities to defend the state against competitors. Not so different than during the agrarian epochs, massive numbers of real persons are shelved, *pro tempore*, in this way. *Their* moral status is one of an ungraceful and undignified shambles, and it is we who bear the moral culpability for this global situation. It does appear, often enough, that the 'care of the self' that Rousseau taught the modern West must indeed come at the expense of all of those who have not yet been taught the self itself.

Saneness

Meaningfuls

The successor to being moral, the state of being sane, is not necessarily an obstacle to feeling good about how one lives, or even, 'living the good life' as if it were a lifestyle choice. The 'healthy' lifestyle is also a slogan that we are all familiar with, and even the great villains of anti-nutrition, the fast food empires, have had to bend at least one ear to it. Given our liberal market, there are always sardonic alternatives, such as eating establishments that go out of their way to serve the most dangerous fats and even advertise them as risky. Throwing moral caution to the wind is never entirely out of style. It speaks to our Janus-faced relationship with morality in general. The Orwellian sexuality of adored adolescence in every media—look but don't touch, or, don't even look but thoughts are, after all, free—the paradigmatic aesthetic of health *as* beauty—Hitler's very own assignation of it—and the further facile fetishes of youth in all of its aspects—as something to be disciplined sexually and otherwise; as something to be envied and resented to the point of *ressentiment*; as the sole source of original and thus innocent love, and on and on—is enough to question the maturity of our collective sanities. But we must first inquire as to the meaningfulness of this Gordian mess: "The meaning component gives us the first and most important clue as to whether a given set of phenomena is a congeries or a system" (Sorokin 1956, 269). To identify sanity as a formal and crucial aspect of human health is but the first step in understanding it as a system of related but still conflicted signs and assignations. One can step outside of the rational-legal authorities as a matter of course, as in consuming dangerous fats in this or that fast food, or in viewing underage erotic performances on the net, and these transgressions, the first against the body and the second supposedly against one's conscience, for instance, are related through their shifting moral grounds. Rationality and morality are not intimate siblings, but they are still kindred. They relate to one another on a need to know basis rather than as perpetual confidantes. This is necessary due to the fact that "... there is no neat, fixed, and formal criterion by which we can deem any of our explanations rationally satisfying or not. We take up a question when we have some sense of malaise or incompleteness in things as they confront us ..." (Barrett 1979, 176). Even so, rationality cannot afford to keep morality too close to itself. Whatever rationales are offered for the content of moral prescriptions and proscriptions, the idea that one can set up timeless principles adjudicating all human behavior in all contexts is surely one of the most irrational ideas ever conjured.

Like cultures, persons also cannot be relied upon to rationally recall their histories. Sanity itself would not allow it. Not only is there too much detail to remember in any fixed fashion, like our rubrics for the evaluation of ideas, we too have changed, sometimes radically, over the life-course. This is a good thing, and not something to be mourned. It is a different way of thinking about health than the moral version, which also contains prescriptions and proscriptions. As Nietzsche famously exhorted, it is a healthy and sane thing to do simply to forget things as they were and perhaps especially as they might have been. In any case, "People do not just remember what happened to them. Deep and intricate processes of recall involve selection, formation, and re-formation of the original experience" (Thomson 1990, 204). Our ideals regarding memory are often Platonic. The sense that there could be an 'original' is actually sabotaged from the start, given that upon first reflection—we do not think in simultaneity with the act—we have already begun this selective process. It is even more transparent if there occurs a context with more than ourselves having experienced it. Thought always accesses human reason, more or less, while action can notoriously leave it behind. Even the word 'spiritual' has been used to refer to 'perfect men endowed with reason' (cf. Jung, op. cit., 212). Presumably, the also rather Platonic notion of perfection is hitched into the sense that reason makes us not merely unique amongst living things but also superior, closing in on an ideal. But why should the use of reason be seen as such a perfect vision? Consciousness appears to us to have a kind of 'leverage' in ordinary life. When reflected upon, it also immediately takes center stage as the only way in which to make sense of human construction and the social world (cf. Barrett, op. cit., 335). When human triumphs are cited, in the arts, the history of thought, the letters and in social reform, reason and the intellect are touted as their source and inspiration. Dr. Westlake's commentaries are full of such praise, directed at his antecedents and those he feels have been left out of the mainstream of medical discourse (cf. Westlake, op. cit., 24). Such paeans can go yet further: "The most harmonious and mysterious creations are those of nature, and to my mind, it is the highest cultural aim of the professional scientist to interpret them so that others may share in their enjoyment" (Selye 1956, 292). But surely there is more than shared pleasure at stake? Wonder and awe, but also utility and the construction of indices that concern themselves with a general quality of life must also be included in the word 'enjoy'. In the same vein, 'behavior' needs must include a much wider ambit than is favored by the utility of behaviorist science: "In attempting to dispel the ghost from the machine, we have banished more than we wanted to. We have become behaving organisms rather than conscious subjects" (Barrett, op. cit., 79). Did the great majority in fact desire to 'banish' this ghost? What did *we* want, and who is 'we', after all? It is more likely that we have set the machine up side by side the spirit, both in the external world and within ourselves. Sometimes it pays us to ignore either our intuition, conscience, or even reason, but never all three at once.

The most grave threat to us taking leave of our senses is the experience of suffering. As Sigerist notes, to suffer meaningfully is the exeunt of experiencing only the twofold path of suffering itself, that of being 'passive' and having 'discomfort' (cf. Sigerist 1977, 389). But there is another facet to ill health that levers these other two characteristics: "The sick man, therefore, lives differently than the rest of society—from the healthy. In short, sickness isolates" (ibid). This isolation, like the technical quarantine mentioned above, provokes in us a fear of the confrontation with death. Death's whole mandate, so to speak, is to separate us from the living, for those with whom we once were kin. All illness, no matter how slight, is a rehearsal for this final production. If the guise of death makes but a cameo appearance in most of our lives until much later on, it nevertheless is able to walk the stage with ease, filling in any minute part that it has been offered. It seems to us that death, personified relatively early on in Western agrarian consciousness, knows that its 'time will come', and that it indeed has control over this time ahead of time, as it were. The fatalist predeterminism of the Greeks and others has of late given way to a more abstract sensibility regarding finitude. Even so, the presentiment of death walks with us as the shadow of mortal life. It is still something more than a mere companion, and many would rather be rid of it entirely. If the whole purpose of health discourses in their competitive variety is to overcome the shadow of mortality, to banish its spirit and the ghost it will produce in the same way that our technology seems to be boundless in spirit even if no specific piece or element of it lasts forever, then we have at least attained the pitch of 'perfection' to imagine immortality and thrust its mortal guise into the world of things.

Means

But in order to have attained this, every possible threat to such an ideal within our own lives must be challenged. This includes the sense that memory could be lost, or that we should be wary of any sign that we cannot recall this or that, however trivial. Like law, memory lives through its spirit, and not so much its letter. That we can recall anything at all is something of a mystery, and even at the level of neuro-chemistry it is not certain how this operation effects itself. The spirit of a concernful-being-able-to-remember is part of Dasein's authenticity. But it can be turned away from the world of lived experience inauthentically as well. To recall to the letter all things, the so-called 'eidetic' memory, is to avoid the necessary confrontation with one's own tradition—akin to the 'horizonal' confrontation with tradition in hermeneutics—and to concentrate instead on total recall, as if one's past never occurred because it remains as it was in the present. In this way, our medical discourse has also been attracted to the letter of things: "Contemporary medicine suffers from one delusion that distinguishes it from all predecessors. It assumes that all ills ought to be treated, whatever the predictable outcome" (Illich 1975, 80). The letter of health could be used as a weapon against the spirit of disease. Increasingly, the territory of one does gain on that of the other, but in the end, there is a limit, at least within the current species, as we have noted above, beyond which the letter cannot resolve the problem: "But in these scientific times we seem to have forgotten this elementary fact, so bemused are we by modern 'progress'" (Westlake, op. cit., 25). This 'fact' is more about the facticity of Dasein in the world as an ontological being. Coherent only in the sense that we are born, live and die, and that all of us do so, means that the 'life force', as Westlake refers to it, can only be managed for the time being, aided, yes, but enhanced only artificially. From our point of view, and from the point of view of our specific consciousness, more particularly, this always appears to be an entropic condition. But this is not objective. The degradation that affects our corpus is part of a larger process of regeneration, though one in which we have assumed some modicum of passing control. The 'forces of life' in general to not degrade, but rather transfer, transmute, and translate themselves into other myriad forms over time. We mourn for ourselves, but cannot be said to mourn the process of living and dying *per se*. This second kind of memory, participating as it does in the letter of things and not the spirit, would certainly be irrational. Yet how rational is it to recall by way of mourning? Even though it is likely that Durkheim was correct about the origin of all human memory in the mourning process, and hence also the origin of human history, this manner of coming to know the experience of being and world no longer takes hold of us. We 'manage' it when we become the 'knower of what is to be known': "The meanings of question and answer themselves become less and less separable from the experimental conditions that the scientist has already fabricated" (Barrett 1979, 383). The human predicament of not being able to predict the future is the only thing that has taken hold in us. It confronts us like an ultimatum, and induces all kinds of avoidance behaviors. Laboratory science may well be one of these, at least in terms of providing an outlet for those who seek to control their destinies and those of the species. The serious questions of existence, however, cannot be asked in this manner. All of the 'whats' and 'hows' of life do not ascertain the meanings of *why* we find ourselves in the situatedness that we do. Situated between cosmic wonder and the trivially otiose, humanity strains its significance by craning in both directions at once. The day to day that is an elemental part of Dasein's being in the world is taken over, rather than taken up, with the petty, and though our turning toward the phantasms of inauthentic desire is accomplished with our fullest beings, as Heidegger takes pains to point out, it serves itself to us as does the decoy to the prey. Science too, whether grasping tentatively the cosmic origins of what is or closer to home, the origins of life as we know it, is an authentic turning towards Being in beings, but it too can be 'perverted' into a form of entertainment or hubris. The material 'focus' of the human spirit is what is truly at issue at both ends of our worldly action (cf. Westlake 1973, 143).

There are many infamous examples of both ends mistranslated as means in medicine. The 'miracle' of birth and its attendant ideas of both innocence and undespoilt humanity, either ready to be nurtured into mature being or already predestined to be so, is savaged by a drug that had as its ends an easement of this trial: "Most people still do not realize that thalidomide was originally marketed as a minor tranquillizer to control the nausea often associated with pregnancy" (Harding 1987, 551). Drugs that alter brain and/or body chemistry are mainly cast into two categories: those that ease the pain of living, pregnancy being only one of the extremities of this ubiquitous class of existentialities, or those that extend the performance of human life. Either way, we are taken away from the vicissitudes of beings, as well as perhaps from authentic Being as we can understand it in ourselves, by their use. Yet in no way can we construct a 'naturalist' argument, whereby the drug free person is somehow the most genuine example of humanity. No, not in material terms. But the efforts involved in self-understanding are sometimes so treacherous that external aids are employed to circumlocute them.

They may even be seen as a way in which to gain a kind of freedom, that from values or from one's social location. The amphetamines and even caffeine might be said to have this effect, as they make us more alert and willing to keep working, even if such work is only labor and the goal we have is to earn a wage. The ability to do so in the face of its apparent meaninglessness is surely a feat notwithstanding. More than this, we also have in our own time the sense that values, apparently the source of much conflict in the world, should themselves be overcome: "This is the ideal of the disengaged self, capable of objectifying not only the surrounding world but also his own emotions and inclinations, fears and compulsions, and achieving thereby a kind of distance and self-possession which hallows him to act 'rationally'" (Taylor 1989, 21). Drugs are one ironic means to this ideal. They can erase pain and discomfort, give one a sense of contentment and calm, relax aching parts of the body and help one sleep at night. We can be said to be 'self-possessed' when we are possessed of ourselves in this new way. We indeed are 'distanced' from our own humanity. It tends to get in the way in any case, either with regard to work, relationships, planning for the future, or simply enjoying the day as it is or the wider world as it is. If drug use/abuse is not quite a form of non-being, it does bear the hallmark of para-being. Its effect is to annul what authentically stupefies us. The advent of large scale industrial manufacture and use of such substances heralds an age in which we no longer imagine suffering as a means to understanding or as a creditable way to transcend the human condition. At the same time, it is a testament to our anxiety that concernful being as a mode of Dasein's authentic existence would make us care *too* much for ourselves and others. This odd situation has arisen precisely because science and its technological progeny short-circuit the task of self-understanding by providing means that can masquerade as ends. It is a kind of overcoming made automatic by, on the one hand, contemporary conceptions of what it means to be healthy—that is, in a 'natural' undrugged state or at the very least, in a drugged state through the use of a substance that aids the body's own health-producing capabilities; vitamins are often cited as being mildly effective in this manner- or, on the other, the sheer availability of any kind of decoy behavior known to the world. Either way, we judge ourselves to have 'overcome the misapprehensions of the past', our own, or that of the history of the science that made our new lives possible (cf. Gadamer 2003, 82–3ff [1935]). A physical 'perception' has been transmuted more or less chemically into an 'intuition' (*Anschauung*). In phenomenology, this term, which can mean both perception of the hyletic and intuition of the eidetic, is sometimes taken to be a means to the essence of things, an ontological device. It does not separate form and representation so much as it provides itself as a means toward both, pending one's context and problem. But the health science or general consumptive culture of drugs, as well as the decoys that abound in the criminal as well as the pharmaceutical market, allow *Anschauung* to be sidestepped in both realms: "The question 'What is Man?' blocks its own view of what it is really after with an object foreign to it" (Heidegger 1999, 21).

Science, and specifically that related to medicine is, however, not exhausted by the production of decoy maneuvers. Like the difference between the ethics of the great religious world systems and the acts of those who claim to adhere to them, science too has its effects and its ideals. Its self-perception is not necessarily a self-understanding as a human endeavor given that most research is consumed and taken over fully by the para-being of inauthentic market. Even so, its origins are those of the human desire to make itself independent of both the world and the world of merely world-denying means. It is both an affirmation of the will and of the world as it stands. It nevertheless is also a new soteriological doctrine which requires believers and agents in that self-same world: "The scientific will, which is theoretical, is first a will to exist in sovereignty" (Lingis 1989, 19). This autonomy is broken free from both the social world of values—it becomes the new highest value—as well as from the otherworld of evaluation—it is its own self-evaluation and self-correction by virtue of its method. But most importantly, it is the act of being in the world that becomes responsible to and for itself: "Universal rational science is the activity by which subjectivity determines itself as absolutely responsible, free—spontaneous and autonomous" (ibid).

Meanings

If this is so, we must surely view its co-option by consumptive affairs as a subversion of its ideals and even a perversion of its human mandate. Yet it is easy to see why this has occurred. As with any salvation doctrine, the effect of one's faith is to absolve one, not of suffering *per se*, but of having to confront the possibility that suffering is one's lot in life and only one's lot. In a word, it gives meaning to human suffering, even if we today often suggest that those our ancestors were presumably content with were mere rationalizations. It is equally too much to say that to be human is to suffer. Suffering is but one of many human outcomes, and most of it, we *can* affirm with the new scientific ethic, is in our own day needless and contrived. But the idea that we have not only the means to overcome it in this world but that it is of the highest and most moral inclination to do so is something we ourselves have invented quite recently. It is very much part of a new idea of what culture should be and do. *This* understanding, which includes medicine as the highest art of life, comes to us as part of the anthropological self-understanding that culture and humanity are not separate nor are they separable. This is viewed most transparently by observing the medical practices of mechanical societies, seemingly so alien to our own. It was noticed "… first, that primitive medical *practices* follow from and make sense in terms of underlying medical *beliefs*, and, secondly, that both are best conceived not as quaint folklorisms but as integral *parts of culture*" (Wellin 1977, 49, italics in the original). Since we live in a culture dominated by technical achievement but at the same time producing an existence sullied by the sense that technique can overcome any existential issue, it is quite understandable that medical practices mimic most closely our ideal that we should be able to *fix* ourselves as one fixes anything in the object world that is broken or even that has lost its function—the collectibles market, for instance, which has translated once purely utilitarian items into valuable artifacts: "Disease breaks away from the metaphysic of evil, to which it had been related for centuries, and it finds in the visibility of death the full form in which its content appears in positive terms" (Foucault 1973, 196). Evil, when imagined as an otherworldly apparition that intrudes into the social world of humans, cannot be 'fixed' in this way, at least not by ourselves. But when recast as a simple cause and effect function which may or may not give the patient an 'evil' experience, it becomes a mere metaphor for suffering. And most suffering *can* be fixed by human beings. This is why disease, even manifesting itself in the patient's demise, takes on a 'positive' content. It has *done* something in the world and more than this, it has its source in that self-same world.

The causes of death can be known. Speculation has been consigned to the antecedent sharps of historical thought. Yes, reductionism continues to be a problem for anyone who is interested in symbolic behavior and hermeneutics. Even so, neuro-science, for instance, has been at the forefront of the investigation not so much into the study of cognition and consciousness but in the dispelling of archaic moral notions. The spirits of another age have been vanquished by the structures of the brain. We do not know how they work, not exactly, but we understand their presence in a manner which differs utterly from the 'presence' of the other-world in our own. If the cognitive sciences are naively reductive in their conclusions and in their search for origins, they do have the merit of making human life more transparent to itself. They are basic in this sense: elemental structures may not have the capability cognitivists claim, but they are something to build from, something that allows for a fuller self-understanding of our being-in-the-world-as-it-is. Even in the midst of the previous century this was acknowledged (cf. Sorokin 1956, 186–7 where he holds that the sociological mainstream was 'obsolescent' with regard to then current theories of cognition adapted from the natural sciences). At the same time, and by the same token, any such prescription for the understanding of consciousness and its detriments that ignores the effects of encultured morality and what have you on the individual agent is bound to be incomplete: "We act as though we understood the purpose of life, and hence could classify routes according to the speed with which they lend to its goal" (Lösch 1967, 225 [1945]). The structures of consciousness are not the structures of the life-world. At most, they might delineate our abilities to comprehend our situatedness of being amongst others, our discriminative powers regarding the differences between being alone and being lonely, or acting with conscience or without it according to the norms of the time and place, but they do not precisely dictate the specific contents of these norms nor the character of the conscience that follows from them. To travel too far down this route is to attribute instinctual behavior to a reasoning consciousness or at the very least to give it too much elemental sway. Perhaps this is the most dangerous aspect of allopathic medical discourse and its scientific relatives. Perhaps this was inevitable, given the dual task of science in general: "On the one hand it aims to represent the hugely complex facts of the world. On the other, it aims at clarity, and for that it needs formal simplicity" (Midgely 2004, 129). Kindred to the organizations that scientists themselves have constructed to sort out who does what and how they do so (cf. Kelleher, Gabe, and Williams 1994a, xii concerning the phenomenon of the hasty professionalization of medical bodies and boards), details are subsumed within unified theories, with cosmology being the candidate touted to embrace 'everything'. But a theory of everything is always an overstatement. At best, it would account for the origins of the universe and how that universe hangs together. It can tell us how human beings think and work only in the most basic sense. What is more interesting than the smugness which might emanate from such a 'grand' theory is that such knowing would reconstruct the mystery of creation. It begs the question of ultimate origins, positing a cyclical series of multi-verses with neither beginning nor end. Now it may well be the case that this is correct, and it is merely our mortal consciousness that finds it difficult to grasp given our own paltry and serial experience of things and of others. Nevertheless, our ability to plumb the depths, either of our own bodies or the cosmos as a whole, presents both a new way of knowing but also a new manner of confronting what is unknown as well as redefining what the unknowable may contain. It is his last aspect that is the challenge to the prevailing moral conscience: "The moral obstacle was experienced only when the epistemological need had emerged; scientific necessity revealed the prohibition for what it was: Knowledge invents the Secret" (Foucault 1973, 163). Indeed, we may construct a mystery simply to enjoy the chasing of it. If we witness the myriad of such entertainment fictions enjoyed by millions and recycled over and over again, we are left with less doubt about the enduring appeal of what is as yet unknown. To suggest to human beings, with their primate curiosity and their reasoned confidence bordering as it often does on arrogance, that there should be something beyond our ability to know in the cosmos is to certainly wave the red flag. Like the fictional whodunits, there is always a moral rider involved: in the cosmological sense, Reason is the greatest detective, and anything that threatens this semi-personified gloss of our species as a whole is more or less evil. Whether it is addiction or compulsion, loneliness or social anxiety, the distractions of lust or fame, all of which are given supernumerary presence in popular detective fictions, the hero must battle not only external forces in the criminals and sometimes also in the official institutions of justice, but also the demons within. Triumph means to not only defeat the perpetrator—to find the cause or origin of things at the cosmological level—but to vanquish, however temporarily, all of those threats that have their source in the hero's own life and lifestyle.

The detective is also a doctor. Reason animates both social roles from the beginning. Curiosity and confidence walk the line with incompetence and arrogance alike. The one who sees through the veil, the one who attains truth, once again in the Greek sense of making something visible, of clarifying a concept in the philosophical role, is the one who is super-endowed with the gift of reason. He is the contrasting character to the magician, who once made the visible invisible, or produced visibility out of the void where none even thought there was a mystery in the first place. Even so, magic has not entirely deserted our metastasized detective, for it still has a symbolic and Durkheimian function even in its latter days of disuse and disdain: "Magic readapts the group to predefined problems through the patient, while psychoanalysis readapts the patient to the group by means of the solutions reached" (Lévi-Strauss 1977, 453). In each *case*—and is it a coincidence that the term 'case' is employed equally by both detectives and doctors, as well as, for that matter, lawyers?—there is presented a problem to be solved. One might well seek a solution simply to prove one's abilities, but proving something to oneself is tantamount to accepting the 'predefined' as both category and course of action. The solution to any *actual* case is one in which the transgression of what should *be* the case is exposed. Disease must yield to health, at least morally, just as crime must yield to justice. So the solutions reached do not demand that we always adhere to the ideals or the norms of the day, only that we recognize them as what we should always do even if we do not in fact do so. Stating this, however vehemently, serves only to remind us that what one can do in fact includes the region of the diseased, the immoral, and the criminal: "The actual must be contained in the possible" (Lösch, op. cit., 123). How it has been possible for medical discourse to both arise and claim ownership of all of the possibilities with regard to consciousness and its assailants presents to us the problem of science and of history in combination. For to understand the incarnative force of medical knowing is to make clear the most important application of the scientific method in human history. It has also been applied *to* that very history, dissecting it as it falls to pieces before our very eyes.

References

Barrett, William. 1979. *The Illusion of Technique: A Search for Meaning in a Technological Civilization.* New York: Anchors Books.

Derrida, Jacques. 1995. *On the Name.* Stanford: Stanford University Press [1993].

Foucault, Michel. 1973. *The Birth of the Clinic.* New York: Vintage Books [1963].

Foucault, Michel. 1980. *The History of Sexuality Volume One: Introduction.* New York: Vintage Books [1978].

Frankel, B. Gail, Mark Speechley, and Terrance J. Wade. 1996. *The Sociology of Health and Health Care: A Canadian Perspective.* Toronto: Copp Clark.

Freund, Peter E. S., and Meredith B. McGuire. 1999. *Health, Illness, and the Social Body: A Critical Sociology.* New York: Prentice-Hall.

Gadamer, Hans-Georg. 1935. "Ancient Atomic Theory." In *The Beginning of Knowledge*, 82–101. New York: Continuum [2003].

Gadamer, Hans-Georg. 1974. "On the Tradition of Heraclitus." In *The Beginning of Knowledge*, 21–34. New York: Continuum [2003].

Gadamer, Hans-Georg. 1978. "Greek Philosophy and Modern Thought." In *The Beginning of Knowledge*, 119–126. New York: Continuum [2003].

Gadamer, Hans-Georg. 1991. "On the Enigmatic Character of Health." In *The Enigma of Health: The Art of Healing in a Scientific Age*, 103–16. Stanford: Stanford University Press [1996].

Gadamer, Hans-Georg. 1995. "Natural Science and the Concept of Nature." In *The Beginning of Knowledge*, 127–40. New York: Continuum [2003].

Gadamer, Hans-Georg. 1998. *The Beginning of Philosophy.* New York: Continuum [1996].

Hall, John A. 2005. *How Homogenous Must We Be? Reflections on the Theory of Nationalism.* Saskatoon: University of Saskatchewan.

Harding, Jim. 1987. "The Pharmaceutical Industry as a Public-Health Hazard and as an Institution of Social Control." In *Health and Canadian Society: Sociological Perspectives, Second Edition*, edited by George Torrance, 545–67. Toronto: Fitzhenry and Whiteside.

Heidegger, Martin. 1999. *Ontology—The Hermeneutics of Facticity*. Bloomington: Indiana University Press [1988].

Illich, Ivan. 1975. *Medical Nemesis: The Expropriation of Health*. Toronto: McClelland and Stewart.

Jung, Carl G. 1959. *Aion: Researches into the Phenomenology of the Self*. Princeton: Princeton University Press [1951].

Kelleher, David, Jonathan Gabe, and Gareth Williams. 1994a. "Understanding Medical Dominance in the Modern World." In *Challenging Medicine*, edited by Jonathan Gabe, David Kelleher, and Gareth Williams, xi–xxix. London: Routledge.

Kelleher, David, Jonathan Gabe, and Gareth Williams. 1994b. "Epilogue: The Last Days of Doctor Power." In *Challenging Medicine*, edited by Jonathan Gabe, David Kelleher and Gareth Williams, 181–87. London: Routledge.

Lévi-Strauss, Claude. 1977. "The Sorcerer and His Magic." In David Landy, ed. *Culture, Disease, and Healing: Studies in Medical Anthropology*, 445–53. New York: Macmillan.

Lilburn, Tim. 1999. *Living in the World as If It Were Home: Essays*. Dunvegen, Ontario: Cormorant Books.

Lingis, Alphonso. 1989. *Deathbound Subjectivity*. Bloomington: Indiana University Press.

Lösch, August. 1967. *The Economics of Location*. New York: Wiley Science Editions, John Wiley and Sons [1945].

Midgely, Mary. 2004. *The Myths We Live By*. London: Routledge.

Neumann, Erich. 1970. *The Origins and History of Consciousness*. Princeton: Princeton University Press [1949].

Peneff, Jean. 1990. "Myths in Life Stores." In *The Myths We Live By*, edited by Raphael Samuel and Paul Thompson, 36–48. London: Routledge.

Samuel, Raphael, and Paul Thompson, eds. 1990a. *The Myths We Live By*. London: Routledge.

Samuel, Raphael, and Paul Thompson, eds. 1990b. "Introduction." In *The Myths We Live By*, edited by Raphael Samuel and Paul Thompson, 1–22. London: Routledge.

Selye, Hans. 1956. *The Stress of Life: A New Theory of Disease*. New York: McGraw-Hill.

Sigerist, Henry E. 1977. "The Special Position of the Sick." In *Culture, Disease, and Healing: Studies in Medical Anthropology*, edited by David Landy, 388–93. New York: Macmillan.

Sontag, Susan. 1978. *Illness as Metaphor*. New York: Vintage Books.

Sorokin, Pitirim. 1956. *Fads and Foibles in Modern Sociology and Related Sciences*. Chicago: Henry Regnery Company.

Taylor, Charles. 1989. *Sources of the Self: The Making of Modern Identity*. Cambridge, MA: Harvard University Press.

Thomson, Alistair. 1990. "The Anzac Legend: Exploring National Myth and Memory in Australia." In *The Myths We Live By*, edited by Raphael Samuel and Paul Thompson, 73–82. London: Routledge.

Wellin, Edward. 1977. “Theoretical Orientations in Medical Anthropology: Continuity and Change Over the Past Half-Century.” In *Culture, Disease, and Healing: Studies in Medical Anthropology*, 47–57. New York: Macmillan.

Westlake, Aubrey T. 1973. *The Pattern of Health: A Search for a Greater Understanding of the Life Force in Health and Disease.* London: Shambhalla and Routledge and Kegan Paul.

Williams, Gareth, and Jennie Popay. 1994. “Lay Knowledge and the Privilege of Experience.” In *Challenging Medicine*, edited by Jonathan Gabe, David Kelleher and Gareth Williams, 118–39. London: Routledge.

CHAPTER ONE

Opening Up the Corpuscular Corpus

> The social origin of disease entities is the need industrialized people have to exonerate their institutions.
>
> —ILLICH (1975, 118)

Being social, possessing language and reason, being interested in both the past and the future, tolerating or criticizing our political organizations, and seeking thrills, pleasures, or the 'simple life' are all normative characteristics of the human condition. Each thought takes place in the culture of its upbringing, then has a chance to take its place in a discourse of understanding both in the sense of self-concern and that of the wider cosmos. Each social group constructs its own language, kindred to the marriage conversation, into which one must be admitted. The hoops of bourgeois culture include university accreditations, professional society markers, as well as certain kinds of real estate and mates or companions, and on top of this, the ability and willingness to pass these acquired traits down the generational line. Middle class children are both the most and least responsible of our youthful citizens, in that they have to bear the burden of upholding the ideal norms of Western industrial societies as well as having the extended leisure to dither within them.

Health is, as well, mostly a bourgeois construct. It was first imagined as a new social contract for those who were never part of the evil of the old order, never either elites or peasants. The middle classes were *new*, like the politics, industry, and intellect of the new age. From the eighteenth century onwards, the gradient of 'eugenic' self-regard took to ever greater esthetic heights, from which one could gaze out onto the frontiers of culture, both future and past. The future was seen as being owned by the new wealth and social capital. The past, grim and grimy both, was the detritus of a breed in its death throes. Precisely, what was old was decayed, unhealthy, diseased, and had thus treated in the most scurvy fashion the aspirations of the healthy ones, the *embourgoisiement* of those who still worked for a living while at the same time not slaving for it. Theirs was the paragon of health in a social world surrounded by illness. To educate the masses whilst tearing down the misbegotten elites was the order of the day, from the French Revolution through to the First World War. The tragic irony of bourgeois culture, as has been cited many times, was the development of the nation-state and the colonial empire. Such a politics of enslaving the remainder of the world while preaching the gospel of human freedom and individual free will was too much for any cultural group to stomach. So the middle classes turned inward, began to live to work, train themselves to both produce and consume, and eventually, in our own day, began to wither on their own vine.

Even so, their idea of health remains our own. The correct definition of exercise, for instance: something that gets the blood flowing and the heart pumping without denigrating the body—that is, no manual labor, but no endless leisure either. Protestant ethic driven bourgeois culture has created the 'new man', as the Nazis had sought to, but it is contained in a universalizing discourse that seeks to reproduce itself across cultures and classes. It is not reserved for 'Aryans', but does take the European type as an ideal. It follows in the shadow of capital in general, as it has globalized itself to the nth degree. That it is assumed to be the best thing is of course, taken for granted at the outset. Yet it is tolerant in a way that the nineteenth century could never be. It takes in many comers and respondents. In our medical ambit, all of the alternative therapies that have graduated into the academy of official and dominant medical discourse slowly grow in number, with chiropractors and psychoanalysts being two of the more vanilla choices readily available for those disenchanted with the usual fare. In its democracy, much like that of its parent politics, Western medicine accedes to alternatives as long as those confine themselves to certain kinds of claims and exhort a mutual recognition within their professional circles. Like capital, which seems to function under many a diverse regime, or education, which is more or less militaristic wherever one travels, medicine is a worldly character with a confident stride, flashing its obsidian credit card and taking the pretty smile in return.

In this first of four substantive chapters, we will review and interpret the history, epistemology, and ethics of the mainstream medical discourse, as well as take a brief look at its social organization, its professionalization and professionalisms, its mores and its mysteries, its inequities and inequalities. The problem of the self-conscious subjectivity of science is discussed, as well as the challenge that the enduring fetish of objectivity presents to the medical practitioner, whose mandate always also includes the patient's own experience as both a clue and a distraction to the matters at hand. By its close, we should be able to understand the ideal of a better practice and ethical outlook that is, often in spite of itself, contained within the larger picture of institutional and scientific practices. To this end, then, it is imagined that we each of us have something to contribute the better functioning of health care as both a cultural construct and a social virtue.

1.1 Recent Histories

The idea that science is nothing but its method is attractive for a number of reasons. First and foremost, it separates science from its parent religion. Most of us seek to at least be somewhat different and hopefully better, especially at parenting, than were our own parents. Method in science does eventually involve a leap of faith, but it is one that must rest for the time being only, in lieu of further data or contradictory evidence. It is ideally open to both, whereas the history of at least much religious behavior, if not belief, is closed in these ways. Faith is ultimately always demanded in the religious worldview, and while a healthy faith in modernity is seen as something that one questions regularly, even to the point of doubting the source of faith itself, this is distinctly a modern view.

1.1.1 The 'Selfhood' of Scientific Healing

Such a viewpoint was carried over by the contemporary need religion has to defend its dwindling franchise of believers and shrinking explanatory territories: "This is connected with the fact that the philosophy of modernity has erected its philosophical self-grounding upon the concept of self-consciousness" (Gadamer 2003, 34 [1990]). It is just that self who practices the science of medicine while flirting with the art of healing. This self is the vehicle for a specific application of scientific method. He or she applies it also to oneself, at least in matters of physiological well-being, and is thus both an educator of his or her clientele or case load, and an exemplar, ideally, of the results of the careful attentiveness to what the pedagogic authority of medicine has to say about the body and the mind in the world: "The physician no longer appears as the kind of medicine man mysteriously shrouded with special powers that we find in other cultures. He is a man with a body of knowledge" (Gadamer 1996, 31 [1967]). As well, the doctor is someone who is trained more or less publicly, on the public dole, and is mostly paid in the same way for his services. The shaman's whole being is *private* or, if not quite so in the modern sense of the term, it is nonetheless 'privy' to another world and thus not entirely of this one.

That being said, we also know that professionalization within the health care fields is carried out within its own shrouds of technical languages, status differentiations, and the use of high technology that, to a layperson, looks sometimes rather like magic, especially if it actually works. Not so different from the shaman, a patient becomes a believer all the more strongly if the treatment has what is judged to be a salutary effect on one's outlook. One's own objectivity as a scientific end is being called into question, perhaps in a radical manner, and the methods applied to understanding it and thus curing its ailments are so directed as to be at least kindred with the attentiveness the shaman gives to his charge. Indeed, "… the meaning of scientific rigor needs rather to be drawn from the kind of object being investigated and the mode of access appropriate to it" (Heidegger 1999, 56–57). Just before this, Heidegger states unequivocally that mathematically based rigor in thinking is a 'mistake' and cannot be sustained. So it is also in medicine. Any investigation that requires 'access' to a phenomenologically constituted object such as the human person—just as in a different way, Dasein is the situated thrownness of the human *being*—must forsake the logic of mathematics, starting with the movement from certainty to probability. Indeed, the shaman's potpourri of sleights of hand, smoke and mirrors, and rhetorical flourish gives way to a kind of intimate pedagogy wherein the diseased or lost member of the culture at hand comes to know his own culture in an entirely different way; from the point of view of what both underlies it—the structures of his cultural consciousness that are veiled over by norms—and envelopes it as a mode of being—the conceptualizations of what lies beyond culture and adjudicates one's ultimate fate. Modern medicine has not, in fact, left these traditions behind them: "A way of teaching and *saying* became a way of learning and *seeing*" (Foucault 1973, 64, italics in the original). What the shaman makes invisible is the truth of the diseased state or the loss of the soul. But he does not simply cover it up, as if his ministrations were a mere analgesic maneuver. Rather, he takes away the profundity of its presence and replaces this with the reinvigorated understanding of both the presence of community—after all, the shaman, though often a feared and mysterious figure, is still one of *us*—and the overarching presence of Being. Even in ultimate failure when concerned with a truly physiognomical malady, magic prefigures the transfiguration of the spirit and, in social contract societies, its imminent return through the birth of another.

It is true that, where still legal, the priest or minister appears at the bedside inside the hospital. The doctor is no longer deemed responsible for the apparently speculative devices of the magician. Mathematical rigor is, if not ever achieved, still a goal in modern medicine in spite of an equal understanding that healing is both an art and the outcomes of treatment are always measurable only in series probabilities: "Sickness was placed in the center of the medical system, a sickness that could be subjected to a) operational verification by measurement, b) clinical study and experiment, and c) evaluation according to engineering norms" (Illich 1975, 112). The applied science of medicine had even more impetus to distance itself from both philosophy proper as the study of consciousness as well as the research sciences of nature given that both of these older discourses at once impinged upon its authority and autonomy but also evaluated it from without. Professional societies, of which more below, took on as their mandate the improving of their practical 'lead' as against these other bodies. The more evidence that could be cited with reference to successful *practice* of science, rather than simple gesticulating about it in philosophy or the use of its method in abstruse and arcane ways, as if the undead alchemist had slipped through the back door of the modern laboratory, the better: "Increasingly sophisticated pathological anatomy meant that diseases were conceptualized in terms of alternations in tissues that were visible upon opening the body, such as during autopsy. This mode of conceptualizing disease had a profound effect in splitting body and mind in the practice of clinical medicine" (Freund and McGuire 1999, 213). But these new definitions regarding how illness manifested itself—the autopsy was both a procedure to identify the autograph of the disease as well as an autohagiographical valediction of the life that it had claimed—did not by themselves offer medicine to the history of science as a liberated form of objectivity in the literal sense. One is still dealing with signs. For the better part of this history, diseases 'themselves' could not be made visible in any other way. At the same time, such new knowledge did not present to its parent discourse any more insight into how medicine could itself be reconstructed in this manner: "What occurred was not a 'psychoanalysis" of medical knowledge, nor any more or less spontaneous break with imaginary investments; 'positive" medicine is not a medicine that has made an 'objectal" choice in favour of objectivity itself" (Foucault 1973, x). Instead, as Foucault relates, such distinctions were localized in the body as deemed to be a kind of essential vehicle for the manifestation of disease. One could simply argue that disease entities, whatever may be their 'character'—and we have already seen how they continue to be disdained in a moralizing and scapegoating rhetoric—only became relevant at all when contracted by a human being, or some other source of human nourishment or context necessary for human survival. This kind of vision never gives up the essence of things to its sight or within the ambit of objectivity. Everything continues to be seen from the perspective of a threatened humanity.

Including the illnesses that are home grown, as it were. Self-inflicted injuries, either as inherited from familial relations in this or that cultural milieu, or those that have identifiable genetic predispositions or yet sudden and positive triggers, or addictions invented by a combination of stressors and choices made in response to them, such a catalogue claims many lives both living and dead. Thus the new corpus of the body as the textuality upon which is written the signature of disease and hang-up alike begins to look very much like a localized version of the pre-modern idea of the 'world as text', wherein one can discover the autograph of the creator writ into the surrounding nature. The augury of signage is not discarded, and hence the compulsive interest the hormonal and peer induced ululations of the body electric: "The power which thus took charge of sexuality set about contacting bodies, caressing them with its eyes, intensifying areas, electrifying surfaces, dramatizing troubled moments. It wrapped the sexual body in its embrace" (Foucault 1980, 44). Even the most dedicated vision must find a way to maintain its longitudinal focus. Interest must be reignited, much like that regarding sex in marriage, another favorite topic of this discourse, and as such, *interest* itself becomes the object of the language of application and control. As it is most convenient to maintain self-interest, it is relatively easy to understand why self-inflicted injuries—committed compulsively or, as many depressed persons proverbially explicate it, 'so I could feel something rather than nothing'—have become the order of the day. They provide the objectifying link between the subject at hand and its readiness to hand in the realm of discourse, aside from locating the body in the world of things. But more than this, the autohagiographic similitude of submitting oneself to becoming one's own objectifying force in the world and as a case in a practical science study has the ironic effect of making everyone into a lay scientist: "What is negated, then, is the person acting in the role of observer; he has *become* his role. The reality of the person as an individual remains, though it has been set off to the side. In the history of science we are witnesses to a methodological death which, far from interfering with the glory of individual scientists, hardly effects the lives of astronomers, physicists, or anatomists" (Natanson 1970, 135, italics in the original). The loss of personhood that we expect to be normative within the clinical spaces of treatment and health care is due just as much to our own interest in what is happening to us than in any autocratic diktat emanating from a white-robed institution.

1.1.2 Social Groups

This said, it is equally clear that the professional drama of health care workers and authorities welcomes this self-interest with open arms. It could hardly do otherwise, for, akin to the social worker who would lose her job if the failings of society that produced her oversize case load were ever actually addressed at their source, the health care professional as we know her today would become as extinct in a brave new world of indefinitudinal cybernetic consciousness. The status of the human within reach of clinical discourse—or, for that matter, any other discourse that centers itself on the pathology of the present whilst casting an anchor out to windward regarding the sense that what the future holds is both objectively better but also morally superior; criminology, social services, and sometimes even welfare policy comes to mind—is subject to a transmigration, though one less focused upon the archaism of the soul (another *remanant* put 'off to the side') than on the body 'itself': "For clinical experience to become possible as a form of knowledge, a reorganization of the hospital field, a new definition of the status of the patient in society [ ] became necessary" (Foucault 1973, 196). The 'sick role' became more of an exacting human resource in the literal sense. Littered with still warm bodies, not unlike the university classrooms that benefit from matching public funding reckoned on enrollment, hospitals and clinics could manage themselves as did any other service sector with a rotating clientele. Their littoral scene was plain spoken: pending class background, payment accepted in full a priori services rendered: "The first groups to demand access to the new style of care were the middle classes of industrializing societies. They favoured the insurance principle …" (Torrance 1987, 8). No socialist style reforms were necessary to provide care in this prepaid manner. Other classes continued to pay per diem. Gradually, this system evolved into universal tax based or employee contribution based access, which is common enough today cross culturally. The major weakness of these systems, as has been pointed out on innumerable occasions, depending on the age of the total population served and the amount of political will at regional levels to channel monies into the system, is wait times. Even in otherwise emergency situations, there may be lengthy waits that give the subject the impression he or she might have descended into a kind of purgatory. Just as the extension of explicatory territories is occasioned by the imaginative use of clinical discourse—especially in reference to psychopathology and like-minded disciplines, for instance, and the mutability of the DSM manuals edition to edition testifies to their culture-bound diagnostics—what constitutes an 'emergency' or something that is 'critical' is symptomatic of a larger social and political scene. But all of this was already old hat within the burgeoning medical fields: "… moral entrepreneurs were establishing a specialized professional territory for themselves by creating illness labels" (Freund and McGuire 1999, 201). Indeed, moralizing, so richly rewarded in the old language of practical religion, could not be simply dismissed by the new one of applied science. As long as illness remains 'metaphoric', as in Sontag's famous analysis, we will feel compelled at a deeper level to 'look after ourselves'. As long as life is considered to be 'sacred' in this way—and perhaps more than any other concept, the Durkheimian sacred has shown itself to be resilient even across mode of production boundaries—we will do, and pay, anything to be healthy, in spite of many of our lifestyle choices.

Even so, this impulse to well-being, while it speaks of the interiority of a Dasein that cannot afford to turn away from the thrownness which is its lot for too great lengths of time, is magnified out of all subjective proportions by the *industry* of health and its denizens. Its objectifying evaluations began to take the authoritative mantle once the preserve of the priestly caste: "… the doctor began to play a decisive role in the organization of assistance. At the social level at which help was distributed, it was the doctor who discovered where it was needed and judged the nature and degree of the assistance to be given" (Foucault 1973, 41). Certainly into the nineteenth century, all of the symbolic elements were in place that led to both universal health care and to the Holocaust alike. In the now well-known film *The Architecture of Doom*, we are reminded, in deadpan tones, how it was 'the doctors' who judged who would live and die, it was they who turned on the gas taps, and it was they who checked if the people 'were really dead' after all, that the 'treatment' had been successful in 'curing' the world of ugliness and decay. Hard to live down as a profession, one imagines. Nevertheless, the doctor, while not as trustworthy as he might have been before Nuremberg, is still the 'go to' social role when we are feeling ill, or even ironically, ill at ease. This *Ungeheuer* that is sometimes promoted by the corpus collossum of medical institutions and personnel—over the counter neurochemicals must be the most obvious vehicle of surveillance available to subject and object likewise—perpetuates the sense that in any social group, the scourge of illness can afflict us at any time. If 'taking a pill', from an analgesic to a prophylactic to a gastro-enteric etc. is considered a point by point remedy for our ailments, then the sundry species of addictions that sometimes results from our use and abuse of 'the pill' is also an opportunity for the clinic and its moralists: "Increasingly, the doctor is working with two groups of drugs addicts: in one he prescribes addictive drugs, and in the other he is responsible for the care of people who are suffering the consequences of having drugged themselves" (Illich 1975, 44). Irony tends to know no bounds *within* rational organizations, but in the health sector, it has spilled out into the streets. So much so, that persons in day to day life take on the aspect of patients well before they darken the doors of their nearest hospital or clinic. Like homework and 'after school' activities such as team sports and clubs, the surveillance devices of contemporary medicine attempt to keep an eye on our beings-in-the-world, or better, beings-at-large. The translucent extension of what within the physical confines of this or that rational organization, 'total institution' or otherwise remains opaque to the outsider, subverts the sense that there is a clear boundedness to these arenas, and that one can be either inside them or outside them, but never both at once.

And it is discourse itself that provides the leverage for such extensions into the world at large. One its most potent examples is the simple statistic, a kind of meteorological tool for health professionals to use during the in-take and diagnostic phases of clinical process. Ultimately however, and within these very stages, such a rubric finds itself in moments of utter impotency as well: "The picture of the individual which his constructed on the basis of standardized values is an extremely precarious and unreliable one. It is only when we start out from the recognition that the distinction between health and illness cannot be so clearly defined that we can remind ourselves that even today medical interns must still begin by asking patients in what way they are feeling unwell" (Gadamer 1996, 160–61 [1990]). Yet here, one might protest, is merely the beginning of the space where standard values and their ensuing prescriptive implications begin. But at each stage of the treatment process, the individuality of the 'case' reasserts itself. It is true that there are observable variables that may or may not come into play during diagnosis, the proverbial line regarding commonplace contexts of such observation "… it embraces the behavior of some men in almost all situations and the behavior of almost all men in some situations …" (Lösch 1967, 184 [1945]) is one such rendition of it—has been extended back *into* the space of specificity.

1.1.3 Critical Implications

Social role behavior aside for the moment, the person become patient has a lengthy list of expectations of the clinical space, the most important one being that she feels 'better' after having entered therein, and especially after having left. It is always a disappointment to experience no change at all in either context, even if the entirety of such alterations are put down to 'mere' psychosomaticism by the professional themselves. At every level, the model of progress, militarism and capital are maintained, even in the usually invisible spaces of where the real action is, as it were, the cellular and molecular arenas (cf. Martin 1994, 219ff, regarding her analysis of textbook descriptions of cellular function and command sequences). This use of language and its implications stem from the architecture of the base metaphors that associate the inability to function in a consumptive-productive situation as pathological. Speaking of menopause, Martin suggests "… that the tenacity of this view comes not only from the negative stereotype associated with aging women in our society, but as a logical outgrowth of seeing the body as a hierarchical information-processing system in the first place" (ibid, 222). And not merely women, but the entire idea of aging is translated into the problem of *agedness*. Once again, the sense that decay is upon us, our society, our morality etc., is a sensitivity—though not necessarily a sensibility—that seems to die hard. Like the concept of the sacred, to which it is not unrelated given our fetish for the 'good life' and for life 'itself', 'decay' is felt as a withering wind of decrepitude, either in physically real episodes of bodily dysfunction or outright failure, or as a symbolic apparatus designed to decoy us from the confrontation with human finitude. It may be taken as an existential sign, though usually it is taken with angst instead of a more insightful understanding, but discursively and ideological it is taken as an enemy in its own right: "As the health-care system responds with increasing intensity to the needs of the elderly, the projected impact of aging on overall utilization rates also increases. But this is not a genuine external or exogenous effect, it is an outcome of the behavior of the health-care system itself" (Evans 1987, 621). This 'behavior' concerns the inauthenticity of one's turning toward the world which appears to never end. That is, such care of the self extends from the notion that we pass into and out of a world that continues along with or without us. The 'withness' of the world is not then for us, or for us alone. It is rather we who are with the world, having fallen into it or fallen at it in Heidegger's sense of *Verfallen*. Such a *Mitwelt* makes us ironically uncomfortable, giving us a feeling that we, because we appear to be with the world only in the interim as it were, are actually and authentically without a home. But unless we posit some other place or even space wherein humanity dwells eternally or authentically, then our understanding of *Mitwelt* must be renovated or salvaged in some manner. Modernity does not make claims regarding these other possible worlds or dimensions, aside from theories concerning the 'multiverse', so that we are prone to disdain any failure regarding our own self-understanding as being-in-the-world while without the longitudinal ability to remain a being-with-the-world.

This sense of ongoing failure animates the behavior of health systems of all kinds, whether out in that very world which might not be our home after all, like institutions and other facilities where our health is at issue—it is interesting that making *facile*, convenient or easy, simplifying a problem, giving one's thought some 'facility' with it, and the term used to designate these spaces are intimately related—or within our bodies: "... just as seeing menopause as a kind of failure of the authority structure in the body contributes to our negative view of it, so does seeing menstruation as failed production contribute to our negative view of it" (Martin 1994, 224). When we are conscious of failure, when this failure is seen as our own and thus consciousness means a self-consciousness of being self-conscious, as in shyness or having some species of social anxiety with others or with the world, we are more readily 'taken in' by the idea of homelessness and thus we imagine ourselves yet more susceptible to decay. Insulated within the envelope of a home-place, decay must work harder to get at us, to bring us down, or tempt us to 'cast ourselves down', to use an older but still relevant language. The inner workings of the body that signify moments or phases in the life-cycle become signs of its impending demise. Like illness, the life-cycle of bodily functions which are in themselves quite 'natural' and expected—indeed, their *absence* would be, ironically, a sign of further and more radical illness—such as menses, menstruation, menopause in women and general pubescence and impotence in men, need not be taken as failures but as manifestations of the normal functioning of the human body over time. But it is precisely that 'normal' functioning over time that is so disturbing for us. For to function as a living organism means not only to have been born but also to die. It means having both a beginning and an end, which is precisely what the world does *not* appear to have.

As against this, artificial 'homes' have been developed to help us turn away from our existential situatedness within the world envelope. Insulating us against the forces of decay and entropy, which always appear to come out of the world and into us—and perhaps *this* is the ontological reason that structures our destruction of the world's environment and biosphere; we are resentful towards a world that lives on without us, a kind of 'if I can't live then no one can' kind of attitude—and never thus emanating from us and altering the ontology of the world, these artifices are most noticeable in the health care system as pharmaceuticals. Yet these are not merely marketed and manipulated by their source distributors and originators, our willingness to live with them and perhaps even decline to live without them has another more important discursive source: "… this acceptance has coincided with changes in the nature of 'illness" as presented to physicians today, with the precedence taken by chronic and ill-defined illnesses …" (Cooperstock and Lennard 1987, 315). Ill health must redefine itself as always and already the gravest threat, lest our conception of what it means to be healthy begins to actually include illness. Such a definition would be considered 'regressive' and even inauthentic, though of course it cannot be the second existentially, as inauthenticity remains a mode of Dasein in the world and a very common place one. The artifices of medical ideology aid this commonality because they turn us away from the world as it is and towards a world that looks more like us, and thus we are more comfortable living within it due to our dislocated sense that this world too shall pas away in a manner like myself. This too is inauthentic but yet it belongs to our very being. The problem then, is to begin to understand why our self-understanding has been misdirected in this way just at the moment that our understanding of other worlds—those of the previous metaphysics, for instance—has been discarded.

1.2 Epistemologies

To do so, we must first examine what those other worlds have been surmised as being, not in relation to themselves, for that would make the study of health into a theological enterprise, but in relation to this world and those who live in it, the originators of the ideas concerning other worlds as other-worlds.

1.2.1 Ontogenesis?

Heraclitus begins this tradition in the West. He ushers in a lengthy process of demythology, that is, of taking the other worlds into this one and uniting them in a kind of basic sociological worldview: "… it is not special knowledge that he makes his theme, but rather a new way of seeing the world—that is, thinking the *logoi*" (Gadamer 2003, 68 [1990]). The *Logos*, the Word, is a construction of the language of the Gods. It is not human language, though we can always bend our ears to it if we try. But languages, plural, diverse, and Babel-like, are very much the province of humankind and we must, if we are to survive at all, lend them our collective and equally diverse ears. *Logoi* therefore presents an immediacy that the *Logos* does not. *Logos* speaks of what we may become and what we are to existence, but *logoi* speaks to what we already are and what we mean to one another as human beings. Thinking the world as plural, and what better metaphor to use than what sets us apart from the other animals and life on earth, the use of language, is the beginning of all demythology. Couple this with the invention of history, occurring more or less at the same moment in Greek thought, allows what had been considered to be timeless to be placed *in* time. This was a crucial development in conscious self-circumspection, for *history is the ultimate argument against morality.*

Such a development had fundamental implications for notions of what could constitute a reasoned being that knew its own goods, including what it meant to be healthy rather than to be ill, or mad. Ultimately, for our own time: "The rationality in question is now procedural: in practical affairs, instrumental; in theoretical, involving the careful, disengaged scrutiny of our ideas and their assembly according to the canons of mathematical deduction …" (Taylor 1989, 243). A lengthy process separates Heraclitus from Frege, for instance, but nevertheless they remain linked. They are part of the same consciousness no less than the rest of us, and even though we are not aggrandized in the history of thought writ large, we thus remain within it. Demythology has, throughout the length and breadth of this now historical process, continued apace, to the point that we might even imagine that the passing of our world as the one that we are enveloped within as an existential facticality does indeed end with us. It might as well do so, we could casually, and quite irresponsibly add. Yet this would be to disavow the authentic existence of the human being as a wholly mutable and historical form of life and indeed, obviate the very manner through which we distinguish our kind of being from all known others: "… the sociologist turns to a 'sample" whose prime characteristic is that it has already 'become", is already in a state of 'becoming" before the social scientist looks into or at it" (Natanson 1970, 72). Furthermore, this object which is also a subject, already and always possesses approximately the same kind of capability as does the scientist or medical professional. We too know what it feels like to be in an 'unhealthy' situation' perhaps all the more when we feel we cannot escape it. This too is fundamental for human self-understanding: "The human being investigated by the sociologist has a reality which not only permits the scientist to look 'into" it but which enables the 'subject" to look 'out" or 'into" his observer" (ibid).

Perhaps the abyss truly is 'other people'. The experience of meaningless comes and goes with context, but health, and its feeling of 'well-being' is surely one of those contexts wherein while the proximal meaning of the day to day may be grasped more fully—one is not distracted, as it were, by one's ill-feeling or even by one's potential ill-will against oneself or others—it is equally clear that the existentiality of meaningfulness proper more readily escapes us. For the experience of ill heath is, as stated, a kind of dress rehearsal for finitude. It reconstructs the space of death, which we cannot experience for ourselves, within the ambient interiority of being. In fact, it lets us know that our inner space is not merely a physiological manifold, but an existential one, the kind of space filled with dreams and anxieties alike.

Foucault suggests that physiology proper was the vector upon which the space of disease was opened up, but specifically, the physiology of the disease 'entity' (cf. 1973, 188–9ff). The separation between the body as a naturally occurring phenomenon and the imputed intrusiveness of an externality in the form of another kind of being, and a vastly inferior one at that, provides the sensibility that it is within the spatiality of the arena in which both beings find themselves interlocked that disease can 'exist'. It exists *here* before it exists for sight. (ibid). Yet if it is taken as a given that the intrusive entity is so far inferior to ourselves, then how is it that it can infect us and distract us both from our daily round and from our noble purposes? It is because the inferiority of the being as it may have existed originally 'in nature' is given a geometric boost in power and fortune by interacting with our bodies. As we mentioned above, it is only due to this interaction that the being of disease comes within our purview as something to be seriously reckoned with at all: "Disease is now no more than a certain complex movement of tissues in reaction to an irritating cause: it is in this that the whole essence of the pathological lies, for there are no longer either essential diseases or essences of diseases" (ibid, 189). This overcoming of form is part of the demythologizing process that begins two and a half millennia earlier. The spatiality of the effects of disease is now the focus. There can be a topology of it, but no ontology proper to this space. And topological insights abound; their irony is, and continues to be, the manner in which they reach around the intervening epochs and cast our glances back into the aura and mystery of shamanic devices. To be sure, it is no longer a case of believing in the idea of magic *per se*. But the surgeon's sleight of hand is as well known as the sorcerer's, and the former's status leans upon that of the latter. A slight error and one is lost, whether it is a case of a brain tumor or a soul that plunges back into the darkness and possible dread of the tunnel which can only lead to the other world. Even so, our latter day medicine men are not mere conjurers, they fill too many social roles to be cast into this corner. Their mode of being-understanding may ultimately, though sometimes circuitously, be traced back to the logic of sorcery—two objects once brought into contact remain connected, for instance, and though this is true for objects, it is likely even more true for persons—but at the same time, their analytic abilities borrow as much from the sense of the commoner or layperson, for it is that very sense that the shaman attempts to expose to a parallax. For the steady hand of the quotidian worker encounters health in the following way: "… first, that pathological conditions have a cause that may be discovered and second, that a system of interpretations in which personal inventiveness is important structures the phases of illness, from the diagnosis to the cure" (Lévi-Strauss, op. cit., 451). But what exactly is this 'cause' that may be discoverable? Can it truly be recovered by working backwards from the scene or space of what is *presumed*—though nothing more, for the moment—to be its effects? If the human sciences continually are faced with parsing out complex multivariate analyses that offer themselves as explications for events or behaviors, observed and interpreted, of what order of validity do we speak when we link an effect with a primordiality? For it may be argued that "… pathology deals only with the gross final results of the disease process; it can tell us nothing of the causes which operated before the first pathological changes began to manifest" (Westlake, op. cit., 115). The 'inventiveness' of the subject and object alike, on the one hand, the response to the ubiquity of 'how does one feel?', and on the other, the experience of the doctor or specialist, general or more narrow, broader or deeper, each bringing with it a set of injunctions that work in the world more like conjunctions, gives interpretation and perhaps even creativity a major role to play. It is an ongoing challenge to present oneself as both a layperson who also feels pain, who also suffers in similar ways as does the patient, as well as someone who, unlike the patient, can overcome suffering. This amalgam of the subjectivity of common humanity and the objectivity of discursive accoutrement and technique links the doctor with his earliest progenitors.

1.2.2 Languages

Both doctor and patient throughout the phases of an illness which, as was implied, must also hold that the end of the illness is part of the health issue itself, rest their ability to negotiate this end on the fact that health as an abstract is something that both agree upon both in its form and as a goal. Its *ontos* must replicate it *telos*, or at least, the former must be replicated in the latter. Just as an illness no longer is conceived of as having an essence apart from what it is doing to us, so health as well can only be known through its presence in us. The archetype from religious language for the one is grace, for the other the absence of grace. Illness is still a sign of the damned. It is a condemnation. Since hell has long switched addresses to the world as we know it, the social stigmata facing those with ill health also finds itself right at home. Health, and not merely due to its feeling of being-at-home and lack of discomfort, freedom and the ability to abstract oneself from all present circumstances through diverse phantasms and projects of action, portrays nothing less than heaven on earth. These connections are more or less transparent, because "What at first looks like an abstract idea stands in reality for something that exists and can be experienced, that demonstrates its *a priori* presence spontaneously" (Jung 1959, 31). The method of this concretization, itself a further aspect of the wider process of demythology, consists in being able to describe what is happening to one as part of the world in which one lives. Illness forces us to reckon with the forces of the world, and moves its worldhood from welcome to judgement. Illness is always evaluator in this basic sense, and one need not employ theological metaphors to understand this as part of the general human condition. And 'descriptivity', what language is in fact doing in making something 'real' in this way, works both ways: "It is description, or, rather, the implicit labour of language in description, that authorizes the transformation of symptom into sign and the passage from patient to disease and from the individual to the conceptual" (Foucault, op. cit., 114). At once we are placed on a surface that stretches before and behind us, the one from the case to the cause, and the other from the idea to the object. Signification does not point anywhere specific by itself. We must cast ourselves into the workings of 'what is happening'. We are, existentially speaking, never aloof to this concernfulness of being, but we can use the inauthenticity of anxiety—if we are the patient, for instance—or that of discourse or even ideology—if we are the medical professional—to distract us from emplacing oneself in the midst of the topos of illness. The illness of one may well become the illness of another. Her malady may become my own. And it is within *this* abstracted sense of ipssissimosity that description begins its joint task: to rid ourselves of the dis-ease of having to confront the amorphous—kindred to the encounter with death which can only become an inexistence, a place of finality, and never may stay 'encountered' in the sense of it being a passing thing; passing on cannot be in passing—as well as pointing us in the direction of what is to be done: "… the particular symptom [ ] is not a local sign; on the contrary, it is an index of generalization" (ibid, 186). Given that working language is always language in use—here we do not speak of *Langage* in the synthetic Saussurean sense—*parole et langue* must have a symbiotic relationship. It is never a case of simply deciding upon a concept and then giving it and identifying voice. Speaking is not quite the same thing as an utterance; we do not presume, as the poet might, to 'speak into being' a new world. Diagnosis, treatment, and potential cure are moments in a discourse that had previously abandoned description as a mere indulgence of either the writer or teacher as well as merely a way in which to communicate with the blind: "One would simply have to give up the notion that the relation between language and fact is one of simple picturing. That logic has atomic forms of statement [ ] would carry no implication about the nature of the world" (Barrett 1979, 53). Such a picture was already itself uncertain. Similarly, the 'multiplication of uncertainties' cannot be said to produce something other than more of itself (cf. Sorokin, op. cit., 283). At the same time, one cannot, equally simply, dismiss numeric measures and the statistics they generate in principle, for though they do not approximate any specific case nor describe any particular subject, they do allow diagnosis to predict treatment and treatment to thus predict outcome. These predictions are also partly predications. They protect us against the confrontation with potential failure. Kindred with other failures that might assail us during life—those which have little long-term consequence we present to our children as rehearsals for the more adult disappointments of later life; a three week post-pubescent encounter will serve as a touchstone for a three year marriage etc.—we may predicate our future existence on the idea that within the curve constructed by these data or those we might yet live on to see it. So "... numbers and the relationships between the numbers are more than mere tools for the construction and reconstruction of matter. They are actual bearers of the order of reality ..." (Gadamer 1998, 73). It matters much then just exactly which reality we may speak of here. There is a human transpersonal reality of social norm and existential 'grace', and we must come to terms with 'both' of them. Numbers 'themselves' seem distant from this, but nevertheless we can use them as arbiters, not of our socially sanctioned grace *per se*, but of our ability to enter into the complex of relationships that *swirl* around mature being in the world. This 'tumult', of which Heidegger famously speaks in *Being and Time*, carries us off into the world and away from being. The solid curve of the statistic emplaces us in a slightly altered symbolic order where we can 'see' where we stand, both as against the others who were told they had contracted similar illnesses, but also against the historical facts of actuarial tables, survivor rates, recovery times and the like. Add into this heady mixture the evolution of medications or operations and the possibility of expanded options for treatment and what is actually constructed is the architecture of a 'new lease on life', as is said. So we may say as much as this for the moment: that statistical 'reality' in medical discourse does bear an uncanny relationship with our expectations of an ideal subjectivity within the world. This may not be our own lot in life. There may be a more or less severe disconnect between our state of affairs and what the curve produces as its model citizen, its cured 'new man' or its 'maturity' of beingness. But at least we know approximately where we stand. This kind of knowledge is worth a great deal in a world that is by its very definition uncertain and has its staying power in the ambiguous.

The mental constructs that we project into the world are both psychogenetic and psychosomatic. We know, for example, that long periods of depression alter our neuro-chemistry. There is a feedback effect between the grease of the brain's wheels and our liquid moods. If our life and the way we feel about it really are oil and water, we are in for a challenging time. We might even think that alternatively, one or the other is always the cause or the effect. Even so, "The fundamental difficulty in discussing psychogenesis lies in applying the idea of causality to mental phenomena, when the subject-predicate grammar of Aryan types of language constrains us to think of mind as a *substance*, but one without position and spatial extension" (Yap 1977, 341, italics in the original). What, then, is the 'substance' of an experience? The sum of human experiences? How can either be calculated? We have a mind to not only reify the source of thought as if we could construct a home to which we can return in times of need and threat, but we can think of such threats as they appear before us and thence enter into us as only enemies rather than merely another kind of experience of the living: "Not only is the clinical course of the disease and its medical treatment thus described, but the disease itself is conceived as the enemy on which society wages war" (Sontag 1978, 65). Disease too is given back not its essence, not what it actually is as an object in the anonymous world of objects and of 'nature', but a mind like our own, though one bent on evil and one that cannot be altered by rehabilitation. It is as if all of the vile veils that cover over human evils are dislocated from *our* minds and transferred over to the unthought of the illness.

Such a transference would not be possible without mind-like analogues strewn around the various discourses. Each of the sciences has its reified fetish. Whether culture, society, mind, space, the market, even the cosmos or 'life', etc., we presume to need an ultimate umbrella for the objects within our discursive ambit. Often enough, one's fetish gets subsumed within that of someone else, but we can always return the favor. Reductionism versus anthropism aside, there is something to be noted regarding the structure of a language which has invented philosophy and science. Some other culture's science might not be asking the same epistemological questions, or even be coming up with the same 'orders of reality'. Nonetheless, there does seem to be a basic empiricism to human existence. Experience, and the knowledge gleaned therefrom, is mostly golden. We need to know where the flash floods flow from, where the herds go to and when, that some of the big cats hunt at night, and others during the day, that this plant grows well here and this one does not. And if these particular experiences seem interminably archaic, we need to remind ourselves that *who* we are, as an essential mode of existence in this world, means statistically at least, the more than 99 percent of our tenure on earth as small groups of mobile hunter-gatherers, living the most uncertain lives of all.

1.2.3 Subject and Object

To distinguish a disease only by its terrifying capacity to sabotage human life is to advance a narrow reification upon another existing form of life. Its otherness is no doubt quite alien, though it remains terrestrial and related to us. This evolutionary relation, now grown cold and distant over the eons, might give us the sense that we are being assailed by a long-lost relative to whom we have certain duties, and from whom we can expect the odd visitation in times of crisis. Like those family members whose appearance on our doorsteps does indeed provoke its own crisis, disease 'vectors'—for we must recall that for the time being and in our own time, disease cannot be its own essence or 'its own thing'—and the contracting of an illness throws everything but the illness itself into an unwanted uncertainty. It exacerbates the ambiguity that is already and always present in everyday life. Certain steps must be taken to avert the impending chaos. Science has been our response to such a menacing figure for some time now, but the purposes of science are not the same as those we hold subjectively dear to us. To use science as our stand-in is to court their loss, for to do so, "… impoverishes the object of all qualities except those relevant to its own purposes. It considers the object only what is measurable, numerable, an calculatable. In this way it guarantees the certainty and exactness of its own thought" (Barrett, op. cit., 212), and just as certainly guarantees the continuing uncertainty of any thought concerning ourselves. In the health care process, it is not 'we' ourselves who are being measured in a scientific manner. It is the interaction between rather specific parts of our body and a foreign life form, the disease 'agent'. Only through this interaction does the 'existence' of disease come about in the first place. But the more disturbing obverse to this sudden relevance of what otherwise would be something no one would be concerned about, is that our existence too comes into focus only within the clinical setting. A person alone is of no interest to medical discourse. A person who has been sick and is now recovered may have a certain control group merit, as well as being part of a past data stream that may be in the future useful.

But a patient is another matter entirely. She has all of a sudden become the center for an interaction that really is the object. The space of this objectification is, as stated above, the combination of a body inside a clinic and a disease inside a body. The person has, most likely not of her own volition, become the very existence of medicine as a human invention. She is at once the reason for its origin and the goal of its attention. The alpha and omega of medical science is to be found within her presence. Of course, we are not speaking of the person. Whoever she may be, this otherness of the human being external to the clinic is not of import. Our way of knowing, our epistemological druthers, object to any subjectivity that carries a human being beyond the subjectitude of a discursive relationship. This must be so, because "For modern science to objectify something means to 'measure" it. [ ] we are even so bold as to establish so-called standard values, clearly one of the principal sources of error in established medicine" (Gadamer 1996, 98 [1990]). So, while standardization rationalizes our sudden predicament of being ill and its subsequent experience of being ill at ease, such statistics and numerics depersonalize to the extent that we can never locate our experiences within the broader community of either human reason or compassion.

It is part and parcel of the history of anxiety that we correspond with one another within the technique of rubric and method. If misery loves company, anxiety loves society. It loves itself just that much to eschew intimacy, but, to give it some credit, it is also anxious about the other's feelings. So much so, that it cannot truly share itself even though it is a general feature of our shared condition. The more objectifying term associated with the being-anxious-in-the-world-of-forms is 'stress'. This term is much less existential sounding than anxiety, but like it, we hear it stated that there can be 'good stress' as well as that negative. Even further down the road to the object lies treatments, palliatives, and prescriptions such as 'exercise' or 'diet', which also can be good or bad. The former holds within its spectrum differences such as swimming, on the healthy side, and ditch-digging, on that unhealthy. The latter's range is too obvious to detail here, but suffice it to say that 'diet' has become in the last few decades an element of fashionable concern even at the state level. All of these experiences and the feelings that come from our participation in them dissuade anxieties but can do nothing to alter the course of anxiety itself, as part of the thrownness of our human projects. But as Heidegger reminds us, we are only anxious because we care about things, others, and about ourselves. Our entire being is one of concernful-being-for either towards the world or towards another, though we can never be concerned about objects in the world *per se*. This is perhaps the reason why the process of objectification has steadily taken hold over the investigations into the life function and animating force of human health: "The givens of natural life, which were at hand, within reach, involved life, now become *objects*, objectives that can never be anything but objectives, terms that remain themes and tasks and never become termini" (Lingis 1989, 16, italics in the original). That is, we can no longer attain what is given because we have excerpted it from our subjectivity and placed it into the world of forms. Doing so with one another and oneself can only follow along with this impetus. Focusing on the world as an environment is an inauthentic, though not lesser, form of being-in-the-world. It is what we are most of the time, but it also has the effect of turning us away from the authentic encounter with beings and with Being. All of this is old hat, but when it comes to the encounter with one's own health, the tonality of this projection is reflected back upon us. It rings in our ears while at the same time facing us, looking into our eyes. It is not a mixed metaphor, but a holistic one. In pre-scientific cultures, we have assumed this kind of *volte face* never occurred, could never be necessary given that "The subjective reaction to the object always takes precedence historically, while the objective qualities of the object remain in the background" (Neumann 1970, 294). It is only within science, its technique, technologies, and method that the world is opened up to consciousness in its own manner of being. We discover, far more than any specific object of interest, from ganglia to quasars and everything in between, that the cosmos has its own way of being that has nothing whatsoever to do with us or, for that matter, our knowledge of it. We realized, as a rider to this discovery, that the true arrogance of human history lay not in its belief in other forms of being—from gods to extraterrestrials and everything in between—but in the idea that any of these other beings had a human interest, would willingly become our mascots. The solitude of solicitude became rapidly our lot.

It is within solicitous being that we approach and encounter the other. We are concerned for ourselves and thus also for the other due to the potential he has for either allaying our anxiety or increasing it. We might well be fearful *about* the other while we fear *for* him. But fear and anxiety are not at all the same. A fear is palpable and more given to the object, since it is extant only within relation to an object, and since "… there could be objective facts about subjective experience, that an appearance is itself a fact, and that some appearances—for instance the experience of pain or grief, delight or trouble of mind—can be centrally important parts of the facts that affect us" (Midgely 2004, 34), we must pay them the most objective heed possible even in the subjective condition we find ourselves in experiencing them. As Midgely immediately states: "These things do not just appear to matter, they do matter" (ibid). Beyond this, however, still lies the problem of our experience of anonymity and aloneness, to which solicitude addresses itself but is also tasked with confronting its own subjectitude. Anxieties take hold of us as facts, but anxiety never does so. Like stressors versus stress, specific anxieties may be talked about, as in therapy, and may even be overcome, as in the canonical phobias or complexes that lead to neuroses. But only in death may we be said to 'overcome' anxiety, or rather, it may perhaps be said that it has overcome us in the end. In death too, we are 'free' from all worldly viewpoints and from all worldviews. Once again, in the pre-scientific epochs of human tenure in the world, what lay 'beyond' the grave wasn't so much beyond life but part of its greater arc. Souls returned in other hosts, or lived on in some other world aloof but still attached, and *interested*, in this one. Only in our own time can we truly speak about what lies 'beyond' the grave, as the grave itself remains part of our world, as do its contents, the more or less discontented remains of our ancestors.

This new kind of freedom, which we imagine percolates within a consciousness that is no longer swaddled in the great arc of cosmic destiny but is rather one locally available view out upon a minute fraction thereof, cannot effectively either embrace all standpoints or escape its own. What it can do, and for the first time, is acknowledge just exactly *where* it does stand: "If the term is to mean anything at all, '*freedom from standpoints*" is nothing other than an explicit *appropriation of our position of looking*. This position is something historical, i.e. bound up with Dasein, and not a chimerical in-itself outside of time" (Heidegger 1999, 64 [1995], italics in the original). It is plausible that Heidegger has recognized in Weber's 'value-free' methods something that the new phenomenology could use. In the text cited, it is only Weber who emerges unscathed by the early Heidegger's searching and insightful critique of epistemology. To identify how one is going to confront the problem at hand and why one chooses to do so in this or that manner before one embarks on the task of science is to vouchsafe any attempt at objectivity. It is not that there exists a value-free position in human experience, but that one's values can, and should be enumerated ahead of the game. We need to know where we stand. And it is precisely *this* that cannot be known in tables of standard values.

Such 'values', as the name ironically implies, are also not at all value-free. But the process of standardizing cases by operational numeric gives us the impression that we have constructed an object that can be studied outside of the sphere of values. It can be evaluated, in other words, without being valued or even valuated: "By putting these ideas into practice, medicine gives the disease categories a reality of their own" (Freund and McGuire 1999, 192–93). So on the one hand, diseases have no reality in themselves—they are objects insofar as they interact with our body, its 'tissues', and our abreactions to their 'presence'—but the categories into which they fall are somehow real. This new order of reality contained two major elements: "… the first was that of individual, concrete perceptions mapped out in accordance with the nosological table of morbid species, the second, that of the continuous, over-all, quantitative registration of a medicine of climates and places" (Foucault 1973, 51). Note that nothing can be said of either the person in this individuation of perception or of her experience of the illness, even though it is this experience that first brings it to the attention of clinical discourse and thus *makes it real*, given that it can have no other reality as an entity apart from that self-same discourse. The uncanniness of ill-health confronts us with such an authenticity of being through its pointed anxiety producing effects—though we rapidly parry, turning to the world to communicate this existential moment in terms of a specific class of *anxieties*, thus avoiding much of its thrust—that we become quite willing agents in this standardization and depersonalization of our experience. In short, we are apt to reify both the disease as an intrusive effect *and* ourselves as part of a category of those so affected: "Reification thus entails a certain amount of mystification, as the human roots of the phenomena are veiled. Reification of disease means conveniently forgetting the social processes by which the concept of the disease is produced" (Freund and McGuire, op. cit., 204). Meaning and one's personal expression of humanity are also sidetracked. There results in a too close connection between the 'body and the identity of the individual' (ibid). In contemporary language, the La Mettrie style conceptualization of the human person as a machine that writes some of its own programming but hardly all of it—the autonomic and proprioceptive functions are not controlled consciously, for instance—cannot then be said to be wholly human in the humanistic sense. It is an organism first, human second. Our use of language, however much our genetic makeup predisposes us to learn and learn it in a certain way, looks in this model more like an unexpected disconnect, distracting us from the sober truth of our organismic and evolutionary status. Language in use, on top of all this, pushes the frontier still further away from the mechanical, though the fact that we use so little of each 'natural' language in everyday relations in both vocabulary content, and aesthetic senses, gives us pause regarding how well language is in fact learned by the majority, apart from our general human ability to learn it.

Given this mélange, it is not surprising that in a science that must confront it head on, the use of symbolic forms is subsumed within the ambit of the object to be, the text becomes part of the tissue of this new world, just as it had dwelt within the autographed world of the pre-modern era. It is not that the social functions of language entirely vanish, 'conveniently' or no, "… it is, rather, as if they had been displaced, enclosed within the singularity of the patient, in that region of 'subjective symptoms" that—for the doctor—defines not a mode of knowledge, but the real world of objects to be known" (Foucault 1973, x). This is not quite a reduction in the usual sense. It is more kindred with the idea that the body has a language of its own, more primordial to human existence than consciousness. It is not only preconscious, but speaks beyond the grave, like M. Valdemar who, hypnotized at the point of his death, nevertheless speaks 'back' unto his audience, using the language of what has become conscious but what was originally muted by both physiological primitivity and lack of actual recognizably human speech as distinguished from our primate cousins. It is this language that clinical discourse accesses and to which it gives voice. It does so, however, in the most banal and innocuous manner, as if the primordial tongue of the body human must be duped into speaking, especially in a situation of life, lest it give something away about its own fate: "One has an opaque body that must be taken to a specialist to find out if it contains cancer. What the patient cannot perceive, the specialist will determine by analyzing tissues take from the body" (Sontag 1978, 12). The opacity of the body is not even so much concealing the facts of its potential demise, but that it has a language with which to communicate them. By manufacturing the means to reconnect this primordiality, its union both announced and enunciated by the data of such tests, intrusive or no, modern medicine has overcome its first major hurdle to understanding a living process that yet cannot live on indefinitely. In doing so, however, the connection between consciousness and its vehicle is put aside: "The reified disease identification often assumes primacy; it if conflicts with the patients' subjective illness experience, the objectified disease-thing is often treated as more real than the sick person's feelings" (Freund and McGuire, op. cit., 205).

The authors conclude by stating that such an ascendant identification is 'internalized' and thus begins to change those subjective feelings, not into something more objective 'in themselves', but more in accordance with a discursive definition of what one *will* experience in the context of ill-health.

And what one will ultimately experience is the process of dying, if not death itself. What we have to carry around with us, the shadow of self, the penumbra of personhood, is a 'death-bearing perception'. We, each of us, is our own undertaker, and though we do not elevate the coffin on our own, we take hold of it, using the firmest of grips, in order to hoist ourselves within at the appropriate time. Medical discourse has reconstructed this view of things from mythological narratives, but it has objectified it as the most recent and perhaps most forceful objection to death in general: "From the moment death was introduced into a technical and conceptual organon, disease was able to be both spatialized and individualized. Space and individual, two associated structures deriving necessarily from a death-bearing perception" (Foucault 1973, 159).

1.3 Today

Perhaps what is most convenient about the sidestepping of social processes and meanings built up from the history of symbolic forms is that we have not so much depersonalized our living selves but our shared fate. Death is no longer a figure like ourselves who has found out the secret of mastery over itself, broken open the seventh seal and plunged itself into the abyss where all meanings ultimately mingle and recreate the Babel of the afterlife, but rather an object that can be studied by science. Death cannot be experienced by the self, but our still awkward being self-conscious about it at least allows it to be empirically known as a fact of our condition. Like any other fact, it has its place in specific discourses, and like any other element of discourse, especially that which straddles uneasily the divide between the study of human beings and the study of the objective forces of living organisms, that bearing intimacy and distanciation, compassionate and dispassionate at once, it must be spoken of no longer in the hushed *sotto voce* of incantation but in the stark and glaring light of method and data.

1.3.1 Externality

In this way, our living mastery over death is accomplished: "… yet behind the more-or-less question of mastery achieved lies and absolute question about basic orientation: the disengaged agent has taken a once-and-for-all stance in favour of objectification …" (Taylor 1989, 46). We will see later on that the movement towards alternative health treatments and discourses is not so much a result of this stance being favoured by the dominant clinical science of medicine 'proper' but all the more so as an aspiring complement to the fissures in that discourse's abilities. It often gives the appearance of being a competitor but only with the hope of displacing what is already absent, rather than the system in its entirety. This too is a convenience of sorts, for it is much easier to market oneself and one's view if one gives the sense that one is not an out-and-out revolutionary, radically planning on stripping the entirety of human society as we know it to the bone. Even so, the impetus towards a final sensibility that objectification is the most realistic manner with which to deal with the unreal, the canniest way to confront the uncanny, pushes even the homeopathic discourse's awareness towards some idea of an object to be studied and manipulated, even if the vaguest of notions concerning it have been put into use. On top of this, alternative medicine or treatment may well be able to be taken into that dominant, given the latter's own aspirations: "What now constituted the unity of the medical gaze was not the circle of knowledge in which it was achieved but that open, infinite, moving totality, ceaselessly displaced and enriched by time whose course it began but would never be able to stop …" (Foucault 1973, 29). Such a holistic phenomena already identifies itself with 'holism' in general. It too seeks to be able to know the forces that construct the 'life force', reversing the order of the questioning as compared to homeopathic holism, but nevertheless, taking up the same goal and object. If allopathic medicine has borrowed the structures of religion and inverted them, that homeopathic maintains a more traditional and indeed, conservative approach to those structures. It too, however, cannot be said to have not objectified them in some manner. The 'life force', whatever it may be, is also depersonalized, just as has been death in dominant discourses of medical science. The purpose of both kinds of reidentification and displacement into conscious language concerns our ability to control them: "… the development of this capacity to objectify pain is one of the results of a university education for physicians. By his training the physician is often enabled to focus on those aspects of a concrete person's bodily pain that are accessible to management by an outsider" (Illich 1975, 100). A pedagogic authority which is itself already distanciated from the world and those worlds of *existentia* within it, such as pain and suffering, or equally, joy and intimacy, finds a comfortable home in any discourse that seeks a distance of its own, not to mention those students who flock to such institutions for the sole purpose of finding a career in capital. Labour power classically alienates. It defines the person and, like the reidentification of the individual with her body and thence with her illness, the ability to produce and consume is itself the master identity of all those who live within the proverbial iron cage. The nation state prevaricates this social organization in part through public health advertising. The influenza season is likely to be partly billed as a threat to both person hours at work and to costs incurred against the publically funded health care system. It is the mark of every good citizen to be inoculated. The recent outcry against vaccinations marks the irresponsible citizen as well as the uninformed adult. Given that this criticism had much of its popular origin in a narrative told by an entertainment figure, its source and its claims are dubious. But the idea that one *could* hold an alternative viewpoint to that of the state and other large organizations and institutions is sociologically interesting, no matter its shaky veracity. For all lines of question are generally lined up lock-step with the official discourses of ideological apparatuses, on top of the much lesser known ones of that scientific. There is a kind of entropy within these discourse as well, though, and thus it is understandable that sometimes even outlandish claims can be fostered and spread to the effect of filling in perceived gaps in medical practice and corresponding results: "Medical knowledge often becomes detached and independent of the research on which it is based. Thus, limitations in the original research are not taken into account in the accumulated stock of knowledge" (Freund and McGuire, op. cit., 195). The same weakness is, of course, to be found amongst lay and popular accounts, however contrived and subjective. At least equally so, the critical sensibility that urges us to question authority of all kinds is also lost. Generally, laypersons attempt to account of a negative experience by examining its details in terms of the experience itself without taking the wider context as a source of impinging variables. As well, the 'analysis' is but a snapshot; one peers keenly at 'what happened' and forgets the previous series of events that may have led to any current situatedness. Everything becomes thus a 'situation' or an 'issue', rather than an event or a present-to-hand: "This need for minute explanation is quite symptomatic in non-scientific minds, which claim to neglect nothing and to take into account all aspects of the concrete experience" (Bachelard 1964, 63 [1938]). But the most notorious aspect of the absence of reason in lay arenas is the taking of one's own experience as the norm. This occurs most transparently in introductory social science classes the world over, and, while not entirely vacuous, such a claim turns the claimant away from the world as it is and into oneself. This is the most convenient manner of avoiding the confrontation with either the socius, tradition, or one's ethically charged Dasein as a being-with others.

More importantly still, is the convenience of not having to use one's own imagination. Self-projection into the world as thrown subjectivity is a major aspect of our condition, and it requires of us to task ourselves with a response that engages the space into which we are thrown. Even children are capable of doing so through the play worlds of the imagination. Their subjectivity is often quite miniscule and though they tend to act as if they can overcome all challenges, nevertheless, they in fact *give* themselves such challenges to overcome. Not as many adults can claim as much. And though some children face real challenges of the medical variety, far more adults are confronted with the rehearsals of finitude that dot the haunted landscape of our dreams for a future. To continue the artifice of turning away from the authenticity of such a challenge, medicine is made routine, as is the practice thereof. For after all, doctors and other health care specialists are people too. Thus "… it can be contended that as medical knowledge becomes codified and routinized and subject to audit, less imagination and less space are required for the autonomous physician to use his or her intellectual powers" (Kelleher, Gabe, and Williams 1994, xxi, and cf. Scambler 1982b, 92ff for an example of the problem of dying within an institution that attempts to make death a simple and anonymous routine). At length, even the new concept of the disease as a besetting force is to a certain extent bracketed, made amorphous once again, and, though without being reenchanted, slides into a netherland of hospice and palliation. This speaks not so much of an oversight, but of the disconnect between research and practice just mentioned. If imagination of all kinds is muted in all spaces—at most, it may become a commodity in itself if it can discover new ways to manipulate consumers into 'doing what they do best', or if it can be made to focus on the most devious manner of defeating one's enemy or yet making him suffer in some way—we should not expect this more potently relevant *existential* disenchantment to provide a means of egress from either wage-labour or the reduction of the person to their labour power, however intellectual or artistic it may be.

But the disconnect between thinking and doing is made more palpable in the sciences perhaps more than in any other kind of modern discourse. The question of the species and its future is raised but in some way left to hang before us without eager response. For example, "Health care, as environmental hygienic engineering, works within categories different from those of the clinical scientist. Its focus is on human survival rather than disease" (Illich, op. cit., 82). Needless to say, no one person *must* survive. It is also questionable along one thread that even the species as a whole *needs* to. Where does this idea come from? The obvious case must be made against self-destruction, yes. But what of evolution? Humanity does not exhaust itself in itself. It is surely our own parochial bigotry writ a little larger than what is normative or traditional that *Homo Sapiens Sapiens* continue indefinitely *as* a species in its own right. Why so? If the costs of healthcare are such a sensitive issue, if illness is so dreaded, if the challenge of facing one's own mortality is so hard to bear, if the task of passing on of culture to one's children is so frustrating, why not simply move on? That this is a staple of entertainment fiction presents to us both the imaginary alternative—which gets technologically more real each year—and perhaps the unspoken ideal. As with the now famous studies of mid-twentieth century stay at home mothers, who, in interview, 'confessed' to wishing to harm or even kill their children in a much more serious intonation than what you can overhear at any local hair salon—and no doubt the post-war period was the last 'golden age' of normative and socially sanctioned child abuse in middle class homes in any case—what is being given voice in the fictions is both an aspiration to overcome one's present limitations—in this, it is an essay on self-improvement of a sort—and yet another mode of inauthentic being-away-from-the-world that allows us some succor in the face of reality.

1.3.2 Inequality

Fantasy, however contrived and fictional, is always at base a way in which to think ahead. It casts our being out 'ahead of itself', as in Heidegger's analysis, by imagining 'projects of action'. Schutz's definition of the phantasm, a constructive daydream which may be shared and having the purpose of testing mentally a possible future and thus a possible new world and oneself 'as if' placed within it, is wholly necessary for a species that cannot know the future in the way we can know something that has been studied before. There are limits, however, and these are most notable within the scientific process as being associated with the making routine of the imagination of those who projected their actions into possible futures in the first place: "The substitution of somebody else's opinions for a real study of the phenomena goes so far that many operationalists seldom come in direct touch with facts pertinent to the inquiry" (Sorokin, op. cit., 39). Unlike the layperson, this time it is the scientist who lacks imagination and attempts to borrow the status of a group containing the rest of us to bolster any confidence we might have in his 'findings'. The larger the group the better, of course, hence the statistical version of veridicity that claims to be as close to certainty as one can possibly attain. But more than this, the very question that can be asked within the ambit of the statistic forces an inequality of the imagination upon the respondent. It delineates what is of import before the potential dialogue can get underway, In this, it is also an inauthentic mode of discourse, bearing some resemblance to the 'idle talk' that Heidegger speaks of as being forced upon us by social conventions and institutional authorities. This effect is particularly noticeable in contexts where the existentiality of the individual is threatened to be exposed, or already has been exposed in an unexpected way: "What is the matter with you?", with which the eighteenth-century dialogue between doctor and patient began [ ] was replaced by that other question: 'Where does it hurt?", in which we recognize the operation of the clinic and the principle of its entire discourse" (Foucault 1973, xviii). This 'operation', not unlike the larger umbrella of operationalism to which it is related on the one side, while on the other it nods its head to the actual physical process of surgery, is one that breaks the body up. The person has already been replaced by the body in question, but this corpus is still far too complex and variegated to be of much use in any clinical setting. We need to find the elements of the *corpuscular corpus.* To do so requires not so much an analysis in any philosophical sense, but rather an anti-synthetic gambit: "The great disadvantage of the analytic method is that, as is illustrated so well by modern medicine, it makes for specialization and fragmentation" (Westlake 1973, 71). Dr. Westlake immediately states that the person becomes a 'heart or liver case'. One speaks again of one's case load, or describes one's 'surgery', sending it to other medicos. Even so, it is clear that the analytic method does retain some value if it is not 'abused' or 'misused' by the statistical fetish (cf. Sorokin, op. cit., 172). The idea of precision and probability are fundamentally opposed. The latter attempts to approach the former as closely as possible, but it is oppositely charged from the beginning. One cannot be forced into the other; like magnets, they are repelled. Sorokin the humanist never hesitates to call this point to our attention: "In the raging epidemics of quantophrenia everyone can be a 'researcher" …" (ibid) simply because anyone can generate a question list, code it and run it through a 'tabulating machine' or all the more so, its contemporary equivalent. Still as nonsensical as it always has been, the production of quantitative research results nevertheless has both a valid and an invalid hold upon the scientific imagination. The remarkable feats of space engineering, landing on a comet, for instance, would not be possible without it. But within the realm of the human sciences, its merits deteriorate rapidly. At most one might allow oneself to say that the general failure of statistical methods to provide an authentic account of the variety of human experience in a manner recognizable to living persons provides us with an ongoing reminder of our sophistication as conscious creatures capable of reason and communicating through language. This is a necessary perspective to maintain and statistics can, in spite of itself, help us to maintain it. This is its greatest contribution to the human sciences, though one cannot cast aspersion on its merits elsewhere. This said, however, "… modern science has come to regard the results of such measuring procedures as the real facts which it must seek to order and collect. But the data provided in this way only reflect conventionally established criteria brought to the phenomena from without" (Gadamer 1996, 132 [1989]). And is the source of this 'imposition' really 'merely' the cultural or historical customs of the time, however rationalized or ideologized? Perhaps one may add the further inequality—that is, the disconnect between the object and the process of its objectification—of the professional groups doing the research. Competition amongst research labs, their staff and management, universities and corporations is more sociologically 'real' than is the 'advancement of science', to borrow a stock but nonetheless famous phrase, and one that adorns the motto of more than one equally famous funding agency. In medicine in particular: "Doctors defend their corporate rights on the ground that they should be understood not in the sense of privilege but of collaboration" (Foucault 1973, 45–46). But this defense goes much further than one research location or hospital gaining ground at the expense of another, or even the relative homogeneity of the social group called 'doctors' or 'surgeons', 'researchers' or professors of medicine. It is the case that very often the membership in these elite groups overlaps to some extant. As in all social arenas, one is sorted and winnowed by virtue of one's merits, however standardized the process is by which they may be adjudicated. That there are many other variables in play is, however, well known. Gender 'segregation'—and the word is used advisably by Butter *et al*, given the *statistics* available at the time—was 'most evident across health occupations', but was also quite transparent as segregation "… in the same health occupation into different types of jobs and organizational units" (Butterick et al. 1994, 80). No doubt, pending the cultural region, something similar could be said for ethnic and class backgrounds. Over the past two decades this situation has been somewhat ameliorated, with a sharp rise in female doctors in developed countries, for example, and even the contribution from recent immigration sources such as the subcontinent, where it is no longer taboo for one's daughter to aspire to medicine or the health professions in general. Even so, the inertia of the system of streaming and hiring is one that has persisted, resulting in a wider set of organizations where "… male workers are heavily concentrated in high autonomy, elite occupations whose status often entitles them to control subordinates in usually preponderate female occupations" (ibid, 87). One must immediately note that these 'elites' work far longer hours and may not have the fullest autonomy that lower ranks often imagine them to possess. Certainly, relative autonomy, writ small but of the same kind that the institutions of training and practice themselves have, even under national laws, is in play, but it is in play in every face to face encounter, which is something a statistical report might miss. It is a challenge in itself to challenge inequality through the use of the very methods that tend to promote it. We are reduced, in a word, to speaking the language of the opponent or the competitor, even the enemy.

Such a language bears within it the hallmarks of its own margins. Long ago, Sorokin reported a number of medical studies in which no controls were used, even though they had been analyzed as if such tests and subjects existed (cf. op. cit., 184ff), while more recently Krieger and Fee explain that in vital statistics studies and records more generally, "Data on social class are not collected. At the same time, public health professionals are unable adequately to explain or to change inequalities in health between men and women and between diverse racial/ethnic groups" (1994, 16). We continue to assign an 'objectifier' to each person even in the critical studies of the uncritical studies, the former supposedly more mature and aware than the latter. Yet, as in legal action, it remains case versus case. More cases makes for a greater approximation to reality, so we are told, but the premise required to understand the world in this way does not budge from its most bigoted former application. Behavioral and statistical manuals aside, to imagine the human world, the *lifeworld*, as a series of regions wherein differing and opposing *categories* of humanity are pitted against one another and can only be observed and analyzed by virtue of these categories and attendant variables is to discard at the beginning the sense that people exist. Not merely as 'thrown projects', not merely as the originators of projects of action, but as concernful beings both within and without the truth. Such an intimate and experiential understanding of human living-on-in-the-world is conspicuously absent in almost all health research, where one might hope that it had been able, at length, to find an hospitable home for itself. Instead, what we do discover are both pronouncements and announcements, not only in the 'epidemiological' sense of public health—the flu season is upon us again—or phase of life preventative maintenance—I am fifty so my colon is suddenly susceptible to cancer—and as such we lose the significance of the depth of being encountered; on the one hand, as a potential community that must be cared for, and on the other, myself who will die and thus be forced to leave that community.

Everywhere there are signs that act as detours for Dasein. Discourse itself is appropriated into the 'idle talk' of the daily round, the appointment and the deadline. That it has become, with the ageing population, notoriously difficult in some regions to procure a visit with one's 'own' general practitioner also colours our perception of what medicine is 'for'. When we do arrive, we are met with a trinity of special signs, which in their turn, assign us to a process by which we become the object of further inequalities, that is, a series of moments wherein we are placed and recorded, though we also desire this passivity in the face of our own self-ignorance, at least the level of the body-technique. That being so, our being-without-the-truth as part of the primordial situatedness of Dasein bleeds into another realm, making us think that the truth itself can be found out, uncovered in its own primordial sense of the term, and that we can be moved without our circumspection into the lighted space of being-within-the-truth. This is more than merely facile and unlikely: "The sign announces: the prognostic sign, what will happen, the anamnestic sign, what has happened; the diagnostic sign, what is now taking place" (Foucault 1973, 90). Whatever 'easing of conscience' or 'peace of mind' that can be attained in life glosses over the constitutive character of memory and experience. It is a way to 'take into account', or 'account for', the way in which one has lived or had to live. This accounting principle is older than capital, but it takes on a specific debit and credit structure in our own time. What has occurred is no longer so much the world as it has been, as it was characterized, for instance, in a Pauline existentiality. For us, memory is away of charting the balance sheet of experience. It is an open-ended compendium that points to nowhere in particular and does not, in itself, anticipate its own ending and thus by extension, our own deaths. What is now occurring is the raw data to be taken into account in the shorter term, and one feels the impetus to 'settle accounts', or even 'even the score' in the somewhat old-fashioned sense of settling an old score or having unfinished business with an other to self. Today, the idea of revenge or even avenging something has fallen also out of favour. That the 'best revenge is living well', though claimed by Aristotle, is more our own sensibility than it was for any ancient culture speaks to this depersonalization of revenge, once again part of the larger process of demythologizing with which we opened this discussion. What will happen has the inertia of a 'must' to it, but this is only because we, when facing down the abyss of our own unknowable futures, attempt to take into account beforehand what kind of credit or debit there may be not quite at hand, only just over the horizon. This is where the phantasm of projects of action comes into play, and this is where what we have experienced as inequality elides into imagined inequity.

1.3.3 Inequity

But before we step forward onto that abyssal plain whose horizon seems to get no closer to us the more we tread upon it, we must take stock of just what can be thought about the experiences we have already had. Diagnosis proceeds upon this rite: that the patient recall to the best of their knowledge how they feel given what they had been feeling, for it is only what one has experienced—discomfort, pain, irregularities of various kinds—that brings one into the 'occurring' of the clinic: "What is possible or impossible to remember, or even to say aloud? What are the hidden meanings of silences and sudden changes of subject?" (Thomson 1990, 80). Seen objectively, it is always possible to say anything aloud. Meanings that are hidden may always be possible to uncover. Their very hiddenness is the manner of being that takes the ability to be uncovered as part of its ownmost possibility. Diagnosis proceeds with this assumption intact. As well, though there may be memories which are lost to us—perhaps they had never indeed been 'memorized' either experientially (we did not, in fact, experience what we think we did) or neuro-chemically as archive—what we know to be a memory is, by definition, something we have recalled already. So diagnosis is geared to steer through the inequality extant between what has been and what is, and in doing so thereby enters into the space of inequity. This space is of the future, though it may be within our reach or just moments away. Inequity characterizes the relationship between what is going on now and what is to come. There can be no question of debit or credit here as yet, because we are not able to take into account what has not yet occurred, just as, somewhat more gently, we are not finished taking into account what is happening to us at just this time. We need 'some more time' to reflect upon it, or perhaps, as above, the present-to-hand has about it or within it some 'unfinished business' which cannot be 'dealt with' until further notice. At any rate, the future does not have this same relationship with the present as does the past. Instead, we are carried toward it, impelled by our very existence in the world. Like the proverbial river metaphor, we are carried along and can see the length of what is in front of us only to a certain degree, and sometimes not at all. The hidden meanings—rocks in the riverbed, eddies in the current—of what lies for the moment silent are also pregnant with inequity. Perhaps what is unsaid will forever remain so? Perhaps what the doctor *really* needs to know the patient has had no experience of? Many cancers begin like this, for example, which is why the public health screenings for such early intervention have taken on the profundity they have. Long before giant tumors which can be experienced as pain or otherwise, long before the metastatic inflammation that presages our demise, intervening by virtue of a diagnostic tool that does not rely on the subjectivities of either experience or memory would seem like a platinum manner in which the discourse of objectivity can triumph over its opposing number: "For instance, in medicine, and especially in psychiatry, there is often a choice between viewing patients primarily as physical organisms or as conscious agents. [This] choice can have strong practical consequences for treatment; indeed it can decide the whole fate of the patient" (Midgely 2004, 38). This is clearly an inequity. The difference between both what the subject can or has experienced is pitted against the unspeaking tools of diagnosis as if dialogue were to be avoided. Early cancer screening kits are even sent through the mail and returned through it, without a word spoken by any party. Yet this is still a 'diagnosis', it is still what is currently going on. Discourse, perhaps ironically, is sometimes at its strongest when there is nothing but silence.

As Midgely immediately states, however, our 'conceptions of what is scientific' often predetermine what fates we may look towards (ibid). If we accept that "Modern medicine has thus become largely a question of giving a name to a complaint, and then of treating its signs and symptoms" (Westlake 1973, 122), then we must also accept a new kind of fate, where our very ingratiation to diagnoses that can remain unspoken suggests that there is no need to recall them as part of our experience as human beings. They become something less even than 'idle talk', and in this way, the implications that such tests hold as part of their ownmost possibility are lost to us. Even so, and in spite of this clever subterfuge, "The public acceptance of iatrogenic labeling multiplies patients faster than either doctors or drugs can medicalize them" (Illich 175, 47). Aside from the State's multiple need-to-know basis—biopower, health care cost prediction, regional economic growth or slowdowns, environmental threats to public health, and so on—the census of ailments, a kind of latter day domesday book that once again records the debits and credits of an entire society, rests uneasily on the precipice between diagnosis and prognostication. It attempts to cover over this inequity by constructing an anamnestic signature, a history of the health of 'the people', in which all have been included at least as 'cases' or yet test results. This recording device is the only way that patients can be experienced, for, moving forward within this new medicalization process, "The number of patient relationships outgrows the number of people. As long as the public bows to the professional monopoly in assigning the sick role, it cannot control the multiplication of patients" (ibid, 77). This 'assignation' is of interest. *Consigning* might also be a relevant term. Monopoly or no, medical discourse and its licensed practitioners exert more than a scientific license if they seek to 'assign' something, anything. Though prosaic license follows on the one hand from their own 'licensure'—we have it in the French as a formal degree, but also in the English-speaking world as one who can become a licensed practitioner in various health system roles—and its not so hidden meaning is that it speaks its certificate into being through the giving of license. One can be said to have licenses, or to exercise license with regard to others and decisions about them, just as the attainment of this or that accreditation gives one 'license' to act in a certain way. Much more generally, every social context has its structures and scripts allowing certain limits of license on the part of participants therein, from asking after one's credit rating to sexual intimacy with unspoken consent assumed beforehand.

How 'real' any of this is when compared to the reality of either our experience of pain or discomfort and the test results or diagnostic outcomes is another matter. "Even the problem of 'representative sample" remains an unsolved problem for many mass phenomena" (Sorokin, op. cit., 256–57). The analytic issue, often purely 'academic' in the casual sense of the term, gives way under the diversity of human experience. But a distinct category of those experiences in fact supports the theses associated with quantitative disconnect, that having to do with the difference between codes and behavior, a difference to be found in almost any social context. In institutions of medicine the gap is more or less notorious, though, through patients' bills of rights and related documents, it has closed significantly over the previous generation. Perhaps most profoundly, full disclosure of one's diagnosis and, perhaps most telling, one's prognosis, is something more or les commonplace today. Not so in the recent past, even when policies mandated it: "These statements of policy, however, did not accord with actual medical practice. There were, in fact, *no* disclosures unless they were deemed absolutely necessary: that is, unless patients demanded 'the truth" or went so far as to refuse treatment" (Scambler 1982b, 88). Now this is of interest on two fronts: one, that prognosis is the most dangerous thing to disclose not because of the reaction of the patient, but because it involves the doctor, and by extension, medical discourse as a whole, to predict what cannot be known in advance. Meteorologists and their poorer cousins, the weather people we actually see on the news, can be mocked with more or less resigned playfulness without either rancor or danger. But the doctor is another matter entirely. We end up mocking our own fates when we are the victims of a misdiagnosis or a prognosis that in the end, carried little weight when compared with the events as they unfolded.

In almost every other walk of life we are quite prepared to put up with the ambiguities of 'futurologies' of this or that sort. Their presence plays on the both the primordial primate curiosity developed into a sincere but over-reaching science of prediction and probability—sometimes sophisticated, sometimes mere sophistry—and the fact that it is simply plain fun to try to know what will happen, either to oneself or to the world itself. Fun, yes, but with a streak of desperation. Kindred with the watching of live sporting events, especially if one considers oneself a fan of one side or the other, or even of specific athletes such as in golf or tennis, a benign *frisson* is to be had given the doubts of all such contests. Though it is of cautionary note that the so-called 'sports parents' take this thrill far beyond its benign beginnings—indeed, here one can recall the etymological connection between 'fan' and 'fanatic'—it is also sage to note that the sciences of humanity, including medicine, have developed what some have referred to as a veritable cult of probability and statistical study. Sorokin's now vintage comments still ring as true today: "Until the cult runs it course, and until its sterility and harmfulness become evident to the rank and file of investigators, it will noisily continue to advertise its doubtful virtues, to recruit its devotees, and to obtain large funds from various private and public sources" (op. cit., 186).

But we draw the line when it comes to illness and health. The stakes are too high for mere thrill seekers, and our loyalty to our health, though often obscured by our actual behavior regarding both mind and body—the theologian would want to add 'spirit' to complete this human trinity—makes illness into a patent enemy and not just an opponent, as in sports. The disconnect between our ideal health-profiles and our diets, for instance, as well bears an uncanny resemblance to those found in all quarters of the medical scene. But it is only within the ambit of prediction that the discretion demanded of a professional is predicated upon an elitist pseudo-morality: "Even when doctors are themselves certain about the course of a disease or outcome of therapy, they may deliberately prolong patients' uncertainty. This 'functional uncertainty" serves managerial ends, such as saving staff time and avoiding the emotional scenes with the patients and their families …" (Morgan 1982, 64). There are a variety of perhaps necessary processes that can serve the same general ends, such as 'carrying out tests' that effectively silence the patient for the time being (cf. ibid, 64–5ff). These tests and the technologies associated with them may also incur in the patient a sense of awe, especially if he or she imagines that their life is personally at stake. The subjectivity of technological presence is a sometimes neglected study, but, aside from being famously satired by Monty Python in the pregnancy scene of *The Meaning of Life,* we are deliberately or necessarily left in the dark as to the function of much of this life-focused machinery. At the same time, medical professionals reassure us with their easy talk regarding the purpose and success rates of such objects and their data: "Awe-inspiring medical technology has combined with egalitarian rhetoric to create the dangerous delusion that contemporary medicine is highly effective" (Illich 1975, 19). Not only this, but along with this effectiveness, certainly at the prolongation of human life, though with many sacrifices in its quality, we are led to believe that the development of democracy itself has ridden along with advances in medicine and progress in health outcomes. This *does* have some truth to it, if we consider that longer-lived humans are likely to have a more thorough perspective on political history, having lived through more of it, and might well be less apt to fall for the same old ideological narrative, at least in their iterative and most concise formulations. The polis is improved with age. Even so, the longer we have to live within our social confines the more jaded we may also become. State sponsored health care also has a response for this: "Such medicine is but a device to convince those who are sick and tired of society that it is they who are ill, impotent and in need of technical repair" (ibid, 11). In this outcome, medicine is seen as a source of false consciousness, or an aid to that already present in the wider social world. Even the self-understanding of subjectivity may be highlighted as but a partial misunderstanding. For it is really only in the realm of the object that reality occurs at all, including the reality of being sick or well: "Thus we today have a science of what it is to be healthy which is impersonally available, and in no way requires for its understanding that we assume a first-person stance" (Taylor 1989, 131). Though it is always ourselves who must die—we can already get an objective though not an existential sense of death from observing the demise of others—it is apparently an equal statement to say that it is also always only our bodies which get sick. *The object falls ill while the subject dies.*

1.4 A Better Ethics?

Yet there remains a profound connection between the two: only in death do we fully realize both the completeness of Dasein in the world and the fact that our moment of mortality is never actually experienced. Realization and recognition are, in this end-case, not part of human experience at the level of the subject. This perhaps is the greatest advantage medical discourse has over our general understanding of health and wellness. It can both recognize the symptoms of objective disease and thus state its case regarding the effects that one will or can experience as a person.

1.4.1 'Causalities'

In death, the two are conjoined in a manner that only the doctor can fully understand: "In anatomical perception, death was the point of view from the height of which disease opened up onto truth …" (Foucault 1973, 158). This was due to the fact that "… disease had truth only in symptoms, but it was symptoms given in truth" (ibid, 154). To be given 'in' something other than itself presents a puzzle to the subject. It is part of the aporetic structure of experience that we should be given pause by that which is other to us, including most disturbingly, human others. Aporesis in turn includes within its phenomenological ambit the additional problem of apophasis. The hermeneutics of such radical experiences, the *new* in every sense of the term, pushes us to rename both the world and ourselves. Not unlike the renaming process that the person undergoes when he becomes a patient, then a case, then a disease and thence perhaps ultimately a numbered and temporarily archived corpse, the confrontation with difference that is the world of others as well as the world 'in itself'—not just in Nature as its 'own thing', but in the life-world into which we are but thrown and continue to 'fall'—demands of us a new language. This situatedness of being provokes in us the urge to retire ourselves to the medical gaze. It is another potent manner by which medical discourse can construct its edifice of objects and naming procedures. We are regularly reminded that "Life is not the form of the organism, but the organism is the visible form of life in its resistance to that which does not live and which opposes it" (ibid). In the life sciences, death has not only lost is personified and mythological qualities, both of which we can likely do without, but more importantly, it has lost its necessary connection with life. This latter aspect seems at first to be a mere extension of the demythology that unhinged death from epic narrative and biography alike, but this is a misunderstanding of the history of the conception. Rather, it was deemed to be crucial to medical discourse and its incumbent ideology of survival and longevity that death be set up as an opposite number. Not only did this anonymize it, in the sense of the 'they' or *Das Man* of Heidegger's existential analytic, but it gave the person now become patient a sense that they were now insulated from their personal deaths. If they had to die, dying could be done as part of the 'they' in the inauthentic we-relations of the socius. Even so, this was not done with the fullness of concernful being and the compassion one might seek to share with the dying or even the sick, but to protect the medical discourse itself from its own ultimate failure. With this, modern medicine painted itself into a corner: by removing death from life, it was forced to acknowledge that all of its successes were but temporary; any success was merely the buying of time from a creditor who would finally collect all in the end. Here too, personification and yet myth lurks, ready to steal in the back door of rationalizing discourses by way of the 'idle talk' of everyday experience. To cover over this by assuming that the bar can be raised so high that death cannot overleap it as long as medicine prevails is naïve at best. For objectivity deals strictly with matters it can subject to the methods of science. Death stands outside such an analytic and its proper place, dislodged by science is, if not myth, is at least within the personal existence of each individual: "To raise a standard of objective science to such an extreme is indeed a very one-sided perspective. The criticism, however, of the social and political claims of the experts can in the case of an appeal to 'wisdom" be quite healthy. It defends the ideal of the free society" (Gadamer 1996, 19 [1967]). Indeed, along with the necessary confrontation with one's own mortality as a part of ipsissimous being-in-the-world as thrownness, is the responsibility every individual has regarding the polis in which she lives. Both of these duties are relatively new, but so are their opponents. They are, on the one side, an abstract death that happens to 'everyone and yet no one', and on the other, the 'wisdom' of expertise that claims to be the sole source of knowledge regarding both life *and* death: "By virtue of such criticism citizens make the claim that they will not be disenfranchised by the authority of the experts. All this has a special relevance to the sphere of medical science and art" (ibid). Beyond the series of modern and highly rationalized expert systems designed to take away the responsibility of individuals both as citizens and more profoundly as persons, there are other kinds of objective 'systems' that remain for the most part beyond the control of either individuals or experts (cf. Alland in Wellin, 1977, 55 for the interaction between the human genome and human behavior). And yet further from the observational doxa of allopathic discourse lies the claimed protodoxa of alternative health regimes, including radiesthesia, which supposedly allows, for instance, for cancer to be diagnosed in the pre-cancer stages and as such allow a genuine preventative medicine to take place given that such cancers in this state can be 'completely eliminated' (cf. Westlake 1973, 162ff for the details of such competing claims). And if this is not enough, we have the perhaps more empirically inclined data from ethnographic work to also understand: "In this context, threatening talk and sickness reinforce each other because witchcraft talk without sickness would soon lose its significance, and sickness without threatening talk would only be puzzling" (Turner 1977, 229). But is modern medicine really devoid of threats? Hardly, if we think of the rhetoric of a potentially gloomy prognosis on top of the already threatening context of having to ask the question of oneself, before going to the clinic and seeing the doctor, 'what is wrong with me *now*?', which is always tantamount to asking about one's fate. Sickness is inherently threatening to all we know and can understand about ourselves and our lives. What we live for is called into question, sometimes radically, but at the very least, the 'witchcraft' of the modern medicine man has as well the potent ability to inflame the risk-laden ardour of anxiety concerning the loss of one's health, however temporarily. Indeed, ethnographically known cultures exhibit a finely tuned sophistication regarding the relationship between illness and death, given that sorcery rhetoric provides a rationale for something that otherwise would appear far *too* radical to be in any way reasonable. Human beings as reasoning creatures must have this meaningfulness in order for life to go on at all. Thus what appears to us to be nonsensical and irrelevant is no different in its social function than the medico-technical language of the applied sciences of life.

Both kinds of language, however threatening, insinuate or declaim the fact that one is now to occupy a different social role. But one is still a member of a society. Illness is not the same thing as death, and we also must recognize that in pre-agrarian social organizations at least, to die is also not to leave permanently the social ambit. In inhabiting this new role, one is charged with exhibiting 'illness behavior', which is "… the way in which symptoms are perceived, evaluated and acted upon by the person who recognizes some pain, discomfort or other sign of organic malfunction" (Scambler 1982a, 47). One's duty to the solidarity of the whole group does not lag simply because one is ill. One simply is expected to alter the character of how one fulfils that duty, and not the duty as such. This is why mental illness, however mythological it itself may be critiqued as, is generally far more stigmatized than is 'organic malfunction'. For the hallmark of all auto-psychosomaticism is the refusal to participate in the collective duty, the social bonds that both liberate us from an animal existence but also then join us to the furthering of the general will. Those who claim mental illness may be seen as betraying the rest of us, and though anyone can develop some sort of psychopathology—and many of us train ourselves to hide those we already may have, or that we imagine we have—those who 'give in' to its influence are really no better than addicts relative to the solidarity of the collective. Kindred also with those who do not work or are seen as 'welfare' miscreants, corporate or individual, the 'insane' are nothing but a burden on a society already working within the dual challenge of preserving both its knowledge and its know-how, passing it along to its successors, and at the same time, trying, at least in part, to actually improve it with a view to a more mature future species. This is a monumental task even in times when there is no large-scale crisis to focus upon. The microcosm of crises evident in the mentally ill speaks also its own peculiarly inflammatory brand of 'threatening talk': it calls into question our social maturity—we live in a society where some of its members fall through the cracks on an hourly basis—while at the same time simply being annoying to the general run of things. It both subverts and sabotages simultaneously.

1.4.2 'Mysteries'

Yet no doubt it is far better to have to 'deal with' the mentally ill than to be ill oneself, no matter the risk of 'contagion'. How a society treats its own betrayal is in fact a good gauge of its maturity. At the low end of the scale, such persons are simply liquidated, as in the so-called 'T4' precursor to the main course of the Holocaust. Perhaps at the high end, at least so far, are the retirement villages which attempt to take seriously the claims and talk of those with dementia, instead of the nagging and arrogant 'telling off' that these persons are generally faced with, especially from their own families. How do *we* know that these fellow humans have not had some neuro-chemical alteration that allows them to experience other worlds or other dimensions, time-lines or biographies, either wished for or actual? At any rate, compassion, and not criticism, is the order of the day. The more of it we exhibit, the less like the always present presentiment of the Fourth Reich we become.

Patience with patients is also a daily order, but this specifically takes place within the space of the clinical. Universities and hospitals, long-term care and those palliative, a kind of revolution in morality is portrayed, if not necessarily taken on as part of concernful being. It is almost as if we had realized the art in life but then found it a bit too dangerous to exhibit other than through an artistic representation thereof. We painted the corridors of the power over life the drab green and beige of an undercoat. The person become patient himself would provide the doctor his true palette. Within "… the field of apprenticeships was divided between an enclosed domain of essential truths and a free domain in which truth speaks of itself" (Foucault 1973, 48). Like a guild, the youth of the practitioner was simultaneously caught across the limen of inexperience—but in this, he had the advantage of desiring to learn the truth at all costs to himself—and the energy that in fact allowed him to sacrifice himself to the truth as it was presented in each case. Journeyman doctors had neither of these points and thus such a dynamic was lost to technical and managerial skill sets. It is also thus that those who are in doubt of their abilities in mid-career in all rationalized systems, including universities and government ministries, attempt managerial tracks instead of risking the disappointment that more practice within their discursive domains would reveal but their lack of acumen to accomplish anything important. But in medicine the status of 'enclosure' insulates this potential failure against all but one's immediate colleagues who, given that they share the same risk, have the 'good graces' never to mention it in front of the practitioner in question. The objectivity of reified truth as 'spoken' by the case of the patient also guards against guild-hall subjectivities or emotions such as simple resentment. In all of this "… inauthentic historical consciousness has thought itself through to the end" (Heidegger 1999, 44). The 'they' in this setting is twofold: first and always primary, is the professional society in which the doctor helps to maintain the mystery of his calling. Secondly, and much more available to be convinced while at the same time needing convincing, the general lay public who are at once most likely to become patients and thence cases. In expressing the truths of apprenticeship through the first level of the 'they', doctors and other medical personnel construct a discursive scene. What the truth is and who can speak it straddle the declination between a subjectivity that must itself speak, at first, alone in and perhaps not even aloof to the discourse, and a series of objects which could at any time constitute objections to this first assay regarding the truth of the 'essential domain'. It presents the challenge to any analysis thereof "… to account for the fact that it is spoken about, to discover who does the speaking, the positions and viewpoints from which they speak, the institutions which prompt people to speak about it and which store and distribute the things that are said" (Foucault 1980, 11). Illness as a mark against life, sexuality as a mark against society, and the duet of desire that these produce in the subject; a longing to return to potency in general, including the 'healthy libido' that never turns against the puritanical or even the practical, are the ultimate objectives of the array of objects tasked to build them up in every subject. A return to health has never quite doffed its own doubled overcoat of a rite of passage and a triumph of morality.

For what is being returned to its healthy state is more than the body, but also the 'soul', which represents the moral conscience as an object in its own right. But a new salient feature emerges with the ascendancy of medical discourse, the arbiter of science. In fact, "… just as the moral and religious view of life requires the separation of the soul from the body, mathematical science requires separation from sensory experience" (Gadamer 1998, 41–42). That the 'soul' is diffuse and only coalesces in death in order to leave the spent vessel behind, pushes the theory of science to abandon its focus on a specific moment, event, or space at which or in which truth can be forever located. Instead, one looks to record series of events, looks at a multitude of locations: "In other words, medical experience will substitute the *localization of the fixed point* for the *recording of frequencies*" (Foucault 1973, 138, italics in the original). The risk to this is obvious: we are no longer dealing with the facts of the matter at hand, as well as being forced to desert the person as an individual who experiences her own subjectivity apart from the insertion into a discourse or an institution. We have already had occasion to note that this kind of anterior experience is gradually eroded and replaced by the subject's own version of clinical 'casehood' to the convenience of everyone around them, including perhaps their own kin. But beyond this, "The phenomenological congruence between ourselves and the things of nature is broken" (Barrett 1979, 200). One mystery is resolved—but not solved—by an avoidance of coming to terms with the confrontation of the actuality of authentic distress in a person that redefines their identity as a human being, however temporarily, only to replaced by the official mystery that can contain such questions as 'What is making me ill?', and 'How do I get better?'. Both of these specific and logistical queries can be responded to in almost all cases by the dominant medical discourse. It may be that in some cases, and ultimately, in all cases that exhibit mortality, that the regression inherent in any questioning along the lines of levels theory in science runs into a blank wall, beyond which no questions can either penetrate or have their answers. But almost no patient proceeds to such a place. There are plenty of 'results' which are purely nugatory; that is, the tests that would have 'explained' the malady simply were not done, because the treatment had already effected a cure. To know, for instance, exactly what version of the *Streptococcus* infected me when the drugs have wiped it out after all would be superfluous, or to gaze at the cancerous tumor that had been surgically removed from my body—my *being*, perhaps?—would be a grotesque indulgence and an offense to the spirit of both recovery and the skill of the surgeon who removed it.

Even so, it is also clear that "… doctors often did not appreciate the effect of the condition on the patients' every-day life …" (Morgan 1982, 62). In fact, "… Prolonged uncertainty also enables doctors to maintain their power over patients, for the less uncertain patients become about the nature of their illness and the effects of treatment, the less willing they may be to leave decision-making to the doctor" (ibid, 64). Therefore the doctor's role in making and maintaining mystery includes the theatre of persuasion and sleight of hand. The entire layout of the space of the clinic aids in this, of course, given that it is at once public—and may be in most cases completely constructed through tax dollars—but as well it is private, for only one who has received the 'call' may enter beyond the lobby or waiting room. Thus the character of 'waiting with others' differs existentially from that of 'waiting alone'. The latter marks the traversing of the threshold between public and quasi-private space, as well as remarking upon our anxiety that we carry over the liminality between lobby and office or examination room. Indeed, it would be better said that this anxiety carries *us* over such thresholds, for it is only our concernful being-about-the-self that has pushed us to *undertake* such a dangerous foray into the space of enclosed truths. We cannot apodictically know that we may even return from such a place. In order to sidestep the fundamental ownmost aspect of our Dasein which is anxiety, we are already working within the statistical realm, and the ontic discourses of the clinic and its modes of 'calling out' to us in an involuntary mockery of conscience, anamnesis, diagnosis, and prognosis, perform what is essentially a deontology of selfhood in the world. The symbolic theatre replace the existential mythos-logos with mythic theatre, including the 'kits' medical professionals must wear on-site at all times: "… they distinguish their possessors from lay people, making their role seem more mysterious, shrouded and priestlike" (Haas and Shaffir 1987, 405). Indeed, the anonymization of modern medical procedures and spaces does not merely alter the person who becomes the patient. Long before I have arrived with some complaint, and long after I have been told that it is either petty, profound, or somewhere in between, the professionals who have depersonalized me have themselves been depersonalized, and far more so than I.

It thus constitutes an appendix to the 'mysteries' of the medical temple and its latter day 'priests' that they themselves have left their human individuality somewhere else, outside of the space of mystery yes, but trailing off into an unknown place, a hagiographic hinterland, an anonymous arena. We will not be able to recover either ourselves or the full presence of the medical professional as person until we both take leave of the medical scene entirely. That we seldom know 'our own' medical team members personally is not fatal to this necessary phenomenological task, as there are so many people involved in the state industry of healthcare, we are in fact likely to know someone involved in it. Perhaps the persistently unsolved case in all of this is why we have so little empathy for those whose entire training towards onticity involves them in exercise of dispassionate loss of self.

1.4.3 Solved?

In general, the patient desires to know the future. Specifically, it is her own future that is of greatest concern. That there is a science that attempts this is certainly as extraordinary as it is penultimately primordial in human culture—augury is understood anthropologically as fundamental to social existence because it gives us the sense that we have a future or if not possessed exactly, that it remains an open possibility that is worth exploring with any means at our disposal—but alone and objectifying, it is no guarantor of what we are actually requesting: "… predictability is not a necessary or a sufficient criterion of a theory being scientific …" (Sorokin, op. cit., 251). As well, validity can be had without there being a 'time-factor' associated with this or that statement within the sciences and especially, within its foundational discourse, mathematics (cf. ibid, 250ff). As Gadamer has succinctly put it, 'we can be said to have a future as long as we are unaware that we have no future'. Given that illness is a form of existential authenticity in that it makes us aware of precisely this finitude, this 'being-towards-death', we are all the more anxious to cover it up again. The truth is on the point of being uncovered, once again, in its original Greek sense, as recovered by twentieth century phenomenology. This uncovering also constitutes itself for Dasein as discovery, although as one matures, this attribute becomes a secondary characteristic or rather, *should* become one given that any other reaction to it could be considered duplicitous.

Even so, what cannot be fully uncovered aids us in recovering what threatens to make itself just more completely visible. Prediction in medicine, the prognostic statements that speak of the future as a possibility or in some probabilistic terms based on *recovery* rates—and here is another word that is regnant with its more existential meaning—serve the joint purpose of re-covering the truth of things in general, while also attempting to speak the truth of things about the particular Sometimes, the latter is achieved: "Differences in infant mortality rates between different social groups must now be imputed to environmental and cultural factors which are becoming more significant prognostic indicators than access to medical care" (Illich 1975, 73). Such 'structural' variables such as these are often beyond the control of medical discourse and health care systems, even in wealthy countries.

Illich immediately precedes this description by stating baldly: "... that the mode of U.S. therapeutic consumption lies above the level at which more expenditure can increase well-being" (ibid). A conspiracy 'theorist' might point to the link between the market for fatty diets and the use of anti-cholesterol drugs, or the consumption of sheer amounts of generally healthy food and the rate of heart surgeries later in life, suggesting that it is 'all planned that way'. However unlikely *a priori* consideration for the construction of such links is, they are no doubt real enough and as well, predictive of future cases and orders of cases.

More interesting, however, are the facts that emerge from the medical arena itself. Unlike the relationships between structures that adjudicate life-chances in the society at large and the kinds of diseases that this or that category of person is more likely to suffer from, the statements regarding health discourses and practice cannot be as easily predicted. For example, between 1961 and 1979 a 'complete reversal' occurred concerning doctors divulging their diagnoses to cancer patients (cf. Scambler 1982b, 86–87). Was this due to incessant patient demands? If so, where is their source in society? Did medical school training change during this period? If so, how and why? Cancer rates undoubtedly rose and given this change, diverse rates of their rise were associated with different social groups and their corresponding structural life-chances. Behind all of this lurks something that could also be mistaken for 'conspiratorial'. Given that the Hippocratic vocation attests to its success only when its services are no longer needed, one might well ask, how does one keep the medical industry afloat in light of more and more successful therapies and drugs? If "Genuine success is accomplished in medical practice at just that point where intervention is ultimately rendered superfluous and dispensable" (Gadamer 1996, 37 [1967]), then what are we to make of the burgeoning use of health care systems wherever they are located. An aging demographic is one response to this question, but after all, our ancestors simply didn't live as long and also didn't seem to mind that they did not. Are we then less fatalistic than our forebears? Why would this be, given the technologies that lay at our side and their capability for self-destruction? Is our reaction to our recent capability for utter and complete annihilation a renewed sense that we need to overcome this, at the very least, at the subjective level if not that political? Or is it happenstance that improved living conditions generally meant that people lived longer and only then began to encounter problems and illnesses that never in any significant scale affected previous generations of population? This, stated sociologically and detailed historically, is the most likely response to our use of health care when regarded only from the point of view of demography. But is this the *only* salient set of variables involved in the growth of health care systems and the corresponding growth in their use? Could there as well be a sense that in two-income families—now the norm in most wealthy countries—there is an off-loading of the source of the response to the need for care in general? From childhood onward, the necessity for care, for the assuagement of anxiety and loneliness, and for the ethical justification of concernful being-in-the-world as the ultimate form of Dasein must somehow be 'looked after' or at the very least, 'dealt with'. In a mock dialogue between a doctor and a layperson, we hear the former speak of it this way: "Unlike teachers and social workers, we have always been regarded with respect, if not awe, by our patients. They know that we, unlike the politicians and bureaucrats, have their best interests at heart" (Williams et al. 1994, 184). Though the layperson immediately questions this sentiment given that doctors have always also striven to protect their own professional interests, he is forced to admit that other high profile social positions are much more 'in it for themselves;' than are medical professionals. At the same time, it is surely hyperbolic to cast the doctor as an ultimate emissary or even patent exemplar of compassion and concernful being. Human beings like ourselves populate the health care systems the rest of use. They also themselves use them in times of illness or crisis. They are not exempt from their own humanity simply due to their jobs and social roles. And, as *all* social roles attempt to exempt us in this way, it is incumbent upon each of us to salvage from the 'they' of inauthenticity the truth of our beings, including the *Mitsein* of the presence of others. Those who find themselves 'separated from others by their power and genius' have many other callings aside from medicine within which to work for the common good without the commonness of the 'madding crowd'. (cf. Shem 1978, 351 for a further example of the same kind of hyperbole to this regard). The idea that 'only medicine' could 'take' the outstanding attributes of the hero's mentor in the well-known popular novel *House of God* is no more than a propagandistic crock, although it could also be read as simply the protagonist's own self-indulgence.

Beyond any of this, and yet contributing to all of it, lies the persistent remanant of sheer poverty in the human lifeworld. Throughout historic times, poverty engenders almost all other blights. If taken existentially to include the poverty of community, ethically to include that of compassion, to be impoverished as a human being affects almost all of us in some manner. Once again, predictive statements may be made: "The increase in poverty of children, usually linked to the increase in the number of female-headed families, is actually the result of the increase in poverty among young adult workers …" (Gimenez 1994, 294). Most mysteries may be reduced to poverty: most crime, most illness vectors—unhealthy food is much less expensive than is healthy, for instance, aside from immunity rates and access to health care—and even warfare as competition for resources that are either hoarded or commoditized beyond peoples' means may also be suggested as sourced in a general inequality. But poverty is so general a term as not to be susceptible to operationalizing. Is this a coincidence? We speak here in terms that must adjust themselves to the technique of technical languages. The conceptual must yield to the 'concatenational', consciousness to that which is merely conscious and better still, self-conscious, as it is this state, perhaps more than any other, that allows the 'they' of the public realm, that 'open space' where all things are said to be possible but not all things are made possible, to sway us from our authentic Dasein. We can no longer observe ourselves: "Medical certainty is based not on the *completely observed individuality* but on the *completely scanned multiplicity of individual facts*" (Foucault 1973, 101, italics in the original). This is the essence of the corpuscular corpus. We are neither corpse nor *corps d'esprit*. The spirit and its absence have been negated simultaneously. The facticality of everyday life is reduced or analyzed into the facticity of discursive statement. Convenient analogy is perilously close to becoming permanent homology. As in Shem's 'gomers', who have 'lost what goes into human beings' (op. cit.28), the clinical corpus, the body of facts to be extracted from the vivisection of reduction, we catch a glimpse of our fates before ever we are diagnosed. This is what makes the 'waiting room' so difficult to bear. We share anonymously the destiny of all who have waited there before us. Not that we are waiting to die, but rather that we have been overtaken by our own history. The way in which we have *lived* is what will be evaluated by the doctor—diets, lifestyles, sexual practices, the work life, neuroses and the like—but while this evaluation has the overtones of a true judgement, it lacks the historical consciousness with which to authentically allow us the insight of self-understanding. It stops short of demanding of us that we alter our beings in the world, while at the same time threatening us with the consequences of our inauthenticity and our turning away from the 'care which is in every case my own'. Being and nature cannot be reconciled in this way: "It is an inappropriate interpretation of the historicity of humanity. Human beings cannot be observed from the secure standpoint of a researcher, and it is impossible to reduce them to the objects of evolutionary theory …" (Gadamer 1998, 29). The thrown project of Dasein continues to 'fall', but always in the direction of itself. It very much matters then which direction becomes our own over the life course, and in which way we choose to understand the meaning of this precipitous movement. We can either be moved by our common destines, or we can move to make them all too common, the breathing corpus that avoids both the mysteries of birth and death.

References

Bachelard, Gaston. 1964. *The Psychoanalysis of Fire*. Boston: Beacon Press [1938].

Barrett, William. 1979. *The Illusion of Technique: A Search for Meaning in a Technological Civilization*. New York: Anchors Books.

Butterick, Irene H., E. S. Carpenter, B. J. Kay, and R. S. Simmons. 1994. "Gender Hierarchies in the Health Labor Force." In *Women's Health, Politics, and Power: Essays on Sex/Gender,*

Medicine and Public Health, edited by Elizabeth Fee and Nancy Krieger, 79–96. Amityville, NY: Baywood.

Cooperstock, Ruth, and Henry L. Lennard. 1987. "Role Strains and Tranquillizer Use." In, *Health and Canadian Society: Sociological Perspectives, Second Edition*, edited by George Torrance, 295–313. Toronto: Fitzhenry and Whiteside.

Evans, Robert G. 1987. "Illusions of Necessity: Evading Responsibility for Choice in Health Care." In *Health and Canadian Society: Sociological Perspectives, Second Edition*, edited by George Torrance, 615–36. Toronto: Fitzhenry and Whiteside.

Fee, Elizabeth, and Nancy Krieger, eds. 1994a. *Women's Health, Politics, and Power: Essays on Sex/Gender, Medicine and Public Health.* Amityville, NY: Baywood.

Fee, Elizabeth, and Nancy Krieger, eds. 1994b. "Man-Made Medicine and Women's Health: The Biopolitics of Sex/Gender and Race/Ethnicity." In *Women's Health, Politics, and Power: Essays on Sex/Gender, Medicine and Public Health*, edited by Elizabeth Fee and Nancy Krieger, 11–30. Amityville, NY: Baywood.

Foucault, Michel. 1973. *The Birth of the Clinic.* New York: Vintage Books [1963].

Foucault, Michel. 1980. *The History of Sexuality Volume One: Introduction.* New York: Vintage Books [1978].

Foucault, Michel. 1973. *The Birth of the Clinic.* Vintage Books, New York [1963].

Freund, Peter E. S., and Meredith B. McGuire. 1999. *Health, Illness, and the Social Body: A Critical Sociology.* New York: Prentice-Hall.

Gadamer, Hans-Georg. 1967. "Apologia for the Art of Healing." In *The Enigma of Health: The Art of Healing in a Scientific Age*, 31–44. Stanford: Stanford University Press [1996].

Gadamer, Hans-Georg. 1989. "Hermeneutics and Psychiatry." In *The Enigma of Health: The Art of Healing in a Scientific Age*, 163–73. Stanford: Stanford University Press [1996].

Gadamer, Hans-Georg. 1998. *The Beginning of Philosophy.* New York: Continuum [1996].

Gadamer, Hans-Georg. 1990a. 'Heraclitus Studies." In *The Beginning of Knowledge*, 33–81. New York: Continuum [2003].

Gadamer, Hans-Georg. 1990b. 'Anxiety and Anxieties." In *The Enigma of Health: The Art of Healing in a Scientific Age*, 152–62. Stanford: Stanford University Press [1996].

Gadamer, Hans-Georg. 1990c. 'Philosophy and Practical Medicine." In *The Enigma of Health: The Art of Healing in a Scientific Age*, 92–102. Stanford: Stanford University Press [1996].

Gimenez, Martha E. 1994. "The Feminization of Poverty: Myth or Reality?" In *Women's Health, Politics, and Power: Essays on Sex/Gender, Medicine and Public Health*, edited by Elizabeth Fee and Nancy Krieger, eds. 287–306. Amityville, NY: Baywood.

Haas, Jack, and William Shaffir. 1987. "Taking on the Role of Doctor." In *Health and Canadian Society: Sociological Perspectives, Second Edition*, edited by George Torrance, 399–421. Toronto: Fitzhenry and Whiteside.

Heidegger, Martin. 1999. *Ontology—The Hermeneutics of Facticity.* Bloomington: Indiana University Press [1988].

Illich, Ivan. 1975. *Medical Nemesis: The Expropriation of Health.* Toronto: McClelland and Stewart.

Jung, Carl G. 1959. *Aion: Researches into the Phenomenology of the Self.* Princeton: Princeton University Press [1951].

Kelleher, David, Jonathan Gabe, and Gareth Williams. 1994. "Understanding Medical Dominance in the Modern World." In *Challenging Medicine,* edited by Jonathan Gabe David Kelleher and Gareth Williams, xi–xxix. London: Routledge.

Krieger, Nancy, and Elizabeth Fee. 1994. 'Man-Made Medicine and Women's Health: The Biopolitics of Sex/Gender and Race/Ethnicity." In *Women's Health, Politics, and Power: Essays on Sex/Gender, Medicine and Public Health*, edited by Nancy Krieger and Elizabeth Fee, 11–30. Amityville, NY: Baywood Publishing Company.

Lévi-Strauss, Claude. 1977. 'The Sorcerer and His Magic." In *Culture, Disease, and Healing: Studies in Medical Anthropology*, 445–53. New York: Macmillan.

Lingis, Alphonso. 1989. *Deathbound Subjectivity.* Bloomington: Indiana University Press.

Lösch, August. 1967. *The Economics of Location.* New York: Wiley Science Editions, John Wiley and Sons [1945].

Martin, Emily. 1994. "Medical Metaphors of Women's Bodies: Menstruation and Menopause." In *Women's Health, Politics, and Power: Essays on Sex/Gender, Medicine and Public Health*, edited by Nancy Krieger and Elizabeth Fee 213–32. Amityville, NY: Baywood.

Midgely, Mary. 2004. *The Myths We Live By.* London: Routledge.

Morgan, Myfanwy. 1982. "The Doctor-Patient Relationship." In *Sociology as Applied to Medicine*, edited by Donald L. Patrick and Graham Scambler, 56–70. Bailliére's Concise Medical Textbooks. London: Bailliére Tindall.

Natanson, Maurice. 1970. *The Journeying Self: A Study in Philosophy and Social Role.* Reading, MA: Addison-Wesley Publishing Company.

Neumann, Erich. 1970. *The Origins and History of Consciousness.* Princeton: Princeton University Press, Princeton [1949].

Scambler, Graham. 1982a. "Illness Behaviour." In *Sociology as Applied to Medicine*, edited by Donald L. Patrick and Graham Scambler, 43–55. Bailliére's Concise Medical Textbooks. London: Bailliére Tindall.

Scambler, Graham. 1982b. "Death and Dying." In *Sociology as Applied to Medicine*, edited by Graham Scambler, Donald L. Patrick, and Graham Scambler, 85–97. Bailliére's Concise Medical Textbooks. London: Bailliére Tindall.

Shem, Samuel. 1978. *The House of God.* New York: Berkley Books.

Sontag, Susan. 1978. *Illness as Metaphor.* New York: Vintage Books.

Sorokin, Pitirim. 1956. *Fads and Foibles in Modern Sociology and Related Sciences.* Chicago: Henry Regnery Company.

Taylor, Charles. 1989. *Sources of the Self: The Making of Modern Identity.* Cambridge, MA: Harvard University Press.

Thomson, Alistair. 1990. "The Anzac Legend: Exploring National Myth and Memory in Australia." In *The Myths We Live By*, edited by Raphael Samuel and Paul Thompson, 73–82. London: Routledge.

Torrance, George M. 1987. "Socio-Historical Overview." In *Health and Canadian Society: Sociological Perspectives, Second Edition*, edited by George Torrance, 6–32. Toronto: Fitzhenry and Whiteside.

Turner, Paul. 1977. "Witchcraft as Negative Charisma." In *Culture, Disease, and Healing: Studies in Medical Anthropology*, edited by David Landy, 226–30. New York: Macmillan.

Wellin, Edward. 1977. "Theoretical Orientations in Medical Anthropology: Continuity and Change Over the Past Half-Century." In *Culture, Disease, and Healing: Studies in Medical Anthropology*, edited by David Landy, 47–57. New York: Macmillan.

Westlake, Aubrey T. 1973. *The Pattern of Health: A Search for a Greater Understanding of the Life Force in Health and Disease.* London: Shambhalla and Routledge and Kegan Paul.

Williams, Gareth, and Jennie Popay. 1994. "Lay Knowledge and the Privilege of Experience." In *Challenging Medicine*, edited by Jonathan Gabe, David Kelleher, and Gareth Williams, 118–39. London: Routledge.

Yap, Pow Meng. 1977. 'The Culture-Bound Reactive Syndromes." In *Culture, Disease, and Healing: Studies in Medical Anthropology*, edited by David Landy, 340–8. New York: Macmillan.

CHAPTER TWO

Metaphoric Metastases

> We are inclined to excuse all these naïve beliefs, because we now interpret them only in their metaphorical translation. We forget that they corresponded to psychological realities. Now it often happens that metaphors have not completely lost their *reality,* their *concreteness.*
>
> —Bachelard (1964, 70 [1938])

How does one understand oneself as a being with a fate that is not specifically predestined but is, nonetheless, destined in the general and widest sense? Is human life merely the 'most interesting part of death', as Nietzsche famously commented? If that were so, what would make death so dull that we could remain conscious of it at all? One thing we do take for granted while alive is that everywhere we go and whatever we do, we or some other or both of us will make something of nothing. This is an elemental aspect of human language, to incur, infer, and instigate meaning at all times and places. Even if it is the most otiose moment of the mundane world, with no apparent connection to the existential orbit, such a moment has its own history, apart from our own presence and subsequent understanding or misunderstanding of it. The metaphoric sediment of human tenure rests beneath our feet. And sometimes, indeed, what has been constructed by our forebears has, and may continue to have, a gravity about it that attaches to our soles, 'brings us down to earth', or perhaps 'evens the playing field' for us. Because we can recognize their ebbing force and perhaps, through whim or cruelty, rekindle its fire, the metaphoric meaning and rhetoric of past epochs remains part of our current destinies. We are eager, as we have seen above, to escape this relationship, the unconscious of history, the confrontation with the tradition which is at the same time our own. But until we 'evolve' into a new species entirely, such relationships will continue to be ambient, remanential, and immanent.

In this chapter we will explore the metastatic movement of metaphor throughout medical discourse, from the general to the particular, and from the ingenious sleight of hand that makes its sources appear disingenuous to the attempts to reify our contemporary discursive material, to remake the ground beneath us and to stand upon it in our own day, without being convulsed by the sense that having survived deicide, that we are at any moment the next to go down.

2.1 Disingenuities

At the very heart of the matter at hand, and in the very essence of matter in general, what matters to us is that we understand our presence in a way that is plausible. This does not necessarily include the rationality of the scientists let alone the philosopher, but it must include something of the sedimental sentiments with which we move about in the world at large. We need to imagine that this is 'our world', after all. We tend to shy away from the alien worlds of others, and, though entertained by the idea, we do not let the still obscure probability of the ultimate alien other in any way guide our daily actions on earth. To wrap the entirety of our experience of the world up in the relatively parochial beliefs that have been handed down to each of us whatever our cultural backgrounds is no mean feat, and requires of us our own circus act of petty magic. Our sideshow consists mainly of the following: all action creates reaction and this can be traced, thought precedes human action but thoughts are still free in themselves, and others can and must take care of themselves. Let's examine each of these in turn, and then relate them to the topic at hand; how does medicine ingratiate its abilities, its techniques and technologies to the metaphoric and arbitrary needs of the population it serves?

2.1.1 History

'Direct physical impact' is one way of both describing and adjudicating action in the world. Along with it, mechanism is the image that we hold dear regarding how the world works. Although completely overtaken by the new physics and even other kinds of observational challenges in related sciences, "… a general belief in this kind of clockwork undoubtedly remains today, in spite of the shift to electronic machinery. We still talk of 'mechanisms', and we are still not really happy about action at a distance, as in gravitation" (Midgely 2004, 117). Indeed, *actio in distans* smacks of a kind of outmoded scholasticism. But, just as Bachelard reminded us that we have a paternalistic attitude to the quaint notions of our apparently duller ancestors, we in our own turn are placed in their very situation by the sciences *and* scientists of our own day. And these scientists, research oriented or practicing, include medical doctors and other health personnel. We laypeople are in the same relative position to the scientists as our ancestors are to us.

This is not entirely a bust. We are made aware of what is called *Mitgehen,* or the 'going along with', whether it be with an other, or with history or with the customs of this place or that. It pushes us to think of an other that others us. Its presence will not be overcome simply by our own. We cannot immediately and completely dominate it. Rather, it speaks to us of a kind of 'method' through which we can understand what we are doing here and how we are being-with in this way, as we are always in the midst of something: "This meaning of 'method' as 'going along with' presupposes that we already find ourselves in the middle of the game and can occupy no neutral standpoint—even if we strive very hard for objectivity and put our prejudices at risk" (Gadamer 1998, 30). Dialogue has always its dialectic. The push and pull of the 'talking' throngs is a viscous and penumbraic manner of avoiding, even as a rehearsal, the confrontation with one's own being. The 'resoluteness' of which Heidegger speaks, is something that is certain of itself only in actual or actuated resolution, the facticality of which is presumably a matter for a philosophical anthropology of the lifeworld. Preceding this kind of event, and yet proceeding to it, is the irresolution that must, ironically, accompany resoluteness in its being-with-me. Along with this, the dialectic of dialogue—this is not the logical or systemic process of negation and synthesis, but the resistance one encounters as being thrown into the world; there are no unnoticed landings nor is there to be found a permanence that stifles all further falling—entrusts to the 'players' the quintessential hermeneutic experience: "... hermeneutics is the announcement and making known of the being of a being in its relation to ... (me)" (Heidegger 1999, 7). Note that we do not speak here of a 'pronouncement'. This cannot be the case on at least two counts: one, that one does not know how to pronounce the language of the other, this is something that must be learned and learned at the price of our prejudices, and two, such a pronunciation cannot be based either on the annunciation of a calling or on the enunciation of a properly trained deportment. One must hear the call of the other before any of this can take place, and even then it might not be at all appropriate. Just so, we are prone to minimizing the contributions of others to ourselves—and, for that matter, the vast impetus and inertia of history as such, the structures of the lifeworld that lie for the greater part outside our control—we attempt to balance the ledger by overdoing it on our own parts. Yet we cannot pass over this auto-hyperbolic function, especially when it comes to anxiousness concerning our health and well-being, because it acts as an *Aufklärung*, a 'wake-up call' as well as an enlightenment: "… the exaggeration is already quite obvious. It is a psychological fact that has to be explained. We do not have the right to overlook it, as would a history of science that was systematically devoted to objective results" (Bachelard 1964, 30 [1938]). This exaggeration is precisely the work of a metastatic metaphor. Just as we cannot take things 'too literally', in the manner of those we disdainfully sneer at who read scriptures as if they meant what they said in the plainest manner possible—but why do they not? We who fancy ourselves more culturally and historically literate are in fact avoiding the idea that antique texts *do* speak plainly and thus reveal a world as it was for the people of the time, or at least the few elites, those actually writing and reading; indeed, *that* is what we should be disdaining—we also cannot afford to go 'too far' in the other direction. For this would be tantamount to reinvigorating the mythic and mystical culture of our ancestors, once again, one of the things we moderns disdain about our shared past. We are also most uncomfortable with the notion that the 'literalists' of any specific cultural tradition remain our cousins even so.

2.1.2 General Metaphor

As long as the invisibility of the truth is attested to by clinical practice, that is, the starting point of diagnosis takes the problem of the 'occult' seriously in that the source of the illness is almost always occluded in some way and will take a number of tests to either divulge or at least approach, then we are faced at first with the problem of 'symptom' and thus symptomatology: "The silence of symptoms can be circumvented, but it cannot be overcome. The sign plays precisely this role of a detour: it is not an expressive symptom, but one which is substituted for the fundamental absence of expression in the symptom" (Foucault 1973, 159–60). We do not understand the illness to actually *be* its effects. There is something else that is the 'cause', or perhaps better, the vector, given that we also must shy away from essentializing the disease as an entity 'in itself'. The 'expression' of any malady is, like our first attempt at communication with an other, unpronounceable, unenunciated. But it will not remain unexpressed due to the metaphoric relation between symptom and sign. The latter gives the former a voice, and though it is still not the voice of the illness 'itself', it speaks in a language of complaint. Just as the bodily systems are disrupted in odd ways—indeed, the other 'detour' that must be mentioned here is the meandering and serpentine course of disease ridden bodies, another aspect of the challenge of metastases—indirect tests might hold the key to the source of the problem. An obvious example, cited above, is the test for fecal occult blood. This in itself has little to do with the threat, but it is able to *announce* itself in a quasi-hermeneutic manner. The prejudices that are challenged have to do with the idea that 'I am in fact healthy. I didn't know I was not healthy, and yet here I am'. This is a real threat, in the existential sense of not-being as well as in the more ontical sense of not-being-able-to. But if we stopped there, if we only had the announcement without the pronouncement, the warning sign without the legend that translates for us the implications of this signage, we would fatally rest in the space of our forebears who relied exclusively on metaphor to inform their 'psychological states': "Psychogenic death, however, is more probable *among* primitives who can be plunged into unrestrained terror as a result of the absolute conviction that they are being killed by magical means than it is among others …" (Yap 1977, 348, italics in the original). Apparently in every culture there is a spectrum of what we would today label gullibility, however functional it may have been or may be today.

Yet there is a deeper and more ontological reason for such psychosomatosis. We already know that we do not know what ails us. All we know is that we have symptoms. They could have many differing explanations, most of them, we hope, benign. Even tumors, those grotesque and eldritch lumps of misshapen and misaligned bits of our own bodies, may simply be present, exhibiting no malignancy. This 'malign' and to be maligned stasis suggests to us an *intent*. The personification of illness is one of the prime vehicles for its metaphoric content. Illness can be said to be more 'contented' within this realm than perhaps in any other, because it is given both agency and character, rather than the faceless enemy of military metaphor—the 'war on cancer'—or the abstract microbiology of organismic evolution. As with every character in literature or otherwise, this or that illness can take on specific attributes, almost like a 'personality'. But such an illness once conceived as an identity that has human-like attributes, also infects us with those same characteristics. Certain kinds of people, base, vulgar, sleazy or irresponsible, contract certain kinds of diseases. It is almost as if the moral character of a human being is assailed. Like attracts like. The dirty perversions of the person end up be interiorized through the presence of a disease which in its turn perverts. Today we are more adept at countering these flights of moralizing fancy—the AIDS crisis was instrumental in doing so in the West, but we can note that in Africa morality is still held to be both accountable and held to be the accountant of such illnesses—but the possibility for a metaphoric metastasis remains immanent. This is due primordially to the belief that consciousness includes something other than what can be either announced by a symptom or pronounced by a sign. Examine the following: "Sickness can be caused by soul-loss due to fright. The soul is believed to have such a precarious relationship with the body that any startling event can cause some of the soul to leave the body. This displaced soul substance or power is seized by the earth at the location where the person was frightened" (Turner 1977, 227). Aside from the ethnographic variance in the content of related beliefs, the basic element is that there exists something aetheric that can be, due to its very nature, easily lost. We possess it, but only in the fragile and temporary sense of it being present. It cannot be held onto by sheer will, and events in the world may impinge upon it. But all of this was never a *metaphor* for our forebears and for pre-agrarian peoples the world over. It was a reality kindred, though metaphysically diverging, from our own medical reality. And once one admits to the soul, one enters this other reality. Modern clinical practice might still use the rhetoric of 'spirit', of late transmigrated to self and 'selfhood', as well as various other buttressing motifs such as 'self-esteem' and 'self-confidence', but it does not admit the 'soul' as a serious epistemological candidate. The soul cannot be diagnosed by the doctor. It cannot offer itself as a space of the symptom. It cannot be understood as a sign or as something which speaks to us. Yet, in the hour of ultimate crisis, when existence closes in upon one and everyone can see it without the help of medical tests or doctor's prognoses, the 'soul' slips in the back door of modern ontographic discourse and announces, not itself, but its impending departure. 'Social death' recognizes this and thus must be distinguished from biological death (cf. Scambler 1982b, 94ff). Scambler relates that a certain nurse, when on duty in the ward where dying patients awaited their fates, closed the eyes of her charges, and "… always tried to close them *before* death. This made for greater efficiency when the time came for personnel to wrap the body. It was a matter of consideration toward those workers who preferred to handle dead bodies as little as possible" (ibid, 95). Ironies abound. I have also been told by doctors that hospice workers as well maintain a distance from the dying. Death must be made to resemble sleep. Death does, in fact, already resemble sleep enough for the Greeks to have made them brothers. In sleep, one touches death, lays beside it. When awake, as Heraclitus also reminds us, one touches the living. That hospice nurses are undeniably awake means that they must regularly cross the threshold between the touching of the living *and* the dead, and those that are dying are already stretched across this ultimate limen.

There are many metaphors for death in daily use even in our contemporary culture, as anxious as it is to deny the presence of death. Nietzsche's indictment that we must 'die many times in order to become immortal' is not entirely lost on us, those with oversize ears. We speak of life transitions as a form of dying. Our old selves must be buried, mourned, perhaps, but not for overlong. Recovering addicts, recovering cancer patients, recovering from the loss of a loved one, or even a change of job all fit this bill. The matriculation, perhaps followed presently by the maturation, from child to adult and so on, all speak to us of the death of the old and the birth of the new. From being without children as adults to becoming parents, or becoming parent-less children in later stages of life, the serial roles and cameos we must take on provide ever-fertile ground for the metaphor of death and its various guises or even rehearsals. Intimacy too speaks to us of the uncanniness of living on towards death, or yet being-towards-death as a primordial mode of Dasein. The 'little death' of the French suggests that the 'bigger' one might not be without its joy. But it is of interest to note that metaphor in general opens our beings back out onto the plain of existentiality, removing us for a moment from the *Offentlichkeit* of the 'they' self and selves as aspects of the socius. The creative use of language always has this potential—of course, such possibilities often lie landlocked in other forms of the public selfhood, such as advertising or sloganeering—and as such, provide an *Aufklärung* to Dasein's inauthentic bents.

Metaphor is, in short, a sign of authentic being. If the 'they' 'tranquillizes' us against this more generally, what are we to make of the use of such a term as a metaphor for the closing off of life? Anxiety, not least about death—and, proverbially, we are aware that death is *not* in fact the thing that most people fear the most, let alone their own deaths; public speaking fills that top spot, followed by the death of a loved one—is something to be covered over and ignored as much as possible. They self-recommend to all of us the hospice well before its authentic moment: "... are tranquillizers to be accepted as adequate solutions to social stresses? These are clearly moral and ethical issues that transcend the bounds of the expertise of the medical profession and demand social, not medical, answers" (Cooperstock and Lennard 1987, 329). Indeed, they demand existential responses, no less than ethical. And perhaps these two lines of reflection cannot, in the end, be separated. Given that many other salient facts ride along with the use of medication to dull the challenge of living on—this is not to say that philosophers represent the ideal form of human life, nor that they have a right to evaluate others lives according to their general privilege; what the thinker's role in such contexts is, is to make more clear the whole, the surrounding issues and the relevant variables that impinge upon reasoned and ethical action in the world—facts such as that women receive twice the amount of tranquillizers as do men (ibid, 314), it is crucial that we learn to confront the wider reasons and expose the more elemental sources of anxieties while at the same time, and in order to, preserve *anxiety* as something absolutely necessary to human consciousness. The former is often a perversion of the latter, ringing into our sense of selfhood the false conclusions of the social self. How am I to be taken by others? Do I conform to the marketed ideals of my social role? Am I only that which my social role dictates I be, or become? And why so? What are the stringent limits that engendering myself brings along with it? Why 'do gender' at all?

Metaphor in its most general sense can be used to disclose its uses in specific contexts. Treating gender or other life-chance variables as 'mere' metaphors may in fact help us dislodge their gravitational sway, and thus promote at the very least a more liberated orbit about them. Similarly with death. Though it completes our Dasein and also Dasein in general as our human condition, 'running along towards death', thrown into the existential destiny of not-being, it also serves us well as a way in which to understand life changes, as we have just seen. So it is not at all the case that metaphor is either a vacuous or even a less rigorous manner of self-understanding, let alone an archaic means of self-expression and the understanding of the world, but rather a way to get at the disclosedness of being in the world as it must be, and not only 'as it is' from the perspective of norms.

That said, our use of metaphor also commonly endangers all of this authentic self-understanding as well our ability to take the other seriously as an othering source in my own life, as an hermeneutical object and objection to my subjectivity and perhaps also to my unknowing or unhearing subjectitude. It is especially noticeable when it comes to ill health and our proximity to it: "Contact with someone afflicted with a disease regarded as a mysterious malevolency inevitably feels like a trespass; worse, like the violation of a taboo" (Sontag 1978, 6). Similarly, we often cross the street to avoid the homeless, as if they were the vehicle for a form of contagious magic. In capital, one might say with some sociological veracity, that poverty *is* a constant threat even to the better-heeled, for one can always lose most jobs or other sources of income, the markets could turn sour, or a crisis may render one's home unlivable, as we witness in the effects of a civil war. The metaphor, though damning and cruel, is not without its truth. But such a truth as this should galvanize us to ethical action in the world on behalf of those others who *do* in fact represent an aspect of my being and potentiality to be. In avoiding them, we avoid the anxieties held within us regarding our own mundane fates. Part of the work of keeping up appearances in our kind of social organization is to make others believe that one is immune to things like poverty and even disease. Health is also *our* 'first principle of beauty', as we mentioned it was Hitler. All along with the fetish for youth and cleanliness, health and hygiene represent a metastatic moment; we humans, always at risk for sliding back into our animal-selves, unclean and even unwashed, work hard to promote the sense that it is health and our consciousness that health must be worked towards and maintained that separates us from the lower forms, those whose lives are not worth living, and further, to borrow another Nazi favorite, those who are exemplary of 'life unworthy of life'.

It is also so in any process of professionalization, but all the more so in preparing for a career in the medical sciences or the health care system: "The process depends on convincing other players in the hospital setting that the neophyte has successfully adopted the symbolic interactional and ideological 'cloak of competence'" (Haas and Shaffir 1987, 414). In bourgeois organizations such as the hospital and the university, government ministry and corporation, where almost all middle-class people eventually find work or careers, it is transparently obvious that social capital is of the utmost. Technique and skill levels may be determined and can always be augmented or updated, but the accoutrement and deportment of our contemporary version of 'my fair lady' is more difficult to train for. Couple this with the ongoing use of the very metaphors that Sontag warns us against—those that personify and condemn the victims of ill-health and sort them off from the rest of us, to name a few—by other writers in the medical and health science fields. They are easy, apparently, to slip in and out of rather semi-consciously: "To what extent could we, by learning more about the mechanism of such regressions, help in the fight against this, the most terrible of human ailments?" (Selye 1956, 304). Selye is of course speaking of cancer, and mentions that certain kinds of tumors do not grow well in persons with higher stress levels. The metaphor is here more subtle, but it is still present, keyed by the use words like 'fight', 'regression', and 'terrible'. On top of this, 'we' must 'aid' in such a fight. No war-time poster would be much different. That all language is elementally metaphoric does not absolve us from taking care. Gadamer reminds us that for the ancients, the use and over-use of metaphor could be seen as the reason why their metaphysics seems so unhelpfully naïve to us as moderns. Speaking of 'fire' as a juggernaut of non-being is to say even more than what can be said about it regarding its messianic quality in human evolution, cultural and perhaps also biological, given that its controlled use represents one of the most important moments in human tenure and consciousness: "Indeed, this would not simply be a bad allusion to the to the cosmological problem that fire is supposed to be an elementary component of the world order. To think of the devouring flame that consumes everything and which nothing resists as a part of the existing order of the universe was evidently a particular problem for ancient cosmology" (Gadamer 2003, 30 [1974]). The trope of fire may be seen as one of the archetypes for medical metaphors, both then and now. Disease consumes all that is living, and nothing living can resist it. If something is immune to disease, it cannot be that that something can be called 'life'. In the same way, fire is resisted and indeed doused by water, but water has an inexistence about it. Its liquid being resists in itself the notion of stability, or even the existential 'self-constancy' that in our own time has become an 'elementary' aspect of being.

2.1.3 Health Metaphors

If the effect of this tropic presence is indeed more profound than whatever is imagined as the cause or even the course of it, then we have something that binds the diverse ultimacies of the radical other, whether this other threatens life or existence, matter or form. Of course, we realize that the content of both our gods and our demons is historically and culturally conceived and not merely 'conditioned', as if there were some other source of human knowledge outside of the lifeworld that could be said to be malleable or, as is common enough in our own culture, to think that the 'I' is something whose solidity perambulates and sometimes wholly avoids its history and its sociality. Modern conceptions of disease serve their origins in this way: "TB was a disease in service of the romantic view of the world. Cancer is now in the service of a simplistic view of the world that can turn paranoid" (Sontag 1978, 68). Along with UFOs, the other belief in which Sontag immediately mentions, the cancer metaphor allows us to imagine organizations riddled with conspiratorial tumors, plots and metastatic networks. This is especially so in politics, whereas in fact these kinds of 'invisible' colleges and translucent collages have always existed in bureaucratic and even institutions harboring and marketing non-rational contents, such as the church. The idea that we 'don't know what is going on' may have some perverse charm to it, but its more profound effect is that we allow ourselves to evade our own responsibility for both politics and the polis alike, as citizens and as persons within a community, however wide. The sense that we 'can't do anything about it anyway' follows directly from our understanding of disease metaphors that irresistibly assail us. Even the most trenchant culture critics, analyzing of all of these phenomena can fall into their use: "It is the expropriation of man's coping ability by a maintenance service which keeps him geared up at the service of the industrial system" (Illich 1975, 160). So far, so good. Sontag states the same in almost the exact terms. But then, on the same page, we find that this 'gearing' is "… spawned by a cancerous delusion about life, and manifests itself when this delusion has pervaded a culture. It is a symptom of the mortal sickness of medical civilization" (ibid). Or social scientists studying medicine: "… some serious conditions (e.g.) some cancers) rarely appear in a striking fashion: their onset may be slow and insidious" (Scambler 1982a, 48). Or medical scientists: "Even now a revolt can break out occasionally in a part which forgets the principle of collective altruism. This is what we call *cancer*. It kills the whole as well as itself by its own unrestrained expansion" (Selye 1956, 283, italics in the original). Clearly, Selye is not actually speaking of events at the cellular level, though he says he is. No, what we are diagnosing is the *zeitgeist* of capital, whose expansion is indeed 'unrestrained', like the conception of fire for the ancients, whose politics are 'insidious', and whose delusions are 'cancerous'. There is no need to mince words here or in any other kind of culture critique. But to use medical metaphors 'in the service' of such is to muddy the waters considerably.

Fire was not the only metastasis of our cultural forebears. Medical conditions themselves, especially the one whose onset was not at all insidious and bore a 'striking' resemblance to religious behavior were singled out as something more than what they were: "… the 'sacred illness' of epilepsy connotes a devout awe and forbearance for those affected by it. For one to rob or otherwise harm one who has fallen from it would be nothing less than a sacrilege" (Gadamer 2003, 78 [1990]). This is a far cry from our culture's version of the sick role. The function of sacred illness was to remind people that not only we they connected to a larger order in which primordial forces, natural or no, could intervene in human life and indeed, take an interest in human history—the 'mascot' gods of the Levant had their parallax on Olympus; the Greek gods disdained their human cousins but meddled in the latter's affairs nonetheless, as well as prescribing their fates, while the cultures whose primary enemies in the region *were* the Greek city-states took on a more personal and loyal set of gods to help them resist those very enemies—but as well, to remind humans of their mortality and ultimate weakness, that is, *inability* to resist, in the face of the fires of these cosmological forces. For us, the sick person is not only no longer sacred, he has, all of a sudden, become quite literally a 'human resource': "He was cast in the role of a legitimized deviant; his exemption from his usual responsibilities was tolerated as long as he would consider his illness as an undesirable state and would seek technical assistance from the health-care system" (Illich 1975, 57). This role applied to, and was applied to, more or less a stringent degree. Those ailments that were most distracting to both labor power and biopower were especially targeted. Illegitimacy was inherent in the diseased state, and social sanction could only be given in the manner Illich and others suggest; that is, one needs to *do* something about it and neither wallow nor, as in the case of sexual 'dysfunctions' take both leisure and pleasure in its presence: "It was enough to make one's voice tremble, for an improbable thing was then taking shape in a confessional science, a science which relied on a many-sided extortion, and took for its object what was unmentionable but admitted to nonetheless" (Foucault 1980, 64). Since everyone was at least interested in these forms of 'deviance', even those who sought to objectify them into a surveilling and controlling discourse could take their version—or was it just *here* that things actually became a 'perversion'?—of pleasure therefrom. A kind of smugly sardonic *Schadenfreude* was developing. Smug in that it itself was not afflicted, or fully afflicted if affected, by the malaise or the disorder, and sardonic equally about those who were and the fact that it had somehow resisted this specific fire even if resistance meant that the fire still smoldered within, one's being coughing up the sputum of residual smoke and ashes, signaling the embers of its own interiority.

To avoid recognizing this problem was to find a way to avoid a form of universalizing self-recognition. One did not want to be *like* the others even if one *did* want what the others had apparently got. Akin to those who work within capitalism and yet remain self-styled critics of it, medical professionals and laypeople alike were able to cordon off their interest by further objectifying it. Krafft-Ebing's famous study *Psychopathia Sexualis,* first published in English in 1882, only was fully translated in the late 1960s—the most salacious narratives and diagnoses had remained in Latin for a doctor's eyes only—to be sold as part of the sexual revolution. Now everyone could be party to their culture's marginal affairs, and perhaps even make a party out of them, as the baby-boomers fleetingly accomplished. But more importantly, in order to avoid this self-recognition and turn the blinding light and searing heat of its fires away from oneself, meant that one had to re-imagine its effects as a self-misrecognition. To do this in turn meant that medical discourse had to reconstruct its metaphoric gaze: "Henceforth the medical gaze will be directed only upon a space filled with the forms of composition of the organs. The space of the disease is, without remainder or shift, the very space of the organism" (Foucault 1973, 191). Something has taken over, and we, in an ironic reference to the previous metaphysics, are *possessed* by the disease. It has sparked an ontological turn inwards, our innards may be turned inside out. The 'very space' of our organism has become, in a trice, the plausible *disjecta membra* of our former selves. All of this can exert its presence, can excrete its prescience unto death, not because once ensconced, the disease organism functions as an alien intruder—we are not exactly 'possessed' in the classic sense after all, but rather inhabited, which still smacks of the other as occult, the incubus of olden day—but that our body serves as its vessel, a desacralized temple given over to the rites of the barbarian: "But at a deeper level than this spatial 'metaphor', and in order to make it possible, classificatory medicine presupposes a certain 'configuration' of disease" (ibid, 4). We already have been told that disease 'entities' do not really exist outside of their action within our bodies. Perhaps this is immediately and even more true of the essence of mental illness, which has no basic externality that can be identified by the microscope. Perhaps this is what we would like to think of *all* diseases. Even so, our distrust of action at a distance makes us tremble with morbid anticipation when we turn our own gaze towards the possibility of becoming ill. The spatial metaphor runs deeper not due to its course finding and running through the inner space of our bodies, but instead due to its ability to cut through the interiority of our beings.

2.2 Engendered States

Diseases 'perform' in this way: they understudy their undertakings. They cannot take the stage until the stage itself is set for their entrance. A minor cut and a hot tub, perhaps, or an untreated spider's bite. They are the most unlikely of heroes, and indeed, can never actually be heroic in their action. We have gotten beyond their cultural personification only so far. We no longer imagine that TB is the mark of a 'great soul'. We sneer at this nonsense with the awkward recognition that the romantics would rather die than live in our world. And indeed, the only romance we today allow ourselves is that of the greeting card variety. Even sexual trysts are calculated to the nth degree, and of late, the internet calculates them for us. What has been engendered by the 'paranoid turn' of modern civility is the incivility of constructing scenes about which we may become all the more paranoid.

2.2.1 Examples

All of this has a sense of the apokotropaic about it: "My relation to my name is not that of belief. It has neither the objectivity nor the distance from me of the kinds of things I normally say I believe. I live this relationship, I live within it; I am constantly renewing it and re-creating it" (Barrett 1979, 303). But simply asserting something does not make it so. We can call ourselves anything we want and we still must wait for the looking-glass self to be sponsored by both significant and generalized others. Yet it is true that how we understand ourselves even in the ontical world is categorically different to and discrete from that which is either present-to-hand or ready-to-hand. We cannot be an object to ourselves. The medical gaze constructs this aperture so that we can join the audience and view the unfolding drama of our demise. Mostly, however, and always to a point, what we witness are the rehearsals. Once in a while, the rehearsal shifts into the fullest performance, and it is we who must in the end pay for it.

Nevertheless, the sick role as a socially sanctioned metaphor for both the damned and the elect—we are *to be* saved by the doctor and his or her sacred arts; and thus the mode of being might run as the 'to-be-saved' or 'to-rejoin-the-world' while the sick role itself is the 'to-be-exempt-from-the-world'—performs its own drama on our behalf. Here we cannot do the naming for ourselves. This is the purpose of diagnosis, the 'knowing' that comes from gazing 'across' and unconcealing rather than simply revealing the truth of things. We must 'show' this state of affairs to be at least 'probable': "A scientist's conscience does not permit him to assert things he cannot prove or at least show to be probable. No assertion has ever yet brought anything corresponding into existence" (Jung 1959, 195). The poet's 'speaking into being' aside, the death of God rendered the one source of evocation as enunciation moot. But it is of interest that the technician, the practical scientists, the one whose sole source of value comes from naming the things as they are, must have a 'conscience' in order to evaluate whether he has done this and not something else. How could this be? If the gaze is male, and the glance female, what gender is the conscience, scientific or otherwise, in this milieu? Better, how is the conscience to be engendered given its indissociable links with the previous mode-of-being-evaluated, valued and indeed, judged? And does the disease possess a gender? It does, it turns out, because it has borrowed the status of the body it has invaded. Its gendered state is now subject to the masculinity of the gaze. It must be disciplined, cast out. The disease is the scapegoat rather than the diseased, as it used to be. At a glance, we can see the difference is subtle, But is it not just kindred with our formal femininity that the glance can only know the subtle while the gaze can only know the gross? The glance always comes first in diagnosis and in a way, prognosis as well. We cannot tell what will occur in detail in the future in any tense, therefore our view of what is to come is always feminine. It is compassionate but lacks the information needed to make veridical decisions once and for all. It is open-minded, but its brain, as is sometimes said, is always ready to fall out for lack of concrete material. The past, on the other hand, is indubitably masculine in this view. Our status towards it is of archaeological depths. We can discern its most detailed attributes, that is, those that have survived, and in our maleness, only what is of value survives in any case, so no matter. But what is occurring at the moment requires both of our 'genders' to look abroad and make their best guess. After the *Augenblick* of 'what have we here, aha, another case of …', then it may be the turn of the new discursive scalpel: "The gaze plunges into the space that it has given itself the task of traversing. In its primary form, the clinical reading implied an external, deciphering subject, which, on the basis of and beyond that which it spelt out, ordered and defined kinships" (Foucault 1973, 136). Because of its masculinity, the need for heroism does not abate even when transmuted into the technical sphere. Engineers of all kinds are portrayed as heroic, if somewhat asocial, but their very asociality and vulgarity is forgiven given our sense that one must be somewhat 'ecstatic' to imagine and then design and build their great structures and intricate tools. The Greek for this now over-emphasized term is literally 'standing outside'. This is what the builder does and as well what he builds. It is either new or is quite literally also 'outside' in terms of where it stands on the earth or in the city etc. Disease sits inside. It must be turned out and made, through ecstasis, to stand outside on its own, where it will inevitably perish. We learn, to our relief, that viruses such as HIV are quite fragile and cannot last long in the external environment. Yet it serves us a caution, for we imagine metaphorically at least that the virus thus 'wants' into our bodies, 'needs' us in some perverted sense of lust or even romance, and it will have its way with us if we ever let down our guard. And it is not merely the 'thing from without' that threatens in this way. The more Lovecraftian subversion of our own bodily functions can lay claim to the unnamable name of 'the thing that should not be': "As long as a particular disease is treated as an evil, invincible predator, not just a disease, most people with cancer will indeed be demoralized by learning what disease they have" (Sontag 1978, 6). Better surely to become 'amoralized', more like the engineers of both life and living, because within this transformation lies the promise of distance and dispassionate objectivity. Death too must come round to this interlocutor, and perhaps be made to change it trajectory. If the abyss gazes into us, then finally, but only in the clinical space, we too can return its gaze: "Now, these men who watch over men's lives communicate with death in the fine, rigorous form of the gaze" (Foucault 1973, 166). More than this, this watchfulness, no more the 'night watch' that seeks communion with the infinite but also provides the guard for those who still must live against that which appears as the thief, has the ability to close the gap between life and death, and between the world and the lifeworld. The fundamental ability of culture to disclose this relationship and then close in upon it is of course primordial to human consciousness, but only within the ambit of technical discourse—the naming and engendering not of culture, but the technical feats and statistics of the tools that culture has produced—do we find that we can finally know it as a destiny: "Man is the creature who can annihilate distance and bring far and near together" (Barrett 1979, 152). This is transparently true in technological terms, with results alternatively trivial—a trip to Vegas by air—or profound—the Hubble telescope. But it is more deeply true in the world of discourse, where aspects of being and even structures of consciousness can be brought close to the knowing and experiencing senses and intellect by virtue of the methodological considerations of scientific language. These phenomena are not unrelated. They both stem from the focus on technique, as we have seen. They both generate objects and employ processes of objectification. All of this is pat. Even the most primordially trivial can take on the appearance of being the most historically profound simply by the introduction of the 'long telescopes of the historical neuters' as Nietzsche slyly suggested. For medical discourse and its related bourgeois sensibilities, Foucault famously states that it is sex that was turned into sexuality in just this way: "The essential point is that sex was not only a matter of sensation and pleasure, of law and taboo, but also of truth and falsehood, that the truth of sex became something fundamental, useful, or dangerous, precious or formidable, in short, that sex was constituted as a problem of truth" (1980, 56). Once so constructed, there were no discursive limits. All brackets, boundaries, and frames that had formerly applied to language could now be projected on to the objects of technical language, whether that psychoanalytic, psychopathological, or even 'simply' physiological. To speak of this thing was to bring it under control. Medical 'law' adjudicates healthy behavior even as it sanctions against ill-health. The content which is most exemplary of this speech and this diktat change radically over time. For Victorians, possessed of their national duties towards competing empires and the absolute need for more and more biopower—not so much for the burgeoning and newly minted mode of production *per se* but for military purposes and the economy of production and consumption—onanism was a foremost medical sin, as was homosexuality, which was also highly illegal. Smoking was not considered a big deal, though its effects were well known even in the late nineteenth century. For ourselves, living in a time where there are far too many people for our strategic purposes or for our still limited compassion, masturbation is considered completely healthy and normal from age ten onwards, or even earlier for girls. Smoking costs employers an publically funded health care systems a great deal of money, though we are not that concerned in the West if the vast majority of Chinese smoke. Being gay today is no doubt still a pain for those who are so, but in more and more countries it is not only perfectly legal but fostered through recent marriage laws. But medical discourse, the DSM series, the idea of psychopathology and mental illness and so on, remain unscathed by their former 'errors' of judgement. We simply put these things down to the fact that people are always children of their time and no other. We expect that our successors will judge us similarly, as long as we indeed have them, and one might even hope that they will given how each epoch exists in a fundamental suite of historical blindness about itself.

2.2.2 Categories

However this may be, it is clear that medical discourse takes full advantage of diverse sources of metaphor and finds all kinds of excuses or rationalizations to justify them. Sexuality today is mostly fantasy, including the hallmark romance already alluded to, and the entertainment fictions that portray people of *most* ages—because of the aging baby-boomer market contingent—having all kinds of fun with themselves and others, onanistically or otherwise. The internet coalesces the holy trinity of masculinity—sex, power, and wealth—in a tightly focused discharge of media that allows its users to feel as if they had complete control over perhaps millions of women—and not just women—that this control can be free of charge and still absolutely effective, and that endless sex and sexuality are its purview. That we claim to be so protective of younger people in this regard suggests that we have misgivings about the whole affair, and that these are not merely leftovers from an earlier time when, as Foucault and others have suggested, sexuality was much more liberated, persons were married at twelve and lifespans were, to our imagination, cruelly short in any case. The 'adult' character of the internet and its anatomical-physiological fetish provides the clearest and most recent effort to control the basic human phenomena of sex by making it not only into a commodity and an esthetic competition, but most disturbingly, into something *for* adults. So-called adults, that is. We might suggest sociologically that this is due to the simple logistical problem of two-income families, where work and child-raising take up so much time that people of all ages do not have a moment for sex, let alone the developed and sophisticated sexuality of romance and theatre, burlesque as well as the impassioned displays of ardor and loyalty, all of which we are at the same time told *must* be part of a truly healthy relationship or marriage. This is easily enough to make persons neurotic, which itself feeds back into the loop of clinical discourse. This situation, ontical in the extreme and inauthentic in its ethics, is so well known that even introductory textbooks in sociology attempt to make a churlish or sardonic joke about it, telling readers that their authors live in such families and, 'oops, we tried to have sex but hey, the kiddies interrupted us' with their homework, soccer games, or illnesses.

So much for romance. Yet sociological analyses provide only the most basic description of the problematic categorical imperatives of medical discourse and their objects. For instance, the major reason why onanism disappeared off the pathological map and reappeared as a key to a healthy sexuality was that it simply does not have to involve anyone else. It sells somewhat mischievous artifacts of technology to boot. We can all celebrate the fact that more people of more ages are masturbating than ever before in human history. Kindred to long work and school hours, the idea of freedom being hitched up to financial and logistical access to resources, and the still quite concrete bourgeois notion that 'incest', whatever its form, is somehow still an evil—ethnographers of the imperial period invented the incest taboo for obvious biopower related reasons, Foucault speaks of the pre-industrial extended family engaging in all kinds of rampant intimacies, little enough of which led to 'inbred' pregnancies given that it is difficult to get pregnant and in any case and nobody kept track of these births—today's family and school attempt to model the ideal medical context wherein sexuality is limited, more or less, to adults, and 'education' concerning sexuality is highly technical and seemingly bereft of an existentialist ethic. What does it mean to 'have' sex? How does one 'have' something like this? Why is sex used as a distraction *from* work while at the same time it poses a threat to economic organization because it is a distraction *to* work? Why has work in all its forms taken over the waking life to the exclusion of sex? We hear in all studies of the family that when things get overloaded, people having children or even getting a promotion, or yet working harder to avoid being fired, sex is the first thing out the window. Shouldn't our children be being taught about *these* aspects of sexuality as well as how to do it 'safely'?

On top of this, our Orwellian fetish surrounding sexuality as a medical model of the greatest moment has other iatrogenic effects: "The penultimate blow to the dying miner is the loss of his sexuality. The miners believe that silicosis destroys potency, a belief that is self confirming" (Leyton 1987, 203). Viagra and of late, its female version—'Niagara?'—are touted messianically in marketing. 'We have stolen your best sexual years from middle school onwards, but now that you're retired and no longer directly contributing to the economy, here's something that will help you have as much sex as your cholesterol infarcted hearts can handle!'. Now there's some advertising. Beyond such satire, sociological studies have also revealed that sexual 'pathologies' or other forms of mental disturbance which may or may not have their roots in repression and sexual coyness, are gender sorted by their level of subjectivity in diagnoses. The medical professional's opinion is much more important in prescription and utilization of health services in women's cases than in men's (cf. D'Arcy and Schmitz 1987, 186ff). At the same time, "… by far the greatest number of women and men are seen for neurotic and psychosomatic reasons" (ibid). All of this is also pat. Given that men and women communicate very differently about health and illness, these tactics in turn influence the temporalizing vectors of anamnesis—'when did you begin to feel unwell?', 'how did this feeling come about?'—diagnosis—'you may have contracted or *developed* this or that'—and prognosis—'this is what we can do for you'. This process is almost pre-scripted, if not exactly prescribed in the usual sense: "Once in the doctor's office, women are more likely to display emotions and report indefinite, passive types of discomfort, tension and worries. These non-specific complaints are the very symptoms from which psychiatric diagnoses are made" (D'Arcy and Schmitz 1987, 191). Men, on the other hand, most often point to something specific in their lives which is perceived as stressful. Economists have argued that the 'opportunity structures' associated with mental illness occur more for women because of their relative absence in the labor force. This sounds a little like the 'idle hands, idle mind' shibboleth, but given that specific circumstances in public and work life are the catalyst for most male plaintiffs regarding mental health and perhaps also that physical, there is a grain of truth in it nonetheless. If we update these statement to our own generation, where approximately seventy-percent of women are working in North America, we find that context and event specific complaints regarding health deterioration are much more prominent for females. The shift in workplace policies and human resource management processes to reflect the changing gender balances are also a testament to the growing specificity of complaints and concerns. This is said to also benefit men, as more precisely and rigorously defined 'empirical' events need to be cited as evidence that there is a problem that at least, non-medical personnel must somehow work to resolve.

That there is some wisdom in this should not be divorced from the metaphor of Sophia herself. The presence of women in any social context has been seen as a civilizing factor—the American West is a proverbial example—and the workplace is different only in degree. This does mean, however, that women are not truly being understood as fellow human beings with which one can share a life, a labor, or even an idea, but as rather ethereal vehicles of, on the one hand, desire, which is certainly old hat, but more recently, of wisdom. On top of this, this is the wisdom of the new, of a youthful parallax that has not been sullied by the jaded and perhaps even the cynical experience of others who had passed before her: "Sophia is neither mother nor spouse; she is always the daughter, the symbol of feminine knowledge and intellectuality, eternally young and intact in spite of her vicissitudes" (Passerini 1990, 58). This metaphor is so well known and well-used in literature as well as in popular books in science and philosophy that one need not belabor the point. Suffice to say that in cases where male-dominance has been carved out of institutions or *into* discourses the 'eternal feminine' infinitely rhapsodized at the end of Goethe's *Faust*, takes on infinite variety (cf. Shem 1978, 140ff for an amusing if sardonic example regarding social workers). Though on the face of it the idea of a gender possessing not only civility but also civilization itself would seem to confer irresistible advantage. But this is not really the case. As with many metaphors concerning women, metastasized by the factical representation of women as tokens or present simply as a distraction for men, these are almost exclusively male inventions. Thus women often feel that they must either live up to them—the pedestal effect—or be shunted aside in favor of some other female individual. Given this, it is not surprising some social scientists have referred to women as 'being mad by definition.' (cf. D'Arcy and Schmitz, op. cit., 193). Add to this the transparently negative medical metaphors having to do with the inevitable 'fragility' of their bodies and minds alike, though it is well known that women can take far more pain than can men simply do to pregnancy. Yet further, such fragility was always linked in some manner to other structural variables concerning life-chances, such as class and ethnicity: "This talk of women's delicate constitutions did not, of course, apply to slave women or to working-class women—but it was handy to refute the demands of middle-class women whenever they sought to vote or to gain access to education and professional careers" (Krieger and Fee 1994, 13). The ascendancy of medical discourse gave an apparent cantor to time-honoured claims regarding the difference between males and females, but once again, the technical language of discourse and especially that of the applied sciences was exclusively engendered by men, so much so that it is only recently that we have become publicly aware that medical drug trials for general use had been and have been only tested on white males, as if all other versions of humanity were merely marginal, or worse, aberrant forms when compared to this statistical *and* ideological ideal.

Not merely the bodies and minds of women and men are subject to varieties of metaphor. Another vector of metastasis occurs with the association of disease 'themselves' with genders. TB was essentially female, though the men who contracted it were said to be of artistic and romantic sentiments, two feminine things which partook in wisdom and thus were related to the presence of the youthful Sophia in one's life and heart. TB was 'but a disguised manifestation of the power of love', but cancer has a much more masculine character: "As cancer is now imagined to be the wages of repression, so TB was once explained as the ravages of frustration. What is called a liberated sexual life is believed by some people today to stave off cancer, for virtually the same reason that sex was often prescribed to tuberculosis as therapy" (Sontag 1978, 21). The sexuality in each case bears the hallmarks of the stereotype of engendered sexual states. For cancer, sex must be a virile display of dominance, for TB, sex was to be sensual and compassionate, aesthetically interesting and heartfelt. In short, for the latter, sex was to be incorporated in the life of the lover, for the former, only a sex life was necessary.

Yet another category of medical metaphor whose states are engendered has to do not with the body *per se*, nor that which afflicts, but its actual non-pathological functioning. It appears that nothing can escape the metastatic 'nature' of such metaphors, as even when things are running 'normally' there is something invasively literary to be said about them: "Whereas in the earlier model, male and female ways of secreting were not only analogous but desirable, now the way became open to denigrate [ ] functions that for the first time were seen as uniquely female, without analogue in males" (Martin 1994, 217). This categorization could apply to various instances of such bodily spumata but, of course, it refines itself when it focuses upon sexual reproduction and its vehemently outspoken differences. The physiognomy of mammals has long been overemphasized in what were supposed to be strictly technical manuals, anatomies, and rubrics, but even here the language is unmistakably mythical and hyperbolic. Ova, for example, are always passive. They are forced to conceive by the intrepid spermatozoa, just as, in agrarian period etiquette—sedentism is the catalyst for the ordering of sexuality with the goal to produce high populations needed for both labor and organized warfare on a massive scale—women can simply 'lie back and think of England' or some more archaic empire like Babylon, perhaps—men must force themselves onto and thence into women in order for coitus to be successful. The almost dead 'courtesy;' of men asking women out on dates but not vice-versa is a vestige of this more brutal metaphorically encouraged act that could be now regarded as common assault. More than this, another "… part of the reason ovulation does not merit the enthusiasm that spermatogenesis does may be that all the ovarian follicles containing ova are already present at birth. Far from being *produced* as sperm are, they seem to merely sit on the shelf, as it were, slowly degenerating and aging like overstocked inventory" (Martin, op. cit., 227, italics in the original). No doubt capitalist social organizations have invented their own Dickensian metaphors to take the place of those Augustinian or Hindu alike. But one thing that has not yet been entirely cast off is the idea that a male, even alone, represents not only the group but also its public voice. He speaks for the she in all of us. Other studies have found that small group interaction amongst medical professionals, indeed, all kinds of professionals, "… follow the lead of the male and focus less on problems of role-strains and interpersonal relations …" (Cooperstock and Lennard 1987, 318), and thus, even within therapeutic contexts where men and women are participating not merely for the descriptive purposes of social research and data collection but also to air out their grievances with one another and with the organizations in question themselves, there is a tendency '… to sustain strained social systems. Significantly, these strains within family groups were mentioned as resulting in drug use by female rather than male informants" (Cooperstock and Lennard, op. cit., 318). Clearly, metaphor can present a distraction to critique. Even when metaphor is used rhetorically to appeal to the student, as we saw above, it has the effect of making an injunction seem like it is sourced in emotions rather than in an analytic intellect or a form of rationality that opposes rationalization. Sociology has from almost its outset been centered around probing the structures of the lifeworld, but it inherits this mantelpiece from the philosophical disciplines in general. When metaphysics became demythologized, one could argue that philosophy became sociology.

2.3 Reifications

Yet in the place of metaphysics there appeared a more intimately risky form of consciousness, that of ideology and its attendant neo-discursive languages. The applied sciences, also eager to cut their ties with the former 'queen of disciplines', Sophia herself, also made a bolt over the stern threshold of anti-transcendentalism. Though hermeneutics does not argue for a return to archaic world systems, religious or otherwise, it does take up a critical stance with regard to all that supposes itself a better substitute or more dangerously, an improvement upon the very structure of human consciousness.

2.3.1 Attitudes

Not that such structures themselves are unwavering. They too are historical through and through. There is no one human nature. Each epoch relieves itself upon the altar of its metaphysics, but of late, we have begun to see this oblation as a kind of egress, an escape, or yet, more phenomenologically, a 'turning away' from our beings and from the world as it is. More liquid is this modernity, but at the same time, libation is still an option. In order to maintain a critical distance from these kinds of rituals, we have at once taken health into our own hands—a detailed look at alternative medical practices and their assumptions follows below in Chapter 5—while at the same time reduced our version of what it means to be a conscious human being in the world to a set of statistics and results, as we have also seen above. Our attitude towards living on is one of extremes. One the one hand, we have personalized this 'self-care' to the point of reinventing midwifery and giving birth in once again one's own abode—which might appear as quaint or at worst quirky if it were not for its perhaps overemphasized reliance on the sense that clinics themselves can be medically dangerous—and on the other, we have dully submitted ourselves to the most reckless and shameless shill regarding pharmaceuticals and their purposes. The most glaring effort of the subject to this regard must be the strain to counter our often poor diets with pills that allow us to continue our bad habits or even addictions. Are anti-cholesterol drugs the morphine of the masses?

If metaphor may be said to partially obscure the 'real relations' concerning conceptions of what is healthy and what we can or must do to preserve our health in the face of all of the other kinds of things we also at least can or desire to do to ourselves, then what direction must a critical tack take up in response? First, we can remind ourselves that reification of all kinds is immediately misleading for an historical species. Indeed, all matter, given enough geological or cosmic time, changes into something else. Though we can find our relatively minute lifespans frustrating—perhaps a positive contribution in the search for immortality is the desire to know the cosmos more realistically and intimately—it is handy for us with regard to seeing through any equally human construction that pretends to be timeless. Morality was once the great pretender to this regard, but today moralizing is seen as the mark of a weak mind. To be a moralist may still have some philosophical merit or critical cachet, because it is difficult to imagine culture critique occurring in the prolix paucity of positivism and its recent variants alone. Each literary age as well adds its 'timeless' metaphors for the critical scene. So much so is this immanential within our cultured consciousness that we begin to lose any critical distance necessary for understanding ourselves as historical beings.

But what one *can* salvage from all of this is the sense that movement is the key to both critique and objectivity in the existential sense of the term. And this idea is part of the very beginning of thinking in the West, for the difference between the reality of motion and the appearance of stasis "… came to bear on the analysis of the structure of the *logos* insofar as only an unchangeable motionless object can be an object of knowledge and knowledge, for its part, is not possible without unfolding that which is itself different in being, that is, without change or movement occurring" (Gadamer 2003, 115 [1964]). So at once we have both the process and the ideal outcome. Diagnosis is the process, cure the ideal result. But between the two of them rests uneasily our consciousness of being neither. We are never at rest, yet we feel as if we should be one thing. Duplicity, the Janus of metaphor itself, is generally derided and is certainly mistrusted. Medical bureaucracies and their personnel say one thing and do another. We are told to do one thing and ourselves do another. Quit smoking, mind your heart, stop abusing substances, over-drinking, get more sleep etc. Like many contexts of contemporary consumption, the customer is put to work by the professionals. Even in counseling or psychotherapy, the onus is squarely on the patient, for the subject is only stable, that is motionless, within the narrow lens of the analyst, and the case resides in an even more stable, if stale and disused, archive of such 'cases' that accumulates like the sediment of a receding shoreline. The patient must deal with his movement and indeed, must make himself move to a new place, take on a novel form, alter his body, transmute his mind and transmigrate his very 'soul' or spirit. The metaphysical metaphor of stasis versus ecstasis is embedded in our idea of self-improvement and cultural progress. Though we no longer emblazon the macro level of improvement on our banners as much as we did before 1914, there is still a general belief in modernity, as Taylor has famously mentioned, in the idea that human beings as children of the now global enlightenment and are thus capable of much more than we are currently allowing ourselves to do. More than this, we *should* make every effort to do so. Speaking of moralizing.

Even so, we are also more wary regarding the sense that results should remain one thing. For if one should attain self-mastery through the constant push to improve one's person, mind, body and even spirit—though we are at odds mostly over how this last might be done, or if it can be done at all—then by definition this means perpetual motion. It matters then in what direction we are moving, and these directions become either occluded by specific present-day interests—the continued hierarchies of nation-states and capital, for instance—or they may be partially clarified by a general facing up to certain empirical realities no matter their 'causes'—the coalescing of scientific, public and political opinions regarding the climate is the most obvious current example. We are less aware and hence less wary of the distraction 'single-issue' arguments and debates foster. Surely 'the environment' is a much larger concept than merely the ecosphere. If human beings have altered its course in a way threatening to life, and it certainly seems that we have done so to a certain extent, then the environment cannot be, once again, by definition, something apart from our consciousness. It cannot be, that is, an object which we only 'effect' from the outside. Indeed, there is a great mass of medical discourse that concerns itself with disease vectors that are said to be patently 'environmental'. What can this mean other than the motion and interaction we have within our world, a lifeworld that includes all life? All of this has recently become plausible because "Objective scholarship, observation, and experiment are not only cognitive methods; they determine a form of life" (Lingis 1989, 65). Further, this form is the most heralded of our own times. It receives the greatest investment remuneration—though not the greatest wealth, *per se*—and the highest status with regard to the entire labor force. It is said to be a life "… in whom intellectual conscience is incarnate, [and to] represent an ideal form of life, a form of life determined by ideals" (ibid). If this is truly the case, such sacrifices that we as a culture make to these processes, these movements and their results, are made precisely because their outcomes represent a wider set of ideals to which science and technology above all others contribute. The contributions that are made, however, are hardly of a piece when viewed either critically or ethically. What can be said of 'intellectual conscience' if it conceives the means of self-destruction? The manner of the gradual lifelessness of the planet? The mode of inauthenticity that represents itself in the world as technique, and the technologies of alienation and anonymity, from sexting to commuting?

No, the intellect too is an historical and changeable affair, which can be enthralled to the spirit of this or that age as surely as any of its vaunted techniques.

Let's instead double-over upon itself the idea of metaphor to turn it at once into part of a critical lens. Why cannot our efforts at objectification, specifically within the realm of health and illness, be taken as metaphors for the 'empirical emotions'? That is, the objects we find least objectionable are those who are subjected to the objections of others are well-being, peace of mind, and physical and mental functioning without pain or discomfort. We must remind ourselves that the static sense of object is recent and very much a child of modern discourse: "In fact, the concepts of 'objectivity' and 'object' are so alien to the immediate understanding in which human beings seek to make themselves at home in the world that, characteristically, the Greeks did not even have terms for them" (Gadamer 2003, 122 [1978]). Gadamer also relates that the Greeks could 'barely speak of a thing' in the casual sense that we use regarding the object world. 'Object' itself, quite literally means 'something thrown against', as the editors of *Being and Time* remind us, and this is called to mind most vividly in the courtroom 'objection!'. Thus our notion of object is a reification of a metaphoric relationship between that which has been stated as the case or yet as a belief and something alternate or other to its *being*, that is, not to its 'thinghood'. A discourse that at the outset expresses itself by virtue of this reification is bound to miss the existential quality of consciousness. This is a matter of lesser note in the sciences of nature, but cannot be ignored in the human sciences and the practical sciences that work with human beings. Medicine is the most important of these discourses, and thus the most at risk from rampant reification. Rather, *we ourselves are thrown against the world* in the sense that we must object not only to the arc of our 'fall' or descent into the world but also to the world as we find it. This world is neither our own nor cares for us in the way we must care for ourselves. It provides the perspective of what it is to be dispassionate, and the wider the world we experience the more dispassionate it becomes. Even so, we ourselves may gain compassion by widening the world that we encompass, and it is this experience, brought forth by the encounter with the other and the ensuing conflict of interpretations this hermeneutic experience always brings within it, that allows us to understand more fully the force of the thrown object against which we must object ourselves.

Illness seems to throw itself against us. But what we experience is a conflict that rages within our bodies and one that our beings cannot ignore. The way we have been living has been objected to in some way. Either we have been lax regarding maintaining our well-being or 'good health' or we have been unlucky. Our experience of being objected to as a living being is no more fully wrought than in illness. No insult can endanger us in this way. No slight, no back-handed compliment, no sleight of hand or nor even slightest returns on our investments has the same effect. Illness brings itself to the fore on the horizon of our being-thrown in a manner that reminds us of art. Both of them "… give us reality in a medium which can't be separated from them. That is the nature of epiphany" (Taylor 1989, 428). What do we have to set against this 'object'? Diagnosis gives us the first clue, something to clew up with, a way to become clued in to the situatedness of objectionable being. If illness metastasizes itself as an existential objection to what we have been in the world and to ourselves—perhaps as well, to others, if we think of the diseases of intimacy or even of laziness; not washing one's hands in the workplace etc.—then the process through which we hope to be through with it, beginning with diagnosis, is also a metaphor capable of overleaping its current bounds and questioning the nature of boundedness more generally. For diagnosis, no matter how rationalized, must involve a sincere dialogue of the hermeneutic variety: "What we understand by a conversation is the situation in which two people are genuinely interested in a topic, become absorbed in exploring it, and are held together in the unity of their talk" (Barrett 1979, 184). It may be true that the doctor is only professionally interested. But how is this different from a philosophical conversation or one about home renovation? We have sought out the expertise of the one who speaks this language all the time. He or she is to be considered a professional quite explicitly in this regard: that they are the one who knows something about having this kind of 'talk' in the first place. They practice it regularly, and thus engender their interlocutors to experience its practice. Professional interest cannot be taken for disinterest or even aloofness. It has its own authenticity about it that places itself at a critical distance. In short, it objects to both the objection that has objected to the subject *and* the subject's own objection to his new life situation and the experience of it. In this way, and only in this way, do we confront the existentiality of the challenge offered; we are, so to speak, offered up to the object and we must get some distance from it in order to 'feel ourselves again'.

One of the tensions that is extant in diagnosis is that we, as a person become a patient, expect to be treated with care. There is a filial piety that misplaces itself by yet another metaphoric metastasis into diagnostic procedures. Even medical professional are now taught to be more 'caring' and compassionate, and everyone can tell the difference between an 'old school' practitioner and one who is merely rushed off her feet. It is likely a dubious scene when the doctor acts like a parent and the patient a child, but the cultural template cannot be ignored. For, "… history must have a face: it cannot exist without a form and forms are cues to points of view" (Tonkin 1990, 34). One's experience individuates over time, but structures such as family organization and institutions such as the schools are not necessarily ever breached by personal experience. Like history in general, we are shaped by them more often than the other way round. In diagnosis, the patient is also a student, the doctor a teacher. We supply some information, but it is the expert who must interpret it. That almost all of us have expertise in something or other, this should cause us no real resentment. It is, at base, simply about someone doing his job in the everyday and does not vouchsafe anything personal. But metaphors can be stronger than rationalizations. If "… the meaning and significance of bodily pathology vary according to one's perspective" (Fitzpatrick 1982, 10), there must be viewpoints that are either simply mistaken, partial, or marginal to official discourses. The patient brings all of these into the examination room, and this is already and always a metaphoric vehicle and one that the doctor must parse out. A large part of diagnosis, I have been told in interviews with practicing clinicians, is separating the patient's self-diagnostic bent from the facts of the case. This is never seamless and may have to be accomplished over long periods of time, especially and classically, in the case of mental disorders and the 'talking cure'. Yet this layperson pseudo-discourse cannot be ignored, for embedded in it are in fact the relevant statements that will lead to a cure or at least some form of treatment salutary to the individual in question. Every treatment has it consequences, 'side-effects' in official terms. Indeed, the memory of health that was experienced before the illness took hold is perhaps the greatest consequence of all; it has an existential import for the construction of one's biography and also carries within it the potent portent of autohagiography.

It is certainly acceptable 'to concentrate on the subjectivity of illness', and some of sociological research in the area of health has done just that. It can be succinctly described this way: "… this work has emphasized the importance of understanding the meaning of illness and health for the individual by focusing on the *consequences* of illness for ordinary, everyday life, the *significance* of symptoms and experiences for the person who has them …" (Williams and Popay 1994, 122). But there are limits. We learn little about the social order of health and illness. We have a dazzling array of butterflies, in Leach's critical sense of ethnographic examples reproduced and indefinitely addended to, but we have but a dim sense of why these actions have occurred, why these artifacts exist, and above all, why we ourselves have no interest in using or reliving any of it. Like an illness past, the entirety of human cultural evolution might seem like a bad dream from which we are only now just beginning to awake.

Rather than the pure subjectitude of the one who has been made into an objection to oneself, diagnosis' optimum ethic is to allow the patient to understand that what they are experiencing has an objectivity separate from persons about it. As much as we have been critical of this earlier, we must also allow the discourse some due credit in that it pushes the person become patient to abandon the offense we have taken against this objection to ourselves by objecting to our own subjectitude that it has engender. We have been duped by the illness, once again, metaphorically but also experientially, and we must see through this sleight in order to regain our self-possession as human beings. In an ironic manner, the reduction of our humanity to the statistic allows us to recommence the rebuilding process from the ground up. Part of this includes our concern, inauthentic as it may be, for the social position and organization which we have recently been forced to vacate: "Disease imagery is used to express concern for social order, and health is something everyone is presumed to know about. Such metaphors do not project the modern idea of a specific master illness, in which what is at issue is health itself" (Sontag 1978, 71). Such stake is an aspect of authentic being in the world, and is generally the first thing that disease metaphors, as well as those associated with treatment and cure, attempt to sideline or even occlude. We are told that dwelling upon our own deaths is morbid. True to form, it is a salient variable in a great variety of diagnoses in the DSM fifth edition. 'Suicidal ideation', a related phenomena, marks the depressive context of subjectivity instead of being seen as part of the coping mechanism for different versions of subjectitude. The pre-modern personality archetype of 'melancholia', related as it was to one of the assumed contemporary causes of 'colic' and even the later 'melanoma' as a kind of darkening of things in general, is the most recent major source of metaphors that continue to upbraid us for not at least giving the appearance of being happy. From Mills' 'cheerful robots' to Huxley's 'gram is better than a damn', both literary and human science critics have noted—often with an acerbic irony of their own that the stolid psychopathologist would merely point out as yet another symptom of the case at hand—that though happiness may still be the ultimate human goal, at least at the level of the individual, its corresponding state is promoted by psychology to also be the more or less sole responsibility of the singular self, albeit with some ability to react to others. This too is a reduction of the complexity of the issue. Even Burton notes that social ills are a root cause of melancholia, though they are always personally experienced. More than this, once the metastasis has occurred, whole systems unrelated to the original source become accessible to the metaphor: "The disease itself becomes a metaphor. Then, in the name of the disease [ ] that horror is imposed on other things. Something is said to be disease-like, meaning that it is disgusting or ugly" (ibid, 58). Persons too, no less. Just as Midgely has more recently declared a moratorium on the name-calling associated with abusing animals we experience as dirty or vermin-like—he is a rat, she a pig, the usual thing—are we to think the same of the inanimate and rather more alien families of life-forms of which diseases are a part?

2.3.2 Effects Thereof

Clearly once metastasized illness metaphors might know no bounds. This is curiously fitting given our horror at them and fear about them. The illness 'on its own' presents the gravest threat. Surely anything bearing a resemblance to it must also be equally threatening. Or the more so, as it pretends to be something other than illness and may only be compared with its model analogically. If this is so, then "The first task of the doctor is therefore political: the struggle against disease must begin with a war against bad government. Man will be totally and definitively cured only if he is first liberated" (Foucault 1973, 33). No wonder the Third Reich could make so much grotesque mileage from such metaphors. The 'body of the Volk' is infected. Certain types of human-like creatures are not really what they appear to be. The 'cultured Jew' is only the most notorious exemplar. 'Decay', in art and elsewhere could be the only result. Cultural leprosy was the outcome of miscegenation, and so on. These all too familiar noises echo into our own time given that we still not only fear and disdain the other but are much slower to act on his behalf if this or that plague-like threat developed, such as Ebola or even HIV. The number of Chinese who smoke has already been mentioned, but it too represents a politics of othering, as does the lack of interest in adopting non-white children or even older children in their home countries in the West. All of these others are tainted by the metastasis of one ill-gained metaphor. The homeless, the addicts, the older orphans at home and the dark-skinned ones abroad—the rush to adopt red-headed blue-eyed Rumanian and Bulgarian starlets still resonates with our own version of Nazi eugenics, and one should note that far more girls than boys were adopted in this instance as well—are all of a piece, cut from the same disheveled and mildewed cloth. The only rationalization that bears voicing in this regard is that international and national policies make it very difficult to adopt from abroad, no matter what the 'case' may be like, and most of us have enough on our own plates to not willingly become therapists for someone's else's errors and abuses. This much is part of our factical life-situatedness and as such, is an authentic form of being though the way in which we perceive it may be inauthentic or yet grossly derelict. Yet it cannot be ignored that we as a society must also spend time working on ourselves in some way: "Now that everybody tends to be a patient in some respect, wage labour acquires therapeutic characteristics" (Illich 1975, 60). Just as we often hear from the very children we tend not to adopt that school was no drudge but rather a refuge from a dangerous home life, that the military provides a home for a disproportionate number of abused and neglected persons—the structured communitarian ethic works well for those who grew up in its absence elsewhere—so work in general is often used by parents who do not wish to confront the chaos at home. The standard for two-income middle-class families has been adopted itself from their professional betters from previous generations. Between work, school and other activities such as shopping and kids' hobbies and training, there is quite literally 'no one at home' anyway.

There is an ironic stoical quality to today's conception of a healthy family. The metaphor of well-being seeks egress from its bodily functions into the mechanisms of social organization. Whatever occurs behind the closed doors of suburban neighbourhoods, the hidden abuses and the transference of sexualities, the incompetencies and the neglect, no ultimate value should be placed on it either way. The stigmata with which the Greeks sought to evaluate the sick is too critical a stance to take given the stressors involved. It is simply unfair, we might think, to expect more from the bourgeois family than repression and manipulation, the celebrating of children's achievements only when they mirror our own or are sanctioned by relevant institutions. 'Health' then, can only be understood if we at first shelve the notion that illness is something that should trouble the conscience and bear a mark concerning our characters: "Stoicism sought to go beyond this classic Greek position, in that it understood health and sickness as two sides of the same coin, as two things of equal worth. Only virtue was a genuine good. Vice was the only genuine evil" (Sigerist 1977, 391). This is fine as far as it goes. But what are the contents of virtue and vice? How is the one taught and the other taught to be avoided? If the illness metaphor is blockaded from further metastatic leaps, what virtues are involved in constructing such a defense? How, in other words, do certain actions escape the stigma of disease or ill-health—for example, what exactly is an unhealthy family or person given the generally low standards we attempt to maintain in daily life?—and how are others practiced *as if* they could never be unhealthy or even unwise? No doubt each of us finds his own set of rationalizations, however semi-conscious and *sotto voce*, comfortable most of the time. But if therapy is warranted, so we are told, at the level of the individual and perhaps the family, what of our general social situation? If we compare a traditionalist versus a modernist perspective, we might be tempted to accede immediately to the following point: "Culture was the framework for habits which could become conscious in the personal practice of the virtue of hygeia; medical civilization is the code by which we submit to the instructions of the therapist" (Illich, op. cit., 91). But the ideational quality of such a criticism does not grasp the existentiality of people's cultural situations. Therapy has long been seen as a decoy to authentic political revolution. Capital reduces its problems of structural inadequacies to the responsibilities of individuals. Yet it is also the case, manifestly, that we as persons *do* have a responsibility to our health, as well as to the health of others. The problem might be more adeptly signaled if we take issue with the definitions of what constitutes virtue and vice. We do not fill these categories with exactly the same stuff as do our classical cultural ancestors. Their beliefs reflected their social organization, almost all of which we would cringe at; slavery, women as chattel, children as animals, animals as tools, organized xenophobic warfare, and ruthless politics. Wait a minute—all of this *does* sound eerily familiar after all. The difference of degree between ourselves and the civilizations that gave us science, philosophy and the germs of the modern polis are just that. To what degree then *do* we differ, then, and why? Where are the similarities that we might eschew if they could become clarified for us? The reification of health and illness is an echo of that secured by virtue and vice, stoicism or no. And the thing that is imagined through such reification is no longer merely an 'image' of something else, for reification makes analogs into homologs. Commenting on Sontag's famous argument, Martin suggests: "These images frighten us in part because in our stage of advanced capitalism, they are close to a reality we refuse to see clearly: broken-down hierarchy and organization members who no longer play their designated parts represent nightmare images for us" (op. cit., 223). Blake's critical poetry calls to mind imagery of the pre-modern era, as if Dante and Donne were suddenly transported into the industrial revolution and able to witness a 'hell on earth'. But our fully contemporary visions have replaced the idea of punishment and penitence with simple degeneration and disorder. Of course, our ideal concerns an order that is imposed and maintained by humans and humans alone. Machines, in the modern viewpoint, can and should only be ever more sophisticated tools in our survival. But gradually a new fear began to creep in; what if the machines take over and begin to serve themselves? "Production gone awry is also an image that fills us with dismay and horror. Amid the glorification of machinery common in the nineteenth century were also fears of what machines could do if they went out of control" (ibid, 224). This is such a well-known, even tired trope in entertainment fiction, from *2001* to *Terminator* that it is not worth detailing. But the relevant point for us is that we are seeking, along the stringent lines of this self-same metaphor, human capabilities to mimic those envisaged by intelligent machines. That is, within the interior of our bodies and brains, we should be able to at least hold our own with advancing technologies that also represent these same aspirations toward indefinitude if not positive immortality.

The idea that one's own body could succeed itself is not exactly new. Lineage systems of the most ancient vintage are premised in part upon the notion that one's predecessors and one's successors hold within them a part of the present, and thus a part of ourselves. But all of this was very abstract and symbolic. The sense that in reality we should be able to outlive our original lives and bodies is something that appears with modernity. And it is symptomatic of a specifically new class situation that arises with industrialization and urbanization, but all the more so with a sense that one must search for and attain a new status. The proletarian classes did not immediately feel its pull, especially before mass or universal schooling, and the elites were still ensconced in the older system of symbolic kinship relations, pedigrees and lineages. No, it was the middle classes that first invented the drive for indefinite life, bringing immortality down to earth: "The bourgeoisie's 'blood' was its sex. And this is more than a play on words; many of the themes characteristic of the caste manners of the nobility reappeared in the nineteenth-century bourgeoisie, but in the guise of biological, medical, or eugenic precepts" (Foucault 1980, 124). This desire to over-reach human life by making it more 'worthy of life' than it already had been, given the vicissitudes of uncontrolled historical mis-couplings and mutt-like progeny, comes to a head in the Third Reich's medical programs and marriage laws. By this time, a time we have not yet shaken off, all forms of symbolic accoutrement were entailed and engrossed by the idea of overcoming and the 'New Man'. But equally, there were negative images, present at the very least for historical perspective: "Both clothes (the outer garment of the body) and illness (a kind of interior décor of the body) became tropes for new attitudes toward the self" (Sontag, op. cit., 27). The illnesses of most concern were not those that afflicted the individual. The 'body of the Volk', citizenry of every nation-state bent on military and economic competition with all others, within alliances or singularly, were enlisted in this newly abstracted genealogy of bio-power. Thus the person was reified in two directions: within his interior there became a space for the playing out of negative metaphors, the more intimate the more threatening—hence the aspersion cast on sexual intimacies of all kinds during the age of empires, especially any that involved taking away the power of reproduction from a populace in general—and outside of him, the positive reinforcement of belonging to a group bent on self-improvement, all for one and one for all. Needless to say, such a procedure involves dehumanizing both the friend of self within the ideologically sanctioned relation to 'those like us', and of course all enemies, those outside the circle of worthiness. This is more truly a re-abstraction, because it rehabilitates, writ large, something that we witness more prehistorically in ethnographic analogs the world over: simply put, horticultural humans are more or less xenophobic in their relationships with at least their closest competitors. But this is not the 'original' situation of the social contract society. Population loads were even more slight, and one group might not even know of the existence of any others, let alone consider them to be a threat. Even so, only if we can recall the diversity of how humans organize themselves while at the same time keeping in mind that each of these ways, though distinct, is still indeed human, can we become more objective about metaphor and its abuses: "The process of forgetting the original images, which deadens and flattens our language into counters, is arrested" (Taylor 1989, 473). As always, detail itself counters abstraction. Not to return to the problem of the structuralists, where the general run of things was always preferred and the counting of cases, their comparison and contrasting taking place only within a descriptive level of analysis. Instead, one avails oneself of the models of natural science without the goal being to unify all things and therefore reduce the cosmos to a microcosm of its own processes. To do so would be, in its own way, to repeat the partiality that the unification sought to overcome; it repeals the need for context and history by stating its case in the grandest terms yet with the smallest elements at once. As such, it retains a dual 'partiality'—once again, it does not encompass the whole of its reality while being beholden to the idea that the simplest set of explanations is the most elegant and therefore the most alike with reality—and cannot be said to advance our understanding of how we, as existential consciousness thrown into the world, have come to not only know the cosmos in this specific way but why we have felt the need to do so. In a word, one can say for medicine what has been said about many other sciences, such as economics: "This saw only an *incomplete phenomenon*, whereas the new theory views the *whole process*. The classical writers explained what took place *on the average*, but now it is necessary to show what happens in *detail*.' (Lösch 1967, 313, italics in the original). But how is it that what has been detailed in the most minute manner was able to enthrall us with its arcane and technical rhetoric to such an extent that we can no longer think of our bodily being and its projecting or interacting aspects without a sense of shame or morbidity?

Both this problem and our general response to it has invoked the dubious powers of reification as well as evoked the even more worrisome powers of myth. To overcome the tainted humanity of the present we desire to overcome our very kind of human consciousness. Perhaps this is but one more in a lengthy series of evolutionary moments, but we might pause before rushing headlong into a future that for the first time could be devoid of anything we have known as humans. Sentiments that at first seem to be responsible and ethical can easily take on other tones: "The civilization that is about to be born will be a human civilization in a far higher sense than any has ever been seen before, as it will have overcome important social, national and racial limitations" (Neumann 1970, 393 [1949]). Where is that civilization today?

2.3.3 Examples

Precisely because we feel that we have the strongest evidence that human beings cannot, by the definition we have given our natures, ascend to such a culture may be the brightest impetus for moving on to a new species. But where is the evidence that anything or anyone new would be, by their own self-definitions and *self-understanding*—if this existential hermeneutical term can be applied here—able to attain it? Indeed, if our insight into our own species as it stands is also 'incomplete', partial in the dual sense of the word, and also more deeply, anxious about its prospects, then we do in fact have a medical metaphor to leverage a cultural analysis. It is to be found in psychiatry: "But the psychiatrist must deal above all with cases where the patient's insight into their own illness is disturbed, and even, as with the hypochondriac or someone who simulates an illness, with cases in which all possibility of reaching understanding seems to have been removed" (Gadamer

1996, 168 [1989]). In such contexts, which may be but microcosms of our general cultural malaise, the medical professional is pushed away from the normal dialogue of diagnosis. He is also puzzled by the past, for any anamnestic qualities that a person may bring to the diagnostic table may have also been disturbed by the illness or theatre—and indeed, the theatrical subjectivity of mental illness has not been adequately exposed and analyzed—as the problem of 'what occurred' is merged by the presence of what is occurring in a specific and radical way in psychiatric disorders. On top of this, there are no reified results given the difficulties and mutable quality of such illnesses, so the prognostic frontier is either quite hazy or appears to be ever slipping away from us though we have undoubtedly walked forward. All of this is suggestive for any cultural psychologist. For what is supposed to be a cure for us as individuals actually has the simultaneous effect of obscuring our social conditioning. In terms of mental illness, it is this, rather than any disease vector *per se* that is the root of the disorder. In general, it is sociological old hat to define 'mental illness' as simply being abnormal or demonstrating an inability or unwillingness to behave as others do, specifically, the generalized other, and to pay little or no heed to the looking glass self. This is a solid working definition, and one that has, of late, worked itself into various therapies. Aside from this, however, treatment for both physical and mental illness may be said to be deprived of sociality in itself, for, one the one hand, we are reduced to an object that is relieved of social responsibility in the sick role, and, on the other, we are relieved of our personhood because our behavior and thoughts are so different from the norm. In both of these, Illich's famous 'medical nemesis' raises its head: "Medical nemesis is the experience of people who are largely deprived of any autonomous ability to cope with nature, neighbour, and dreams, and who are technically maintained within environmental, social and symbolic systems" (op. cit., 166). Given that all of us are so maintained as human beings, what Illich is really getting across is that the character of these particular systems of symbols and techniques denudes us of our shared humanity or, at the very least, forces us to share our humanity in denuded form: "Medical nemesis cannot be measured, but it may be shared" (ibid). To keep life going by virtue of technique alone may be the price we must pay to become different from ourselves evolutionarily, but this thought may also be subject to the limitations of what is precisely the human imagination in its self-absorption. We do not know in any certain way the outcome of there being present with us artificial intelligence—and as we have seen, the term 'artificial' is itself a misnomer; according to what 'nature' is cybernetic consciousness less 'natural'?—and we know even less about it if this new form of life evolves without our presence. Just as we have reified the most convenient metaphor regarding our own form of meaningful existence, we have done so, very much ahead of the game, with any potential successors to us. This premature evaluation of what technology can or cannot do for and by itself reflects the somewhat hypocritical and self-conscious manner in which we approach the study of other life forms and the construction of other possible means of becoming or being intelligent. These biases are reflected in how we raise our children—at once, alien life forms that will think along different demographic lines, but as well, those that we have ourselves both created and constructed—and how we give advice to 'developing' countries. We have gotten to the point where human suffering is considered a universal evil; something that brings us together and makes us the same thing. But we have not yet understood that "… different ethnocultural groups do not necessarily reflect similar attitudes to pain, and reactive patterns similar in terms of their manifestations may have different functions in various cultures" (Wolff and Langley 1977, 318). The classic though dated rubric available from anthropology gives us cross-cultural pause, though, as with all such models or lists, we are confronted with the diverse categories of illness construction and must face up to the fact that our own models may be perceived as just as fanciful by others in our own time or those who have preceded us. The arrogance of assuming that the 'oriental, the ancient, and the primitive' are all equally ignorant as to reality is not worth commenting upon. Specifically, contemporary forms of mental illness may well be participating in earlier forms of what was perceived as real illness, given the causation rubric that included "… sorcery, breach of taboo, intrusion by a disease object, intrusion by a spirit, and soul loss" (Wellin 1977, 50). Certainly the second is at work in all cases of psychiatric disorder, even if only as an effect. If the soul is also a social construct—only theology disputes this today—then its loss is part and parcel of the patient's turning away from the social world into a marginal aspect of the lifeworld inhabited only by those others who have othered themselves *away* from culture as a whole.

So we cannot afford to dismiss what appears to be 'merely' metaphoric as a way that those in the dark attempt to find meaning in their illness or their health. In this, the power of metaphor is equally present as it is when it is used by a culture to demonize both disease and their victims. This second type of metaphor, and the one that we have spent the most time analyzing, is also available to work out the problem of having a system of organizations working for the collective but bearing all of the marks of the divided society in which it dwells. Hospital 'castes' and cliques "… with virtually impenetrable status and mobility barriers between them" (Torrance 1987, 491), are suggestive in this manner. More than their having the social function of mirroring the wider hierarchies of our organic solidarity, they portray to those who have turned away from their responsibilities to this solidarity how life is supposed to be lived. There is a moral order to the clinic and the hospital, to the health care system in general, that is meant to provide a therapeutic ambience, an atmosphere unclouded by the delusions of the paranoid or the schizophrenic, and untainted by the intrusion of the 'disease object' germ or virus.

This order is exemplified by the precise hierarchies displayed, and the patient, in order to once again become a fully agentive person in this order, must mimic its standards as if they were rehearsing for their wider social roles and practicing their return to normalcy. *The moral theatre of health care* is thus the most profound metaphor of all.

References

Bachelard, Gaston. 1964. *The Psychoanalysis of Fire*. Boston: Beacon Press [1938].

Barrett, William. 1979. *The Illusion of Technique: A Search for Meaning in a Technological Civilization*. New York: Anchors Books.

Cooperstock, Ruth, and Henry L. Lennard. 1987. "Role Strains and Tranquillizer Use." In *Health and Canadian Society: Sociological Perspectives, Second Edition*, edited by George Torrance, 295–313. Toronto: Fitzhenry and Whiteside.

D'Arcy, Carl, and Janet A. Schmitz. 1987. "Sex Differences in the Utilization of Health Services for Psychiatric Problems in Saskatchewan." In *Health and Canadian Society: Sociological Perspectives, Second Edition*, edited by George Torrance, 185–98. Toronto: Fitzhenry and Whiteside.

Fitzpatrick. 1982. "Social Concepts of Disease and Illness." In *Sociology as Applied to Medicine*, edited by Donald L. Patrick and Graham Scambler, 3–15. Bailliére's Concise Medical Textbooks. London: Bailliére Tindall.

Foucault, Michel. 1973. *The Birth of the Clinic*. New York: Vintage Books [1963].

Foucault, Michel. 1980. *The History of Sexuality Volume One: Introduction*. New York: Vintage Books [1978].

Gadamer, Hans-Georg. 1964. "Plato and Presocratic Cosmology." In *The Beginning of Knowledge*, 102–18. New York: Continuum [2003].

Gadamer, Hans-Georg. 1974. "On the Tradition of Heraclitus." In *The Beginning of Knowledge*, 21–34. New York: Continuum [2003].

Gadamer, Hans-Georg. 1978. "Greek Philosophy and Modern Thought." In *The Beginning of Knowledge*, 119–26. New York: Continuum [2003].

Gadamer, Hans-Georg. 1989. "Hermeneutics and Psychiatry." In *The Enigma of Health: The Art of Healing in a Scientific Age*, 163–73. Stanford: Stanford University Press [1996].

Gadamer, Hans-Georg. 1990. "Heraclitus Studies." In *The Beginning of Knowledge*, 33–81. New York: Continuum [2003].

Gadamer, Hans-Georg. 1998. *The Beginning of Philosophy*. New York: Continuum [1996].

Haas, Jack, and William Shaffir. 1987. "Taking on the Role of Doctor." In *Health and Canadian Society: Sociological Perspectives, Second Edition*, 399–421. Toronto: Fitzhenry and Whiteside.

Heidegger, Martin. 1999. *Ontology—The Hermeneutics of Facticity*. Bloomington: Indiana University Press [1988].

Illich, Ivan. 1975. *Medical Nemesis: The Expropriation of Health*. Toronto: McClelland and Stewart.

Jung, Carl G. 1959. *Aion: Researches into the Phenomenology of the Self.* Princeton, NJ: Princeton University Press [1951].

Krieger, Nancy, and Elizabeth Fee. 1994. "Man-Made Medicine and Women's Health: The Biopolitics of Sex/Gender and Race/Ethnicity." In *Women's Health, Politics, and Power: Essays on Sex/Gender, Medicine and Public Health*, edited by Nancy Krieger and Elizabeth Fee, 11–30. Amityville, NY: Baywood Publishing Company.

Leyton, Elliot. 1987. "Dying Hard: Industrial Carnage and Social Responsibility." In *Health and Canadian Society: Sociological Perspectives, Second Edition*, edited by George Torrance, 199–215. Toronto: Fitzhenry and Whiteside.

Lingis, Alphonso. 1989. *Deathbound Subjectivity.* Bloomington: Indiana University Press.

Lösch, August. 1967. *The Economics of Location.* New York: Wiley Science Editions, John Wiley and Sons [1945].

Martin, Emily. 1994. "Medical Metaphors of Women's Bodies: Menstruation and Menopause." In *Women's Health, Politics, and Power: Essays on Sex/Gender, Medicine and Public Health*, edited by Elizabeth Fee and Nancy Krieger, 213–32. Amityville, NY: Baywood.

Midgely, Mary. 2004. *The Myths We Live By.* London: Routledge.

Neumann, Erich. 1970. *The Origins and History of Consciousness.* Princeton, NJ: Princeton University Press [1949].

Passerini, Luisa. 1990. "Mythbiography in Oral History." In *the Myths We Live By*, edited by Raphael Samuel and Paul Thompson, 49–60. London: Routledge.

Scambler, Graham. 1982a. "Illness Behaviour." In *Sociology as Applied to Medicine*, edited by Donald L. Patrick and Graham Scambler, 43–55. Bailliére's Concise Medical Textbooks. London: Bailliére Tindall.

Scambler, Graham. 1982b. "Death and Dying." In *Sociology as Applied to Medicine*, edited by Donald L. Patrick and Graham Scambler, 85–97. Bailliére's Concise Medical Textbooks. London: Bailliére Tindall.

Selye, Hans. 1956. *The Stress of Life: A New Theory of Disease.* New York: McGraw-Hill.

Shem, Samuel. 1978. *The House of God.* New York: Berkley Books.

Sigerist, Henry E. 1977. "The Special Position of the Sick." In *Culture, Disease, and Healing: Studies in Medical Anthropology*, edited by David Landy, 388–93. New York: Macmillan.

Sontag, Susan. 1978. *Illness as Metaphor.* New York: Vintage Books.

Taylor, Charles. 1989. *Sources of the Self: The Making of Modern Identity.* Cambridge, MA: Harvard University Press.

Tonkin, Elizabeth. 1990. "History and the Myth of Realism." In *The Myths We Live By*, edited by Raphael Samuel and Paul Thompson, 25–35. London: Routledge.

Torrance, George M. 1987. "Hospitals as Health Factories." In *Health and Canadian Society: Sociological Perspectives, Second Edition*, edited by George Torrance, 479–500. Toronto: Fitzhenry and Whiteside.

Turner, Paul. 1977. "Witchcraft as Negative Charisma." In *Culture, Disease, and Healing: Studies in Medical Anthropology*, edited by David Landy, 226–30. New York: Macmillan.

Wellin, Edward. 1977. "Theoretical Orientations in Medical Anthropology: Continuity and Change Over the Past Half-Century." In *Culture, Disease, and Healing: Studies in Medical Anthropology*, edited by David Landy, 47–57. New York: Macmillan.

Williams, Gareth, and Jennie Popay. 1994. "Lay Knowledge and the Privilege of Experience." In *Challenging Medicine*, edited by Jonathan Gabe, David Kelleher, and Gareth Williams, 118–39. London: Routledge.

Wolff, B. Berthold, and Sarah Langley. 1977. "Cultural Factors in Response to Pain." In *Culture, Disease, and Healing: Studies in Medical Anthropology*, edited by David Landy, 313–8. New York: Macmillan.

Yap, Pow Meng. 1977. "The Culture-Bound Reactive Syndromes." In *Culture, Disease, and Healing: Studies in Medical Anthropology*, edited by David Landy, 340–8. New York: Macmillan.

CHAPTER THREE

Detrimental Health

> … how is it possible to describe or rather think this universe without at the same time raising the question of how this universe originated and what was there before it?
>
> —Gadamer (1998, 97)

The universe of health and illness presents the following challenge: once we make the distinction between feeling well and unwell, we must understand how one passes from one to the other and why. To personalize these experiences is to miss the reality of both their happenstance and the procedures by which they are removed or resisted. That one becomes ill often through accident or 'misfortune', that is, in a most uncalculated manner, and that one has to combat this happenstance with something that is calculated in the extreme is itself an interesting paradox. The irony of being forced to work hard to rid oneself of something that came so easily reminds us of both the debits of weight and weight loss as well as actual capital debt. The tension to which one is given over in this process of becoming sick and re-attaining one's wellness we will designate as 'detrimental health'. This phrase also includes all of the over-calculative efforts at becoming well as well as the purely pecuniary products and energies used to sell them that are included in our contemporary health care system. To expose and discuss this series of ironies is to give some sense of what is important to us *aside* from feeling comfortable and functional as a conscious body and agent. Like any cosmos writ larger or smaller, we also must ask after the meaning of cosmogony, that is, the origin myths and narratives we have provided ourselves to explain the problem just raised by Gadamer; does what is now present explain or in any way give a clue to what is not now present, and how can we know this?

3.1 Obscured Motives

Knowing something about how the way things came to be is to understand that the world is not what it appears to be. Its steady and continuous presence is actually neither steady nor continuous. What is it that keeps the appearance of being so from being seen through too often and too radically? This itself appears to be a basic sociological question, and one that can be used to understand the challenge of being healthy not only by physiological means, but to do so also by those at hand in our cultural world.

3.1.1 Structural Masks

To do so, we must remind ourselves that society as a whole is a 'total institution', and, as the protagonist's wife in Shem's famous novel upbraids him with Goffman (cf. Shem 1978, 133), it is also understood that within society there are other versions of the total institution that provide, as we have just stated, a moral mirror for correct behavior, including what is to be considered 'healthy'. That technology is used widely and sometimes indiscriminately 'against' those who do not conform is also well understood. The most obvious example is medication for the purposes of social control, and to "… manage the contradictory socialized expectations that both males and females face through their life cycles within the corporate economy" (Harding 1987, 560). Pharmaceutical usage by women mirrors that of the period previous to the establishment of the FDA in the United States, the so-called 'patent medicine' era. Most of these 'cures' were in their majority ingredient alcohol, but as they were packaged in a medicinal manner, women could partake of them without stigma. Men, meanwhile, continued to frequent the saloons for their drugs of choice, though in essence this 'medication' and its effects were no different. Today, alcohol usage by men trumps women's use by much smaller margins.

It is objectively difficult to say which dominant gender is subject to more stress in developed nations. Certainly, the stressors differ with the 'social expectations' and across demographic group, the younger the more tolerant of dissension and creativity, we sometimes assume. But health itself, as well as physiology and anatomy, has historically been centered on the male model, to the point where the sex organs of females were imagined to simply be the inversion and occlusion of male genitalia. If by definition health is at least paternalistic if not an outright example of patriarchy, then what is to be said about 'being healthy'? Whose standards should we employ, and for what ends? Sociology has for some decades been interested in such questions: "Here the aim has been to discover how women's morbidity and mortality can be explained by the capitalist and patriarchal organization of society, and to develop campaigns to improve their living and working conditions" (Kelleher, Gabe, and Williams, 1994, xix). Yet caution must be exercised. When a social group has for millennia been oppressed, the pendulum always swings hard about. It is one thing to clarify and expose the conditions for oppression, but it is another to assign blame to those who may either be equally oppressed by the same structural forces, or oppressed in a different manner. 'Epistemic privilege' is a very local thing indeed, and cannot be used to condemn those on the 'outside' of this or that specific social location. After all, the cultural imagination may be distinct enough that we are immediately made unaware of how things work and feel for these others. To overemphasize this or that standpoint, even in theory, is to repeat errors of observation long ago noted as plaguing the human sciences: "In a sense they cancel a large part of the knowledge of mental, social, and cultural phenomena accumulated by the experience and study of many generations of observers and thinkers" (Sorokin, op. cit., 20). None of this is to say that critics, feminist or otherwise, have not discovered something real and vital. Health is clearly a social construct that has favored the male anatomy, neurochemistry, and dynamics of outlook. To be male is the base-line of well-being. It was for the greater extant of written history also considered a good in itself. It is likely that Weber was correct in assigning the source of these misconceptions to the displaced intellectual classes who, with increased leisure time as well as access to the ruling castes and the perceived need to maintain at least some modicum of influence over them, catered to the cultural imagination of the masculine archetype, the warrior and hero. It is also likely that without this encouragement from the literati, the warriors and merchants would have been less interested in engendering an apartheid of polis and publicness. The role of religious specialists cannot be forgotten, and surely misogyny numbers amongst the 'calumniations of the priests'.

Even so, in our own time the capitalist model secures favor for those who forward its sacred trusts, the bottom line, the deal, the advantage, the sale, and there is no evidence that females are lesser able in these arenas than are men. The health field may be understood as detrimental not merely through an internal iatrogenesis, but simply by the fact that it functions in a corporate world as a kind of pseudo-corporation when publicly funded, a simple company where it is not: "Not only is science a business, but all work performed in modern life is organized like a business" (Gadamer 1993, 17 [1972]). Each of us is a cog in a larger machine, a part of an organic whole, as Durkheim described. The externality that the healthy individual adheres to mimics—or does it provide the model for?—the internality of the person as a functional body with parts operating as a whole system. "But this means at the same time that the function is one that is discharged without its own orientation to the whole" (ibid). Gadamer reminds us that the 'virtues' of Weber's rational organizations do not include autonomy and the 'formation of one's own judgments'. Hardly so. It is not clear, however, that any social formation, even the most primordial types of the 'social contract', pay much heed to the singular experience and judgement of any specific individual. Though we may ethnographically read of the shaman or chief, or someone who otherwise is an elder or leader in a small group situation, we also understand that mechanical solidarity acts, if anything, against these individuals over the mid-term and flattens them out, as it were, into an existential horizon that we in modern society have long forgotten existed. And today we are not so individuated that one person can either take on such ultimate responsibilities, nor is thus made responsible by other elites, to the point of autocracy. It is a convenient media fiction, and perhaps also a political contrivance, to imagine that one person sits behind the desk where the buck must stop. Truman aside, we know that if blame can be placed on the one, the system itself will survive any crisis. Even in the last desperate months of the Reich, Hitler's orders were being utterly disregarded by his previously most loyal followers, Speer, Guderian, and Doenitz being the most obvious examples. But competitive capitalist nation-states, based on rationalizations of ethnicity or destiny remain in our world today. The conflict that is created amongst them differs not in the slightest from that which led to the cataclysms of the twentieth century, and the concept of detrimental health plays fully into that conflict. The Reich's aesthetic model of the health of the 'body of the *Volk*' provided, post-war, a model upon which to transform and build. Enough has been said about this elsewhere that we will not repeat these analyses here. It is sufficient to remind ourselves that once the polis begins to conceive of itself in terms like 'bio-power', the rest of it is an inevitable consequence.

All of this too hinders the development of personal judgement based on experience and reflection. Making up our own minds is often severely limited to relatively trivial choices regarding consumption, and even though personal relationships count for much more than commodity brand choices, the fact is, at the end of the day, one can pretty much fall in love with almost anyone, so that these 'life crises' of the sentimental variety are overblown, which is also a media and perhaps as well a political convenience. Any distraction, any decoy, to keep our emotional intellects busy allows the politician to maintain his lock, as Hitler himself wrote. We are even told that the concentration of our intelligence on the personal is a form of healthy-mindedness, and that if scientific problems remain the concern of highly trained elites alone, the wider questions that animate human consciousness, its history and its future alike, will likely remain unasked or underexposed:

"The scientific legitimation for detaching the concept of intelligence from the specific substantial problems that we face as human beings is neither self-evident nor beyond question" (Gadamer 1993, 49 [1964]). To imagine that thought is so divorced is to participate in the detrimentality of living being. It is, essentially, to ignore the thrownness of Dasein into the world as well as the worldhood of the world. Phronesis, rather, is the conceptualization of intelligence that allies itself to the most human of efforts; our ongoingness and our 'futural' orientation. This 'practical wisdom' is not detached from specific problems in the world, nor does it exert a theoretical bent in order to so become disattached. Phronesis could be said to be the basic attitude of any applied science that has its purview the human condition or one crucial aspect thereof. It is the opposite of detrimental health in its own conception of what is 'healthy'. Practical science is primordial to the human condition. In some form, it has always existed. The fundamental relationship between experience, observation, and the imagining of projects of action are surely concomitant with at least the 'social contract' and thus the beginning of humanity. Medicine is the most recent form of this science which is both human science in that it is practiced by ourselves and concerns us most intimately in its predictions and projects, its data and experience, and it is also a science of the world and of nature, for it is the *objection* of the world to our human presence—this must be taken as an ontological objection and not one that is agentive in any conscious way; though the elements of nature including its animal life do adapt in the face of human presence; viruses being the most threatening of these 'natural' adaptations and as such bring to a focus medicine's role—that present our human-oriented practical sciences with their most relevant objects of study: "One of the tasks of medicine, therefore, is to rejoin its own condition, but by a path in which it must efface each of its steps, because it attains its aim in a gradual neutralization of itself. The condition of its truth is the necessity that blurs its outlines" (Foucault 1973, 9). This 'condition' is not only human in the proverbial sense, but rests in a situatedness of being that is at once resistant to self-knowledge—our experience does not always capture us in any hermeneutic manner even though each moment has the potential for a new basis of self-understanding—while at the same time knowing that it both must know about itself in some way and that it has already and always been engaged in the search for such knowledge. To have done so means that the concernful being in the world which is our own through circumspection in the world and reflection within the existential envelope develops methods of both adjoining its self-knowledge and avoiding it. Medicine remarks on its own conditionality by partaking in the conditions that give it relevance to human beings who are both ill and healthy at the same time. The majority that beckons us and reassures us falls roost under the term of 'detrimental health'. But because its frame is unfocussed, this 'blurriness' allows us to remain aloof to that aspect of concern that would, if recognized in the day to day, impel us to a much greater caution regarding how we treat our bodies and brain, and perhaps as well those of others in certain contexts; the residue of sanctioned violence against children, or certain adventurous activities such as extreme sports and like sexual recreations, or yet well-known and more directly health oriented phenomena such as second-hand smoke, are possible examples.

All of this is possible as a series of events in the ongoingness of Dasein simply because of the organic structure of our lifeworld. Everything is specialized, as is everyone. We cannot know, then exactly what we are doing to ourselves or others at all times of the day. Some general rubrics certainly can be applied, but in certain contexts they can also easily be forgotten or sidelined. The medical discourses that dominate the health fields in the West and provide the linguistic scaffolding for its institutions reflect this organicity, just as they have cut up the corpus of the body, as we have seen above, into its own system of organic parts and functions. But, given that "… the law of specialization is not confined to the development of modern medical science and medical practice. Scientific research in every discipline finds itself facing the same situation" (Gadamer 1993, 106 [1991]), what are laypeople, also faced with this bewildering array of facets, niches, and apparent choices, to do with each of our knowledge, incomplete and only partially conscious of itself?

3.1.2 Logistical Masks

There is an additional phenomena that makes its presence felt when one does in fact decide to pursue more rigorously a self-understanding through health and wellness that are then taken in tandem as aspects of concernful being in the world. This is the decoy dynamic of fixing secondary effects rather than addressing root causes. This is so well known a cultural dynamic that it would seem to bear little on our discussion of the discursive being of health and health care systems. Yet it too pertains to such an analysis simply by it being such a pervasive force in our society. From individual families to nation-states, whether in the realm of economics—household debt or national debt, the credit system and global labor and consumption—or that of 'moralities'—the question of the 'good citizen' or the 'poor parent' etc.—it is almost always more convenient to respond to an effect rather than a source. "For instance, much of the demand for liver transplants is due to alcohol. But it is a lot harder to think what to do about alcohol than it is to call for research on transplants" (Midgely 2004, 120). There are many such examples, from lung cancer and heart disease to vehicular injury and death to drug addictions of all kinds and other forms of addictive behavior that may have more social or even legal sanction to them besides. If Scheler was correct in thinking that *Ressentiment* lays at the truest source of many of these kinds of issues, then we may take it that an alteration in our existential consciousness is what ultimately must be attained. Perhaps this is yet another reason that compels us, rather in undertones, to search out new life forms with which we can be replaced as a species. One is forced to confront the problem of imagining that I would be better off if I were not merely *someone* else and that this other could well be dead so that I would replace him, the standard practical definition of *Ressentiment* or 'malicious existential envy', but in fact *something* else entirely. This would present itself as both a radical expression of, and antidote to, *Ressentiment*.

Even so, is this the most ethical way to confront the challenge of being human in an elemental sense? It does appear to agree with our general sensibility of feeling that if something is broken we might be better off replacing it, but it also seems to partake in the less empirically verifiable sense that we are simply tired of something, jaded with the worldly challenge of our thrownness, and are constantly, as Heidegger never fails to remind us, searching for ways to escape from it or avoid it. Certainly there are ample examples of this behavior as well, as if we were, at base resentful in that existentially malicious manner for having been born in the first place. The threatening melodrama of rhetoric such as 'making one wish one had never been born', in previous decades oft leveled at children, speaks another kind of meaning when held up in a more general light. It is as if we all *already* wish this, and not because of any punitive action taken against us by other humans. We are all in the same boat regarding our situatedness of unworldly being, and we do not then pretend that some relish their births more than others in this way. Only through the ontic trappings of life-chances variables do we succeed to enjoy life beyond the effect of falling. This 'enjoyment' is considered part of good health, and must be maintained though action that enhances our health and skews the probabilities associated with contracting injury disease and death more in our favor over the majority of the life course. Indeed, philosophical reflection on the meaning of existence might be seen as a mark of an *unhealthy* mind, one that broods and is never satisfied with itself. The lives of the artists, thinkers and writers bear the hallmarks of ill-health, whether of the purely social variety or actual addiction, disease and general marginality. So for the rest of us, the object lesson that emanates from these abject fellow humans is that queries into the ontological fore-structuring of human consciousness ironically leave that fullest consciousness behind in their efforts. This may be ironic but it does serve as a practical caveat against 'thinking too much'.

And organ transplants, donations for research and to save the lives of others, as well as dietary supplements, anti-depressants and a myriad of other 'responses to effects', are still specific examples of something much wider: "In spite of all the brilliant medical research work, in spite of new 'wonder' drugs, there is an almost complete failure to deal with chronic disease and certainly to prevent it. The reason is plain: A true diagnosis is seldom made in the sense that the fundamental or basic cause is ascertained" (Westlake, op. cit., 121–2). This wider horizon that distracts us is itself an effect of something deeper: the flight from mortality. Our evasiveness in the face of a death which is always our own and no one else's is yet positive evidence of the will to life in general and sometimes, the love of a specific life. This is ultimately the reason that lies behind both our conceptions of health as sacred and our willingness to buy into detrimental health. The former represents an ideal; one we believe to be beyond our grasp. The latter represents our inauthentic response to this perceived shortcoming in the ontic realm. The actual problem, however, concerns not our health, real or ideal, but our conception of what the sacred means. We tend to still imagine that if we had 'perfect' health we would not die at all. Perfection is associated with something that is seen as rusticating somewhere beyond the human world and thus beyond humanity itself. So we medicate effects and not so much causes, and we attempt to fix the problems that occur as a result of some other, more structural or existential challenge that we have, as Midgely notes, more difficulty facing. Whether the forces that are ranged against this potential confrontation occurring are political, moral, or merely technical—we *do* wish to cure some of the root causes after all, though which ones have a fashionable ring to them depending on which decades we examine—it is, in the end, *the meaning of the sacred* that must be altered in order for a new conception of health to arise.

There is a kind of indefinite, though not infinite, regress to this suite of problems. Consider Sontag's apt note regarding cancer: "Rich countries have the highest cancer rates, and the rising incidence of the disease is seen as resulting, in part, from a diet rich in fat and proteins and from the toxic effluvia of the industrial economy that creates affluence" (op. cit., 14). It would be a daunting analytical task to trace back each disease 'event' to its environmental, genetic, and perhaps also psychosomatic elements. And how far can we go to change the structure of our mode of production? Contemporary medicine, however much as it has absorbed the older notion of the sacred and attempted to both use it as a tool and yet also live up to it, is surely also but a handmaiden to modern, technical and industrial civilization. It is both an aider to and an abettor of it. This more objective aspect of its 'iatrogenic' function concerns us in the same way we may be disturbed about our political organizations or our rationalized institutions that compete with one another and even sometimes go to war. All of our modern ways of managing ourselves are held enthralled to the system of production and the corresponding system of its objects. We have already seen that ill-health constitutes not only an objection to our continued existence, but as well a more general objection to *how* we live, that is, in the main as producers and consumers. There can be no egress from this version of onticity, and one may suggest that the character of its 'onticality' rests in its ability to not only distract us from existential questions, in the classic phenomenological sense and its accompanying moral analytic, but also to decoy us from constructing a different, and perhaps more authentic version of it itself, without regard to the 'flight from death' so critically celebrated by philosophers. First things first, we might be pardoned for thinking.

Even our most intimate moments are rounded up by theory and corralled by the discourse that emanates from its praxis: "Sex was not something one simply judged; it was a thing one administered. It was in the nature of a public potential; it called for management procedures; it had to be taken charge of by analytical discourses" (Foucault 1980, 24). Human curiosity and adaptive ability, though inspiring, has always been a threat to large–scale organized societies, from intensive horticulture and the first sedentism onwards. We are arguably more intrusive in our surveillance over intimacy than any other culture in history, and yet we continue to try to adapt to this oversight. Sexting by young people is only one example, but like many other inventions, it too plays its own ironic role in heightening the surveillance procedures and the perceptions that 'more management' is indeed necessary. This is the *real* reason why sexting and like activities are part of detrimental health. Privacy, intimacy, authenticity and candor of all kinds and in all places is guarded against. The so-called 'public displays of affection', frowned on in the work place and even banned in certain school districts and schools that have certain religious suasions as their backdrop, represent other examples of healthy mental behavior and action being recast as detrimental to our health in the service of 'public health', which is more a kind of neo-fascist moral hygiene. In order to flee from these equally terrifying prospects, we continue to invent apace. But the content of our inventions becomes more and more desperate. In 1977 the World Health Organization baldly stated for the first time regarding pharmaceuticals that "Promotional activities of the manufacturers have created a demand greater than the actual needs" (in Harding 1987, 546). This was especially so in the case of tranquillizers. Legal alcohol combined with doctor prescribed tranquillizers was found to be the second greatest cause of drug-related deaths at the time, falling behind only the combination of heroin and morphine. This phenomena is now so well-known that citizens have demanded more oversight for such corporations and their relationship with practicing physicians. But laws exist only to a degree and vary widely according to political geography. The curricula of doctor training too is crucial to this regard. The abstract statistics called to mind by such studies are hardly the only exemplification of detrimental health. Neuroleptics have well-recognized and iatrogenically inclined side-effects, but in a very Goffmanesque fashion, certain ideals are seen to be a must while others, ideally looked after in a 'perfect world'—once again, the irresponsibility thesis of maintaining an extra-human standard for the conception of what is either ideal or 'perfect' is exposed—must be sacrificed for the former to hold: "One significant factor in this resistance was that acknowledging the existence and pervasiveness of tardive dyskinesia hurt the economic and political interests of many clinicians. The institutional and professional mandate to control the deviant behaviors of patients often superseded concerns for the drugs' physical risk to patients" (Freund and McGuire 1999, 197). Rationalized organizations seek to reproduce themselves as they are. This neither requires logistical expansion nor demands moral consideration or ethical reflection. Our subjective experience with mental illness also creates the predilection to disdain those afflicted with it. Our inability to understand how much is psychosomatic, theatrical, iatrogenic, or neuro-cognitive in each category and case by case hampers our ability to feel compassion for the individual person. Like the many masks of some of these illnesses, detrimental health utilizes a number of logistical faces to obscure its often more widely held and sometimes even 'sacred' ideological and discursive motives.

3.1.3 Personal Masks

If health is to be considered in an existential way, its holism does not necessarily turn in the direction of 'holistic' conceptions of health—to be examined in detail in the following chapter—nor as the sole responsibility of the individual who 'experiences' his or her health as part of their self-same existence, but rather as a scientific and politico-moral embrace of the social world. We are 'in' health in a different way than the sense we us the word casually in phrase like 'I am *in* good health' or the opposite. From the point of view of an objectifying study, health is 'inside' us and ill-health is a reaction of this inside to generally exterior forces. We are not here speaking of the 'interiority' of phenomenological or even psychoanalytic interpretations, but simply of the idea that we, as human objects, are confronted by objections to our presence that result in threats to our continued existence. Because we do not speak of the depths of either psyche or being, we can treat only the surfaces thereof, and "… regardless of what symptoms are considered, there exists a real and significant *clinical iceberg* [ ] the medical services treat only the tip of the sum total of ill health" (Scambler 1982a, 44, italics in the original). Even this rendition implies or assumes that there is a depth that can be reached through technique alone, or a combination of therapeutics and therapies. Such an iceberg, conceived of in clinical terms, does ultimately float in a larger ocean of discourse. But what if our beings are attached to the ocean floor? What kinds of masks do we invent to free ourselves from the ground of our being, this thrown project over which we originally had no control? Does illness perhaps remind us of our lack of control over being in general? If so, can our detrimentality be explicated along the lines of our general inability to accept this groundedness, so much so that the great bulk of post-war philosophical discourse has attempted to envision being as something that indeed floats free of itself? Or is this another ambuscade, desiring to both evade mortality on the inauthentic side of things, but also, in its equally unerring authenticity, attempts to evade being cloistered by ontic or epistemic languages and associated social arenas?

Masking thus would be essential to both these endeavors. On the one hand, taking on the role of 'iceberg' still gives us both depth and force. We can sink ships, withstand warmer temperatures and waters, move about with the currents of the day, and settle into an imposing presence in front of harbors once presumed to be safe havens. Such a role also, on the other hand, allows us to forget that we are not so free, either culturally or historically, and certainly not legally or by virtue of our respective citizenship. Our faux iceberg is an answer to both failed technologies, and the absurdities of human hubris, most famously exemplified in fatal combination by the foundering of *RMS Titanic*. To be the iceberg rather than the ship is to echo Paul Simon's famous folk lyric concerning the difference between the 'hammer and the nail'. If we could, then we surely would. But a clinical version of the iceberg motif is allows us to avoid the confrontation not so much with our basic existence and condition, but with much more specific historical and cultural institutions and organizations, such as schools and hospitals, governments and families. The so-called 'ADD', which did not exist as a diagnosis when I was in grade school, is characterized by a fundamental inattentiveness: "These behaviors, however, have been frequently observed among schoolchildren, probably since the invention of the institution of the school" (Freund and McGuire 1999, 200–1). It is arguable that it is a contrivance of pharmaceutical companies, though, as mentioned, some tranquillizers prescribed for it have been in use since the mid-1950s. After both Nuremberg and Hiroshima, no doubt the entirety of our culture craved a collective tranquillizer, and we have found more and more subtle means of social control over the intervening decades. The general disapproval and increasingly legal sanction against the physical coercion of children opened up a space for that chemical. Not that we should retreat into barbarism, but the hypocrisy of such a movement is self-evident. It is at least fairly clear that in medical practice, "These entrepreneurs were establishing a specialized territory for themselves by creating illness labels" (ibid, 201). At the same time sociologists are also well aware "… that disapproving cultural and professional *reactions* to deviant behavior can often foster rather than inhibit a continuing commitment to deviance" (Scambler 1982b, 189, italics in the original). Like the weapons used at Hiroshima and Nagasaki, a sanction in the form of a neuro-chemical has lasting effects beyond its application or administration. Kids get over being physically assaulted, especially if it is not too severe, simply because such attacks effected only the external parts of the body that were not usually vital to its long term functioning. Yes, there must have been psychological and emotional tribulations, but almost anyone over thirty in the West likely experienced some form of physical 'discipline' once in a while. This is not at all to make light of such injuries or practices, but drugging children is another matter. The part of the body that is affected is the center of consciousness, the seat of intelligence, rather than the seat of one's pants. Surely both forms of social control are part of detrimental health. "Discipline' is a term of newspeak, but so likely is the conception of ADD. The *actual* problem, the depths of this version of the iceberg as social institution, is the organization of schools, education, our work life, and the family and its schedules.

Once again, how far do we go in adjusting the social structures around us so that authentic mental and physical health is attainable is an open question. People do get used to this or that form of life, however hypocritical or in due course, uncomfortable. One can easily, to quote another famous popular song, become 'comfortably numb'. Tranquillizers, legally prescribed or purchased 'over the counter', picked up in the liquor store, or clandestinely procured on the streets, are a major form of construction of this numbness, the tip of the subjectivity of the clinical iceberg. The clinic no doubt has its cynic as well. This calculated cynicism is found in almost every work place and is a function of the hyper-rationalization of modern organizations, where the 'bottom line' is written in crystallized carbon and employees are forced to compete somewhat ruthlessly with each other in its pursuit. It is no surprise that tranquillizer use amongst adults is more diverse even than that prescribed for children, who have no doubt started to realize that they have been entered into a system of relations that limits their human freedoms. Later on, it is the work life that produces similar tensions, and for many decades, as we have already seen, there was a gendered division of labor that was reflected in the rationale of patients who were put on such drugs: "Most typically, male informants discussed the onset of somatic symptoms in relation to work stresses or new strains brought on by a change in jobs and the continued use of tranquillizing drugs as a means of controlling these symptoms" (Cooperstock and Lennard 1987, 324). The balance of this gendered ledger for approximately the same time period occurred in the home life, where females demanded the same kind of relief but for altogether different, though related, reasons. Such reasons "… are suggestive of the widespread stresses and depression facing women in the child-rearing years in the existing family system" (Harding 1987, 555). As with the schools and workplaces, the families we tend to live in represent focused loci of interpersonal tension. Perhaps it was always so, in various forms and to various degrees, since the rise of organic solidarities. The inertia of history, though an argument against any universalist morality, is equally never an argument that can be leveled against an ethics. Rather, conceptions of health that fail to include a cognizance of the history of such conceptions do us a disservice both intellectually and in terms of physical health. Clinical discourse is its own tranquillizer, ignoring the facts of the case and covering them over with a mind-altering, and thus consciousness dampening, product. To be sure, such drugs are often prescribed in tandem with other forms of therapy, but cannot such therapies also be questioned along the lines of failing to confront our biographical placement in the subjective horizons of historical consciousness?

It is not beside the point to suggest that critical social studies of health and health care do provide an entrance to such existential work. The well-studied use of tranquillizers is an obvious example. Generally, such studies seek to expose, if not always outright critique much less dismantle and replace, our assumptions regarding how we 'must' live in 'our' society: "The prescription rate for young married women shows how legal drugs can function to manage the social and economic problems associated with the nuclear family" (ibid.). Treating the tip of the iceberg, whether conceived in existential or clinical terms, repeats the error of myopia. We observe only effects and imagine that this is what needs to be adjusted. In any case, it is not always certain that effects are the easier to alter than the roots, given the possible side effects of effects, not the least of which is the continued need for such consciousness altering medication. Even the dullest of us can be relied on to usually know, somewhat intuitively, when something is amiss. We are either being hoodwinked or stepped on, or we have failed to recognize the advance signals that others are giving us when we ourselves are in the wrong. Even if we often cannot piece together the puzzle that is interpersonal interaction, the fact that we are aware of some kind of problem means that our consciousness is functioning in a healthy manner. We do *not*, in fact, need to be medicated, though we *do* need to, in some other way and by some other means, become more aware of what is transpiring before us. Getting to the bottom of things is actually and ironically avoided and evaded by the use of any form of 'discipline' for children and drug abuse for adults. Our incipient awareness of *Ungeheuer* is a sign of both authenticity and self-understanding. There is, as Westlake puts it, a 'horrid suspicion that all is not well.' On top of this, there is a further and more specific paradox associated with the canonizing of most self-help work, whether emotional or physical, in the languages of clinical discourses: "… the more we seek health, the less we find it. We talk health but get disease" (Westlake 1973, 171). This realization dovetails with Foucault's famous commentaries on sexual discourse. The more talk, the less real action, as it were. The fact that there exists a somewhat vulgar casual phrase that exhorts us to do the opposite also speaks to this semi-conscious self-understanding that verges upon authenticity. So it is not merely actual physical goods and services, the control of which manipulates the market and extends the networks of detrimental health, but also the way in which language associated with certain social contexts and diagnoses appears before us seemingly bereft of its own respective social and historical sources: "Thus, the control of supply, often masked as improvement in standards, is a crucial contingency in forging professional dominance" (Torrance 1987a, 13). What can be said of products such as pharmaceuticals can also be said equally of discourse. It too has its progressing 'standards' and supply lines, its market—the popularization of self-help through quasi-therapeutic talk shows is an obvious example of the commodification of inauthentic concern and simplified health care—and its professional dominances. For every television program that appears to cast real persons as part of its therapeutic circus, their desperate anxieties and pathetic conditions paraded in front of millions of viewers, as in Peter Gabriel's video parody *The Barry Williams Show*, there are thousands of more educated professional practitioners privately engaging in some resemblance of the same thing. For when one confides one enters into the world of surveillance. Norms hover around one, and the call of judgement, though no longer eternal and sourced in the divine, remains as clarion and perhaps all the more imminent for us. And we have given ourselves over to these desires for a *contretemps* with what we think is already detrimental to our health: "Public support for a nationwide addiction to therapeutic relationships is pathogenic at a much deeper level [ ] More health damages are caused by the belief of people that they cannot cope with illness without modern medicines than by doctors who foist their ministrations on patients" (Illich 1975, 39). In an abstract sense, therapy as entertainment—'I'm so glad I'm not like her, as pathetic as I am'—and the sense that one *can* in fact make do with suffering however unnecessary and unjust—'I thought *I* had problems'—provides viewers with a combination of both alienated and 'false' consciousness not unlike that produced by some actual drug prescription and use: "Over-medicalization changes adaptive ability into passive medical consumer discipline" (ibid). We must then distinguish between the merit of the positions themselves taken by therapeutic discourses and try to separate those from the belief in them, however passive or agentive. To do this would provide one marker as to the whereabouts of the boundary between detrimental health and actual aid to recovering one's authentic well-being and unclouded self-understanding. At some level, we may take umbrage at being told what to do, whether in the ungallant ululation of the talk show or the paternalistic if sometimes well-meaning whispers of the clinic. We may well realize that "Arguments of this kind have no power of conviction. But the fact that such arguments are not only used but undoubtedly believed is something that cannot be disposed of so easily" (Jung 1959, 54). One may not be able to 'kill an idea' but one can sideline it by presenting other ideas, better formulated and more appealing to the conscience. Of course, one assumes, that after all of this other 'idle talk' and idolatrous commodification that one's conscience, as a referee for all evaluation and as a safe harbor for one's sentiments, still exists.

3.2 The Finesse of 'Techniqueness'

If various guises of the mask and its accompanying charades are accounting for part of the manner in which health care slides into detrimentality, there must be spaces in which corresponding techniques also play their part in both assuaging our anxieties about the state of our health as well as managing the resources that the health care system actually receives from governments and private funding sources. We will find that the introduction of new technologies carries within it the potential for manipulation of funds, especially if these are publicly sourced. Professional monopolies that homeopathic and other alternative practitioners have been working to crack for over a century also enter the equation. Not that alternative discourses eschew the setting up of their own version of monopoly, as we will see in the next chapter, but at first, all outsiders are but looking in. Finally, our need to feel at home in the denial of which is something that is a given within systems that have the tendency to depersonalize, gives such systems and their personnel an added advantage. The playing of the card of 'returning home' from being otherwise, that is sick, is something that in fact can be used to cut costs or at least, redistribute salaries and accreditations into an even more steep hierarchy, as with the example of the nascent corps of in-home care workers. In turn, we shall briefly examine the seemingly 'autonomic' effects of techniques and technicians alike and discuss how their organizational structures lend themselves to the production of detrimentality and iatrogenetic issues that the system itself cannot afford to include in its self-diagnostic regimes.

3.2.1 Autonomic Effects

Rational organizations are in constant competition with one another not only for funds, but in order to maintain their very existence. This might suggest that they either grow or perish, but in fact, bureaucracies in the classic sense seek only to reproduce themselves. But whereas we mentioned above that this was their sole purpose as if they could simply recreate their identical situation in the wider social networks of power, this is not exactly the case. Organizations rather, must defend themselves by adapting, not necessarily expanding, but by altering their interiors. This may involve changing the training of those who inhabit them, modulating pay and benefits or playing off certain castes against others, as the university management does with faculty and students. Doctors and patients might perform a similar function, and certainly the tensions, sexual or otherwise, between doctors and nurses are proverbial if overdone in entertainment fictions. But most obviously is the place of actual technologies and techniques within the inner space of medical organizations. There are a number of effects regarding the introduction of updates in both of these arenas: "The argument that costs *must* rise to accommodate the application of new technology is a thinly veiled argument that they *should* do so" (Evans 1987, 626, italics in the original). It is one thing to invent new machinery or treatments that actually increase the rate of recovery of this or that category of patients, but it is patently something else if, as a rider to this innovation, there is assumed that one must pay more simply because of this improvement. It is as if all things old were priced according to their value for life, hence all things new must therefore be better and by definition should cost more, their pre-tested value as equal to their cost. Cost-saving measures in reaction to expenditures on technologies are more often applied to techniques or the technicians themselves rather than objects, which are seen as somehow sacrosanct and beyond the reach of medical managers. Like any commodity, however, one could simply not purchase it en masse, forcing prices down, or government agencies could limit costs by either funding the innovations themselves or simply demanding corporations limit their profits. Though this would certainly be tantamount to heresy with regard our beloved pantheon of capital, it nevertheless represent a real option. Harding cites the 1967 Harley report on the Canadian scene as an example of another kind of cost manipulation that occurs at point of purchase: "… the profit rate of the pharmaceutical industry was twice that of the total manufacturing industry. As antibiotics and birth control pills before them, mood modifiers have opened up a massive and profitable market" (Harding, op. cit., 552). Though we would not like to live in a world without the first two, perhaps tranquillizer use could be curbed to the point of helping people through crises brought on by the human condition more universally, instead of those seen as effects of a specific social organization. Like the Nazis who were charged with particularly heinous crimes against humanity, the euphemistic languages of both certain diagnoses and the effects of certain medications conceal what is really occurring. 'Deployment groups'—literally, 'single movement groups'—could have meant anything, but everyone now knows what the *Einsatzgruppen* were up to. But what of FBP (1961) or MBD (1970)? 'Functional behavior problems' and 'Minimal brain damage' seem characteristically vague, as does our own generation's foci, ADD and even Autism (cf. ibid, 553ff). The sheer amount of drug use, especially of the tranquillizing varieties such as Diazepam—its major trade name is of course, Valium; with uncharacteristic social critique in mind, The Rolling Stones immortalized its true purpose—should give us pause. Whatever is going on in our society is something that we are almost all participating in, unlike the Holocaust. What softer but still in its own way deadly version of auto-genocide are we practicing upon ourselves?

We are perhaps more familiar with the marginalizing of the elderly than with younger people or children. This is due to the physical limitations the aged bring to the field of relocation and concentration. The nursing homes and palliative care facilities. Of course we don't gas them. But they, like those who were unfit during the genocides, are where they are primarily because they are deemed unable to function in both a symbolic and a simple production and consumption order of relations. Is there such a thing as labor-based eugenics? Are our anthropological cleansing factories using human resources in an innovative, if dubious way? Gentler and even compassionate, yes, but the message is still clear enough: abandon life all ye who enter here. Shem notes with poignancy the moment at which his protagonist realizes that it would be better to murder his own father than submit him to such a fate (cf. 1978, 177). But far earlier in the life cycle do we also tend to concentrate our medicative efforts on those who appear to be equally unfit for our social organization, from those who can't seem to pay attention in school to those whose creativity begins to frustrate the rest of us who simply don't have time to even imagine being creative. If a gram is better than a damn, it is still better than a sham. We are a little disturbed that these outsiders might begin to speak what they have noted; that our empire of capital has no clothes, only vestments.

Not only this, but the use of medication for children especially increases both our sense of desperation about and propriety over them. The one due to a lingering bad conscience that we as adults are not providing what they need to grow into healthy human beings—the hours of electronic entertainment is one such guilt trip for those who care—and on the other there is an even stronger residue of an archaic social relations in which children were nothing more than property. Their current status as semi-chattel is confirmed in some political regions by certain laws, including those which allow their coercion. Children must be forced to acculturate. All socialization requires some form of coercion, subtle or no. But detrimental health finesses its way into the milieu of enculturation through contexts where children and even those older quite rightly question the meaning and purpose of what is happening to them. With our hustle directed towards keeping up with both others and with the trends of lifestyle and fiction alike, we are a society, perhaps more than any other, which does not have time for such questions.

Detrimentality sticks. Its labels are difficult to peel off once they adhere. And our adherence to them is something that if oft overlooked. We are more content to assume that we have been labeled. That somebody else has stuck us with something that we do not want or that we do not represent. But there is a self-fulfilling prophecy involved in all such social contexts, from streaming to slavery, that pushes some of the responsibility, warranted or not, back upon us. In medicine, ambiguity of diagnosis and the lack of causal evidence, especially with mental anguishes, obviates the one to one principle that guides the ideal science behind the application. Patients sometimes react to this: "Medical uncertainty, then, proved an incentive to disavow the label" (Scambler 1982b, 190). Symptomatically, medical care, in the face of such ambiguities related to cause or source of illness, or even to the point of what exactly one is diagnosing, must retreat to examining specific effects, related or no. But "The fact that modern medicine has become very effective for specific symptoms does not mean that it has become more beneficial for the health of the patient" (Illich 1975, 45). It is also characteristic of technique in general that it pay rapt attention to what is most technical in the wider world, including that which manifests itself as a treatable or at least, visible and tangible event, emanating from within the body, perhaps, but nevertheless, showing itself as something that should not be present. Whatever its roots—and here we are aware that we could easily fall into an indefinite regression; what actually *causes* certain cancers, or even more so, certain categories of mental illness?—its end results, short of death, may be worked at and at least managed. Not entirely unlike a society that was so anxious about its demise that it culturally lobotomized itself, our own organisms writ small and personal might be at risk for a general 'purification' that leaves little behind in its wake.

3.2.2 Technical Autonomies

Beyond any of this, however, is the reality of the sickness, discomfort, pain or suffering, both to be found in the individual and perhaps the society as a whole. This situatedness of being-not-at-home in the world is more than a restlessness of youth or of the mid-life 'crisis'. It makes one want to jump out of one's own skin in a more literal manner. The body, the vehicle supporting and in some way constructing and reconstructing consciousness, has broken down and must be fixed. It is no surprise then that we are willing to accept the most irascible treatments and the labels that accompany them, in order to 'get well soon'. This inevitably plays into the theatre and rhetoric of technique in general: "A patient's own state of need encourages this tendency to privilege the technical wonders of modern medicine above everything else and to forget that the application of this knowledge is a highly demanding and responsible task of the broadest human and social dimensions" (Gadamer 1993, 164 [1989]). The 'magic bullet' chestnut, which finds its literary kindred in the proverb, is fetishized as sacred. It can provoke miracles of attitude and belief, if not actually produce them on the ground or in the person. 'We've got a pill for that' may well be the dream of certain doctors and pharmacists alike. At the same time, we do increasingly hear a counterpoint to this shrill that in its own way seeks to clear a space of the sacred. This overtone incudes the caveat and thus also the *caveat emptor*. It reminds us that no pill can cure anything by itself, that there may be side effects, that you may have something else 'wrong with you' after all, or that what you have is in fact ultimately incurable. As my own father used to like to quote in his declining years, 'death is after all the cure for everything'.

But are these cautionary tales really an authentic argument against sheer and shallow technique, or are they themselves a citing mere technicalities? "Technique has something of the ring of phoniness to it in this context, a turning on and off which reveals the manipulator, not the person. If the doctor's effort is to cut through the disguises of the patient, what about his own masks? What justifies lies when they become enmeshed with truth?" (Natanson 1970, 86). We might well add, can truth and lie ever fully be parsed? Perhaps the inclusion of the lie is a necessity in exposing the truth of things, if only for comparative purposes. At any rate, it is clear that in cautioning persons about their diagnoses, prescribed treatments, potential outcomes along the way and end results, we are at once not so much showing up the fragility of what we're about as medical practitioners but as well showing off that we are sophisticated thinkers. Having thought our processes through to the end, having experienced the data of past cases, built up over decades, we can tell you that you are not only sick, but that you're sickness is, after all, your own, and we can only do so much because we are human like yourself. This mélange of compassion, candor, caution, and solicitude brings about at least as much awe in the patient as does the miracle pill and its shill of cures. Therefore it is at least plausible to understand sociologically caution itself as a kind of hubris.

This oddly inverse pride in our technical accomplishments—'look, we may not be able to cure you or even find out what's really wrong, but would you rather have been born even twenty years ago?'—contains an especial potency given the wider context of rhetorical flourish and fashion: "Using all the techniques of competitive business, our 'business men of science" also use the techniques of modern advertising, of running down the products of their competitors and enhancing their own" (Sorokin, op. cit., 19). The apparent denial of hubris has the effect of assuaging our doubts about doubt itself. We say to ourselves, 'After all, these experts are like me; they don't have all the answers, I feel much better about them caring for me given that we're all in the same boat'. Not that the denial of perfect expertise is not part of expertise itself. It is certainly an aspect of knowing that we are aware of what we do not yet know. In science, the key word is always 'yet'. This distinguishes its version of confidence and/or arrogance from that of religion, where on the one hand we are told we know all we need to know, and on the other, that there are some things that we cannot or should not know. But the fact that medicine and health are also an industry with a bottom line, and whether public or private it is increasingly the same situation, blurs the distinctions between what should be public knowledge and what could be kept back. Further, such studies that are done have been too careful to mimic the natural science model of laboratory and controlled variables. For many decades it could be said in round terms that "… pharmacological studies on the whole fail to take cognizance of cultural and psychosocial effects, such as the patient's cultural group membership, socioeconomic class and expectations of treatment" (Wolff and Langley 1977, 314). It is surely detrimental to our sense of well-being and our desire to recover our feeling of being at home in the world, however partial and finite this may be, but it is also equally detrimental to suggest that, while drugs and surgeries etc. can only do so much, that information extant should be somehow considered 'dangerous' to the morale of the patient, or even the culture as a whole. This kind of 'Pythagorean' mysteriousness gives rise to paranoia and bizarre conspiracy theories, such as the recent spate of nonsense regarding vaccination and autism. As mentioned, that one of its major sources was an entertainment figure seemed only to give it more mass appeal. No doubt this is due in part to the *our* cultural druthers of distrusting authorities of all kinds and powers, but this distrust can only be affirmed and fostered by the methods through which medical treatment reach the wider society and the claims and caveats that accompany them.

Ultimately, a technical autonomy that rests upon the presumption that technique 'itself' should stand aloof to specific human concerns or subjective sensitivities in order to maintain its scientific authority is doomed to failure. For "In the vast technical structure of our civilization we are all patients. Our personal existence is clearly something which is everywhere denied and yet it is also something that is always involved in the attempt to regain that balance which we need for ourselves …" (Gadamer 1993, 81 [1986]). On balance, the corporeality of organismic systems held within the body and containing its functions presents only the first challenge to health professionals. In our individuated society, filled with semi-autonomous subjects who have partial knowing regarding the objectivity of social structure and almost no knowledge of cosmology and the like, this challenge is seen as profound enough to occupy the vast majority of skills and efforts within any health care system. But the more profound confrontation still awaits us all; we must reconstruct what it means to be human in the face of both a subjectivity that now includes a more detailed understanding of our finitude due to the illness from which we have biologically recovered as well as the social function of returning to the ontic envelope and with that return, the expectation that we put aside this more authentic self-understanding in order to simply 'get on with it'.

3.2.3 Organizational Autonomies

In every profession, there is a significant divide between theory and practice. The 'book-learning' of the classroom must fold back on itself when it meets the 'real world', we are told. Student practica of all kinds, whether law, architecture, engineering, the health professions of education, contain this confrontation as well as exploits it. Students are taught, somewhat clandestinely, that what needs to be known is not so much what specific data or information or practices that will be more or most relevant to this vaunted 'reality', but rather how to decide on relevance in the first place. Medical school must be the archetype for this relationship, though law school might be considered a close second. Arts and science Ph.D.'s have the luxury of never leaving the theoretical space in which they were born. Even so, the recent absence of in-field employment has forced even intellectuals to step timidly into the 'reality' of public affairs, often retraining themselves and thus facing the divide of 'praxis'.

But this gap between potentially 'all knowledge' and what one actually 'needs to know' has another purpose than to winnow the pragmatists from the dreamers. It sets up the discursive barriers needed for organizations to maintain their effective autonomy from one another. The hospital is not the university or even the teaching hospital. The law firm is not the academic corridor nor the courtroom the lecture hall. It is an almost universal observation in the health professions that "The only portion of medical knowledge relevant to doctors is that which relates to conditions they are most likely to encounter in clinical practice" (Freund and McGuire 1999, 190). So the etiology of a disease, for instance, is something that would be an extra. To know the theories of possible causality and the history of the origins of this or that illness is something which, in the examination room, only a patient with a scientific or an historical bent respectively might be interested in. Similarly, if such an etiology contains within in more social factors than those physiological, like diagnoses concerning addictions, doctors, while not likely to moralize in our day and age, "... nevertheless feel irritated about their involvement in a problem where patients often deny their illness and are poorly motivated to cooperate in treatment." (Patrick and Scambler 1982, 9). Here as well, the rubrics of relevancy are fully present. What is the role of the doctor? The medical establishment more generally? No health care system can cure the ills of an entire society. Organizational autonomy has this other rider alongside it; that while the divide between history and science and the practice of both serve to guarantee a certain immunity from what ails the masses for professionals—their relative wealth and privilege are merely symptomatic of this social altitude—when cases arrive at the door of the clinic suffering not so much from an easily identified disease vector—an infection or virus, for instance—then medicine is faced with a quandary. More than ever before, diagnostic manuals of all kinds are filled with references to the ambiguities of case studies and records. Though this serves to quell any particular patient's overcompensatory hero-worship of the doctor—a doctor's vehicle I observed during this study sported the personalized license-plate stating 'ICURU', which surely doesn't help matters—it reminds practitioners that their powers are limited to the institutions in which they serve. Generally, in terms of internal affairs, this does not present a problem. Given that "... public government had ceded to the organized profession many of the powers of 'private government' within the health sphere" (Torrance 1987a, 19), this 'relative autonomy' as Bourdieu has noted, clears a space for those within it to adjudicate not only their practice, but who can practice as well as to whom this practice is administered. The addict has been accepted into this process only with the greatest reluctance, often at the behest from a 'public government' that it must do so. Indeed, the internecine divide between general practitioners and specialists have created tensions that, in order to circle the wagons and protect what are nonetheless common interests, "… were then projected upon the external bogey of government intervention" (ibid, 25). Historically, a residential system compelling all lower rank workers to not only live on the premises as students but also as workers, calling to mind the older model of the religious orders upon which the early hospitals were based, reinforced the ambience of organizational autonomy (cf. Torrance 1987b, 481ff). This tightly woven fabric of training, partial residency—still a requirement during working hours for students and apprentice professionals—and professional exclusivity both in the discursive and legal spheres, as well as the ability to mandate behavior through codes of 'ethics' and simple human resource oriented job roles and rules—this last is shared by all professions and even more widely, of course—maintains to this day a virtually unbreakable boundedness of autonomic function. In the rare case where an insider must somehow act as an outsider, the difficulties are plain. One example: Dr. Westlake's own son was dying, and he was convinced that normal operating procedures would hasten his death. "Someone had to alter the course of events from outside the hospital, and I was the only person in a position to do it. I had to in effect pit myself against the whole vast machinery of a modern hospital, and I may add, it was the hardest thing I have ever done in my life" (Westlake 1973, 86–7). Even medical personnel, when confronted with illnesses of either their own or loved ones, are almost automatically marginalized into the patient role. At first this sounds sage, given that the scientific objectivity needed for treating the patient is sabotaged by the closeness of relation, but at the same time there is a risk of a loss of insight that may be critical to such treatment. Though Oxbridge philosophical writers regularly misinterpret continental thinkers of all stripes, Midgely's point concerning Marxism is well taken if seen in relation to the practical applications of science like medicine and engineering, as well as something that Marx himself sometimes imagined he was doing: "Though it uses science, it is not itself a piece of science but a powerful myth expressing a determination to put ourselves in a relation of control to the nun-human world around us …" (Midgely 2004, 116). The finesse of technique and its own application to the world speaks of this determination. It is almost as if the role of science and technology has been subtly reversed; science is seen as a mere tool, a means to a new and more powerful technology, and technology itself is seen as the paragon of knowing and as such, controlling nature and culture alike.

3.3 The Ghost of Uniqueness

In 'mature capital', an aging population presses hard against a health care system originally designed in periods of rapid economic growth and immigration. The surplus energy of such a society, its 'accursed share', could be harnessed by productive forces and also could afford to pay for public policies such as the care of health and research against disease. It is a different story today for many of these countries. Productive forces have lagged, the laboring population has shrunk, as has the middle-class tax base. It is a new situation for capital and for democracy. In its newness, it nevertheless comes across as uniquely our own. It is its uniqueness rather than its novelty that is a clue to authentically interpreting it at an existential level. Concentrating on its difference rather than trying to adapt to it as if it were an outcome of a rigid sameness, an inevitability given the lives of previous generations—this is a rationalization that helps us avoid the anxiety concerning 'the new' in general—allows us to imagine that we ourselves might have to also be different in order to live within this new world.

3.3.1 Constructing the General

Science that is applied is always applied *to* the world. Instead, we need to work *in* a world. There is a dialogue that is relatively unspoken between cultures and natures, not unlike the authentic conversation of humankind. We know the difference between 'talking to' someone and speaking with them. The first carries the air of demand or even command. The second is the genuine dialogue that accepts the encounter with the new, in this case, another being, and the likelihood of her uttering her difference to our face. For "… where something *strange* presses into the world closest to us and we happen across it, the characteristic of disclosedness nonetheless announces itself precisely there in our exploring the thing in question …" (Heidegger 1999, 72, italics in the original). The burgeoning use of health care in contemporary nation-states is strange in the sense that it is new. We might add that it might seem odd as well if we did not know that wealth has an exogamous iatrogenic effect on consumptive populations. We still suffer from 'consumption', as it were, though its meaning has altered structurally.

Note that Heidegger's language implies that what is new can only be noticed due to its almost intrusive quality. It 'presses' up against us and 'announces' itself when we regard it in almost an askance fashion. He continues: "… such ascertaining of something is not its being, but rather the possibility of its being-an-object …" (ibid, 73). Human curiosity is prior to theory, but there is a difference between disclosing and explicating. The first is more like a presentiment of something to come. This 'something' is a thing in terms of it becoming or being taken for an object or object relation. The demographic that is now retiring, the largest generation in human history, will utilize the health care system like none before or, presumably, after. The entire system will have changed by the time these persons die as a group. We not only do not know what their use will look like as a whole, we do not know what the system will look like afterwards. Such 'things' cannot be disclosed in an existential manner until and unless we ourselves are disclosed by them. They are at once events and objects in the world. They occur and they alter the world of objects around them, including ourselves as interacting physical beings that have become 'present-to-hand' to both others like ourselves and to the machinery and institutions we have developed. Therefore it is the 'encounter' with the other kind of being that is strange to us and perhaps also to itself—in that it is historically a novel occurrence and can be predicted only analogously—that presses us to resist its force. Recall that this newness makes itself known by being against us in some manner; it objects to our presence. It may be that, after our 'exploration', we find that this otherness has the force of a housecat pressing up against our leg just before the dinner hour. If this is the case, such a metaphor allows us to welcome the new, perhaps with a smirk or a groan, but nonetheless it is essentially non-threatening. But what if the pressure against us comes from a puma that has leaped on one's back and started biting one's neck? We must judge the significance of the encounter rightly, lest a misinterpretation carry us astray over the course of time. This "… can only be understood on the basis of disclosedness which is found in it …" (ibid), such within-ness carries an interiority that does not assimilate itself into the known world and bears only an uncanny ambience when placed in relation to objects with which we are already familiar. Akin to adding a friend to one's intimate circle, disclosive encountering discloses itself through the new chemistry of interaction. In the analogy, the social dynamic is altered, sometimes significantly, by the presence of an additional person whose own version of intimacy must be 'explored'. Such an encounter is hermeneutic in the sense of it challenging prior prejudice, but only engages in hermeneutics 'proper' when it is forced to explore and interpret the results of its findings. Even in undertaking this reasoned investigation of the new, structural or personal, historical or scientific, even perhaps visionary, we are not at all guaranteed to understand the truth of things. We are, rather, vouchsafing our willingness to explore and disclose ourselves to this otherness which has been disclosed by its pressing encounter. It is no doubt a matter most pressing that an aging demographic has the potential to seriously overload a health care system and the personnel within it. Will time-honored responses be correct in such a case? More funding, expansion of facilities and services, more education regarding preventative care? What of government restrictions on manufactured food recipes, or altering the tax base to skim funding from consumptive practices that have been evidenced as having more or less serious health risks to them? The so-called 'sin taxes' are a minor example of what could be greatly expanded, given our penchant for sugars, fats and salt. A user-pay system in social democratic countries could be taken as heretical, but it too has its merits. The chief ethical problem is, however, that it tends to make the poor pay twice, as people who are impoverished have worse diets given that fresh ingredients most often cost more than processed food does. The incidence of heart disease and other suites of illness is higher in these social groups due to this relationship from birth. Since there are health fashions as well, marginal social classes who do not follow bourgeois fashions of any genre may be left outside those that actually promote better health, as some do.

All of these possibilities are pregnant within the exploration of what has been encountered as a pressing presence of the new. At the same time, there will be discovered an aspect of being which in its truth is in fact untrue, and this also is inevitable in any historical and human relation: "… since human beings are by necessity exposed to a multitude of influence and distractions, it turns out that untruth inheres in the concept of knowledge itself …" (Gadamer 1998, 108). Untruth is 'inseparable' from and 'constitutive' of knowledge. The discovery of untruth is an elemental moment of truth. There is no worldly context that does not bring what are at first apparent opposites together in some fashion. It is not simply a case of when one comes to know the truth of things one also, by definition, comes to know all that is not true of this case or that. This rather legalistic understanding of truth occupies the space in which only the most basic events of living on have taken place. It is only by applying such a definition—made ever more poplar and ever more distracting by our entertainment fictions; those that feature crime-solving are perennially amongst the most popular—to human contexts that we become frustrated. Our casual language does address this issue by speaking of 'shades of grey' and the world is never 'black and white', but we have a difficult time accepting this. Understandably, when the stakes are at their highest, we cling to the legal definition of truth and untruth and expect medicine to transform an essentially ambiguous world into one dyadic. But the features of a disease resemble not so much an alien landscape but rather those of our own, whether in economics, politics, the arts or even science: "Only in special situations that resemble laboratory conditions do comparable features come together, and they are then regarded in the same way" (Lösch 1967, 333). Behavioral psychology, neuro-science, evolutionary biology, macro-economics and quantitative social science attempt to reorder the human world in order to better glimpse an order presumed implicit. But there is no immediate evidence for such an order as these discourses posit. The occult structure of consciousness is something that is an assumption. Skinner's disdain for cognitive concepts is ironic given that 'the mind' is still a fetish object, however reified, for all of behaviorism's bastard children. But the onus cannot be placed on modern discourses alone. Equally, our age has seen the 'destruction' of metaphysics and the disintegration of the aspiration for a unified science. The Plato of German idealism is probably ultimately to blame, but he is a denizen of a period very close to our own, and is not the Plato of the ancients. No thinker can fail to be most impressed by the ability of human beings to adapt adeptly to the reality of ambiguity and indefinition, and to adopt varying and constantly changing tactics of subsistence and survival. If there is a structure of formal thought it would be the ironically prescient anti-structure of adaptation based on the weighing of experience accumulated but not necessarily undifferentiated. It is this tension between memory and anticipation that may lie at the heart of our realization that the physical and mental aspects of being must not only adapt but face certain limits in their adaptation. One of the first and most famous definitions of stress addresses this sense of limit: "Stress is the sum of all the wear and tear caused by any kind of vital reaction throughout the body at any one time" (Selye 1956, 274). Because the body and brain, or if one prefers, mind, are subject to stress, it suggests that our aspirations and our abilities do not always coincide. Yes, we can amend our world to a certain extent. Our unabridged passion for technology tells us that this is one of our most fervent desires. Technology and the techniques that manipulate it are not merely an expression of the vanity of humanity. Religion alone, as James famously asserted, can serve that more specific purpose. No, the tools we have fabricated over the millions of years of human evolution have not only altered the world at large, they have driven to a reasonable extent that evolution itself.

Even so, our accomplishments are themselves grey in their scale and ambiguous in their eventuality. The phenomenon of the confluence of health and technique is the foremost example of a stressful tension that at once promises more than it can deliver while declining any ultimate responsibility for the return of one's good health. If doctors are said to have a monopoly over the serious discourses of medicine, we cannot neglect that which a certain kinds of technologies, and its producers, have as well: "… social iatrogenesis is not due to the individual behaviour of any number of doctors but to the radical monopoly the profession as such has attained" (Illich 1975, 75). Though the definition of who is an insider has enlarged over the recent decades—mainly because alternative practitioners come more cheaply than do the highly trained and more formally educated doctors—there is still a strong sense that the court of final appeal, short of the aforementioned religion, must be found within the hallowed halls of the hospital. Indeed, one could claim that the recovery from a serious disease state accomplished in the absence of allopathic personnel and machinery suggests that it was more a 'state of mind' that had been overcome through the counseling and rhetorical ritual of alternative medicine and curing, but more on that below. But if the motive force behind the construction of a general sense that through technology and discourse, formal training and relatively high personal remuneration, long work hours and ironically, high stress employment positions, that health can be returned to those who interface with such a system, is simply an unequally general lack of control we have over the world and over our lives within it, then any analysis must turn to the ways and means that such dueling senses become enmeshed with one another and why.

3.3.2 General Certitude

No doubt it is stressful to come to the realization, perhaps in one's early twenties, that one is not only not immortal, but that one will face, from now onward and as an adult, situations over which one can exert little or no influence. No longer do we have the quite valid, if shopworn, excuse that we were but children, and that those whose adulthood had already been attained by biological tenure and social matriculation were in charge. But what is the nature of 'our turn'? Its character too appears to one of a gradual series of attainment. When have we 'arrived', as the consumerist phrase puts it, and how do we know we have? Indeed, such a moment might be but fleeting, as in when one reaches the apogee of one's institutional career and then observes it pass one by. Fortunately, we have several different vectors by which to measure achievement in life, and we are told that the most important one of these is our personal health. Like the 'child' argument or rationale, we are also told that youth confers an automatic good health for the vast majority of us, and the real achievement lies not in mimicking the abilities of our collective youth but in maintaining ever new and ever more mature balances of health throughout the life cycle. To do so is to be more certain of one's general condition, kind of like a more actively conscious knowing that one does not have many or any inherited and deleterious alleles that suddenly sabotage one's apparently top-shelf physiology.

But in order to do so one must excerpt oneself from the general *cultural* certitude that youth is not only the best time of life in terms of its actual non-responsibility and its apparently halcyon attitude, but also from the expectation that one should be able to do all the things one did when one was young. The more so, since we are now, supposedly, so much more mature than we were and an aspect of this maturity is to know when and how to exert oneself, and with whom. That neither of these ideas has much merit, the one because childhood is *not*, in our society, at all carefree and non-responsible—it tends to be stressful and irresponsible at once, given the tensions of becoming a fully social being—and because we find that we patently cannot exert ourselves in any way kindred with our younger selves. We have neither the time nor the energy to do so, and often, we lack the opportunity as well. The rate of adultery must be the proverbial exemplification of how we strain to mimic the constitution of youth while at the same time faced with adult responsibilities. It is more about this cultural tension than with any biological mammalian 'drive' to spread one's 'seed' as widely as possible. This myth is also told more or less explicitly from a male perspective in any case. Biology, relevant or no, is a mere rationale for the occluding of social habits, detrimental to our health or not. Aside from the unwillingness to 'act one's age', something that the social tension between a memory of lost youth and the existential reality of aging and living-on-towards-death confronts us with and that we take pains to avoid, there is the additional challenge that all attempts at replication face: how do we know that we are returning to our youth as it was, or even as it *should* have been? This second being a much more likely idea in most people's minds, it itself is an attempt to restore a general certitude to the effort at reconstructing youth,. We need not and indeed, should not, attempt to regain what we actually were, but rather life as how it should have been, as if we were still children but possessed with the wit and resources of an adult. *This* combination, the adult mind in the physiology of the youth, explains all manner of activities that appeal to those ensconced in the middle of life. It is a way in which to evade the horizon of finitude which each of us must face. It can be given an ethic to a point: why reach ahead towards death when one is still alive, life is for the living after all. In principle, this is correct. The manner in which we live is at issue, and not *that* we must live. And reaching backward, even with the added advantage of pretending that a youth could have the abilities and resources of an adult, is not the same thing as living as a Dasein in the world of the present. To live does not mean to retreat into the once lived or wholly into one's imagination.

That we manufacture the intimacy between our adult selves and our lost and half-forgotten youth is symptomatic of other forms of tortured intimacies, marriages that have lasted too long, perhaps, or friendships from our childhood that we realize cannot stand the test of time. What is ultimately at stake is our sense of being healthy and living a 'healthy life' and not merely a lifestyle. We could consult the experts, but to do so is to also involve ourselves in another kind of forced intimacy: "Any sort of closeness between doctor and patient has become an extremely fragile achievement" (Gadamer 1993, 127 [1989]). Genuine dialogue cannot occur at all if the patient is perceived by medical staff to be ill due to their own immaturity or irresponsibility, such as drunkenness or addictions of other kinds, or even those who have attempted suicide (cf. Morgan 1982, 79ff). The effects of the absence of intimacy in human relationships, with all of its attendant support but also obligation and responsibility of *Mitsein*, pushes the already marginalized, whatever the cause, into the farthest corners. The moral gravity of health care is represented whenever we fail to account for ourselves to the standards of the wider community. It is also well known that those with addictions or serious mental illnesses are like 'black holes', sucking in the life energy of all those who dare to get too close. There is an 'event horizon' associated within the space approaching these individuals past which nothing can escape their pull. It may be that health care personnel, who must deal with their fellow humans in crisis on a daily basis, become both attuned to, and tuned out from, those that cannot be helped let alone cured. The human need for community and intimacy is nonetheless still present, but to attain this, one must also be willing and able to hold up one's end of the bargain, which in this case means acceding to and accepting that very morality which we might otherwise feel is out of place in a science based medical system.

So the morality of medicine has both a detrimental effect on health—it clouds our perception of professional compassion and also opens up the problem of how compassion and intimacy can be achieved along with dialogue, as we have seen, in a outwardly professional social context—and has the effect of setting up an applied science as an arbiter of community values. Yet at the same time, however critical we may be of this dubious tandem of effects, it is also clear that part of the 'cure' for many ailments is not only based upon the general values of human community and interpersonal intimacies but as well that medical professionals themselves believe in these values and have chosen to represent and uphold them in dispensing their duties towards the sick. These assumptions dovetail with a wider set of increasingly shared beliefs concerning the value of health care as well as what kinds of treatments should be valued, and finally, the value of being healthy in general. In our time, "… there is an acceptance of modern medical science as the basis of valid knowledge in health; a high valuation placed on personal health; a less fatalistic acceptance of disease, illness and injury; a desire for active intervention in illness episodes; and high expectations for good health care" (Torrance, op. cit., 7). This suite of aspirations and desires is quite recent. The earliest signs of a post-war shift in expectations can be traced to the 'pain' studies of the 1950s and 1960s wherein ethnic and gender specific samples were told ahead of the experiment which 'kinds' of people could take more or less pain. Knowing this, or at least, accepting what the researchers told them, the experimental subjects to a tee began to demonstrate much higher or lower pain thresholds during the experiments (cf. Wolff and Langley 1977, 316ff). The expectations we have of our contemporary health care systems and those who work within them come, in part, from the rising sense of what a good society should look like in the wake of the world crisis. At the same time, individuals, no matter of what ethnic or gendered stripe, *should* be able to foster these higher standards through their own dutiful and collectively oriented behavior and endurance. This is why we see the abreaction of those responsible for caring for those who have denuded themselves of responsibility; this kind of care appears to be foisted upon them and is deemed to be unfair as a result. There are, of course, certain social groups more at risk for such aberrant and marginalizing encounters with health care than others, including the elderly in our society and increasingly globally. The true poignancy here is that getting old is in fact no one's fault. Nevertheless, aging itself is, as we have seen above, seen as an existential threat, and there is a kind of latter day contagious magic assigned to it. Like the black hole effect of mental illness or addiction, the aged also have a boundary around them that the rest of do not wish to cross. But unlike the other marginalized and lowered value groups, we all *must* cross this boundary at some point, and what is more, we know this. As Heidegger famously reiterates, 'my death is in every case my own'. So while addicts and the mentally disturbed are not necessarily ourselves in the future, the aged always are, and thus they ironically present an even greater source of resentment to health care workers and to others in their immediate community. Once again, it is more convenient to prescribe a pill than to adjust social structures to make living on to historically unheard of ages for human beings more tolerable and existentially acceptable: "This suggests that the social isolation that comes with aging in the nuclear family is largely responsible for the depression and anxiety that is being managed by these drugs" (Harding, op. cit., 556).

It is surely profoundly ironic that the more we age, the more we disdain our mortality. We seek the immortal, but all signs that society is producing more closely analogous likenesses of longevity are shunned. This tension is symptomatic of more than the obvious sense that our ideals of immortality do *not* include a lapse in quality of life. The sense that we are working towards an ideal and yet along the way there are a great number of apparent martyrs to this cause is mindful more of the shifts in consciousness associated with religious visions. It is this that disturbs us, I think, because science, especially that geared towards the preservation and enhancement of the quality of human life, should not appear to fall foul of the snares of morality and the entanglements of existence as it is. From the outside, these are the truer detriments of health, and they present the desired uniqueness of our historical epoch in a wider temporal light. We are more like our ancestors than we would wish to be: "Thus today one sees science itself in conflict with our human consciousness of value" (Gadamer 1993, 9 [1972]). Gadamer specifically has in mind the planned obsolescence of aging and thus the aged as well. He says that while it does not have the 'power to shock' us as Darwinism once had for our recent predecessors, it is still disturbing. Mainly, due to the potential for *ressentiment* given that most of us today desire longer and more fulfilling lives, but only those generations down the road will have the technological opportunity to experiment with such avenues and thence make those kinds of choices. If one believes that the cure for mortality means the end of the human species, which it surely does at least as we have known it in historical periods, then one must accept the alteration of both consciousness and the values emanating therefrom that will just as assuredly come about through this new version of human evolution.

3.3.3 Best Practices?

Martyrdom aside, such a goal is alternatively afar and close at hand. It sidles up to us, in the way of the strange, in a hermeneutic or what at first might appear to be an uncanny encounter. But it also, especially at the level of technique, seems unimaginable. Health itself would have to fall by the wayside. Trading health for functionality might seem mere semantics, but to function as a human being is something quite different from how a machine functions. Strikingly, this idea of indefinite extension of consciousness is not as new as we might believe. During the enlightenment and after the French revolution there was widespread medical opinionating on the topic: "There must be an ideal state in which the human being would no longer know exhaustion from hard labour or the hospital that leads to death" (Foucault 1973, 44). Such remains our ideal, though we are woefully lapse regarding the quality of life of those who produce worldwide so that locally we can enjoy something closer to this revolutionary ideal. And we conveniently also forget that what the enlightenment radicality proposed is still just as radical for us, as almost willing unbelievers in our own cultural heritage and our modernity, that such a life was destined for *all* human beings. To our general detriment, the passing path towards indefinitude is also as fragile as the community it is supposed to engender between ourselves and our personal health and that of others. In the main, this is due to the sense that health can be not only recovered, but actually and actively 'produced'. Health is certainly a hot commodity for our society, and we do pay attention when a threatening plague develops in the nether regions of the human lifeworld, though we are neither particularly attentive nor compassionate unless there is an alarm to be sounded down the street, as it were.

But such chickens do not only cross roads, they 'come home' to roost: "Soon the typical patient will come to understand that he is forced to pay more, not simply for less care, but for worse torts, for evil that he is the victim of, for damaging 'health production'—however well intentioned" (Illich 1975, 33, cf. also Evans 1987, 633 for the relationship between expanding budgets and levels of care observed). Though there can be direct relationships between the value of a commodity and the money spent not only to produce it but also to procure it, it is not a necessary relation. This logistical interaction is a subspecies of that which exists between objectivity and best practice. Sometimes distanciation and a dispassionate stance, as well as the experimental methods used in the research sciences aid the cultural expectation of valuable health care, though they must be seen as coming at the price of other kinds of relationships. But increasing objectivity for its own sake is kindred with the idea that an expanding budget can cure all ills: "A dentist or psychiatrist who decides to become more objective by ignoring the pain of his patients will not thereby become more skilled or more successful in his profession" (Midgely 2004, 24). These are the more obvious categorical examples, but there are also existential contexts wherein the doctor is called upon to confront the dilemma of easing pain without erasing the humanity of the patient, without 'taking away his person'. Gadamer reminds us that in cases of chronic and terminal illnesses the most objective thing to do is also seen as the most inhumane, and calls to mind the notorious beginnings of the Holocaust, given the rationalizations surrounding the murder of those with mental illness. The end of life presents to medicine not only its limit situation, a true 'event horizon', but also the ethical conundrum of to what degree of palliative care is either necessary or desired: "Here the contribution of those factors which cannot be objectified is even more important. The doctor is burdened with terrible problems, especially treating the dying" (Gadamer 1993, 172 [1989]). Objectivity cannot lessen these kinds of burdens, but may indeed increase them over the longer term for others such as family members. Just as minors cannot legally give consent but can 'assent' to treatment, the dying or otherwise incapacitated adult is often not taken to be a fully consenting being. Various legal agreements can be put in place ahead of time, kind of like 'pre-nuptials' before one is to betroth death. In an era hedging up to a point where legal jurisdictions seem poised to write and defend 'right to die' legislation, it is regularly recommended that persons do enter into these kinds of agreements, the most common one being the so-called 'do not resuscitate' clause, which is actually carried on one's person. In these incipient contexts whereby the personhood of the potentially incapacitated person is maintained by a kind of future-oriented archive, a 'dying will' so to speak, "… the very notion of compliance would be altered to one of therapeutic co-operation or alliance" (Cooperstock and Lennard, op. cit., 315). Since such limit situations 'cannot be taken away', as Gadamer puts it, and since we are all of us part of the human category of 'potentially incapacitated', one can only speculate about the effects of having enshrined in charter or constitutional legislation the absolute right over one's own life. This latter day child of enlightenment thinking might also be viewed as a step closer to the time when human beings no longer exist as a species in the way we know ourselves today.

In the meanwhile, our challenge as collective humanity is not altered by the ability to predicate the locus and means of our individual fates through the law: "In fact the most chronic of all illness is the path which leads towards death. To learn to accept this is the highest task of humankind" (Gadamer 1993, 90 [1987]). And such an acceptance, even in the face of the aspiration to transcend our bodily limits and reconstruct human consciousness in a manner which may well also transcend itself, need not be done entirely alone. A Shem exhorts in his recent afterword to his famous novel concerning the training of doctors, the fact that illness dislocates and isolates us is its most deadly effect. Like institutional protocols, isolation is the most dangerous result, one begins to think that rather than the situation being out of whack, it is oneself (cf. Shem 2010, 376). Perhaps better practices begin with the ability to question all comers, whether it be organizational structures, the need for certain styles of budgeting or management, hierarchies that exist based on tenure alone, and certain union requirements that protect incompetence. Indeed, just as we do not face death entirely alone, though its experience is 'in every case mine' and there are those who die alone and lonely in spite of having lived, once, within the human ambit, we also do not encounter our personal limits entirely as the person we once were. The transformation wrought by the healthy detrimentality that is death in its immanence is assuaged only by the experience of the fullest health that came before it and as such cannot be taken away.

References

Cooperstock, Ruth, and Henry L. Lennard. 1987. "Role Strains and Tranquillizer Use." In *Health and Canadian Society: Sociological Perspectives, Second Edition*, edited by George Torrance, 295–313. Toronto: Fitzhenry and Whiteside.

Evans, Robert G. 1987. "Illusions of Necessity: Evading Responsibility for Choice in Health Care." In *Health and Canadian Society: Sociological Perspectives, Second Edition*, edited by George Torrance, 615–36. Toronto: Fitzhenry and Whiteside.

Foucault, Michel. 1973. *The Birth of the Clinic.* New York: Vintage Books [1963].

Foucault, Michel. 1980. *The History of Sexuality Volume One: Introduction.* New York: Vintage Books [1978].

Freund, Peter E. S., and Meredith B. McGuire. 1999. *Health, Illness, and the Social Body: A Critical Sociology.* New York: Prentice-Hall.

Gadamer, Hans-Georg. 1964. "The Problem of Intelligence." In *The Enigma of Health: The Art of Healing in a Scientific Age*, 45–60. Stanford: Stanford University Press [1993].

Gadamer, Hans-Georg. 1972. "Theory, Technology, Praxis." In *The Enigma of Health: The Art of Healing in a Scientific Age*, 1–30. Stanford: Stanford University Press [1993].

Gadamer, Hans-Georg. 1986. "Bodily Experience and the Limits of Objectification." In *The Enigma of Health: The Art of Healing in a Scientific Age*, 70–82. Stanford: Stanford University Press [1993].

Gadamer, Hans-Georg. 1987. "Between Nature and Art." In *The Enigma of Health: The Art of Healing in a Scientific Age*, 83–91. Stanford: Stanford University Press [1993].

Gadamer, Hans-Georg. 1989. "Hermeneutics and Psychiatry." In *The Enigma of Health: The Art of Healing in a Scientific Age*, 163–73. Stanford: Stanford University Press [1993].

Gadamer, Hans-Georg. 1991. "On the Enigmatic Character of Health." In *The Enigma of Health: The Art of healing in a Scientific Age*, 103–16. Stanford: Stanford University Press [1996].

Gadamer, Hans-Georg. 1998. *The Beginning of Philosophy.* New York: Continuum [1996].

Harding, Jim. 1987. "The Pharmaceutical Industry as a Public-Health Hazard and as an Institution of Social Control." In *Health and Canadian Society: Sociological Perspectives, Second Edition*, edited by George Torrance, 545–67. Toronto: Fitzhenry and Whiteside.

Heidegger, Martin. 1999. *Ontology—The Hermeneutics of Facticity.* Bloomington: Indiana University Press [1988].
Illich, Ivan. 1975. *Medical Nemesis: The Expropriation of Health.* Toronto: McClelland and Stewart.
Jung, Carl G. 1959. *Aion: Researches into the Phenomenology of the Self.* Princeton, NJ: Princeton University Press [1951].
Kelleher, David, Jonathan Gabe, and Gareth Williams. 1994. "Understanding Medical Dominance in the Modern World." In *Challenging Medicine*, edited by Jonathan Gabe, David Kelleher and Gareth Williams, xi–xxix. London: Routledge.
Lösch, August. 1967. *The Economics of Location.* New York: Wiley Science Editions, John Wiley and Sons [1945].
Midgely, Mary. 2004. *The Myths We Live By.* London: Routledge.
Morgan, Myfanwy. 1982. "The Doctor-Patient Relationship." In *Sociology as Applied to Medicine*, edited by Donald L. Patrick and Graham Scambler, 56–70. Bailliére's Concise Medical textbooks. London: Bailliére Tindall.
Natanson, Maurice. 1970. *The Journeying Self: A Study in Philosophy and Social Role.* Reading, MA: Addison-Wesley Publishing Company.
Patrick, Donald L., and Graham Scambler, eds. 1982. *Sociology as Applied to Medicine.* Bailliére's Concise Medical Textbooks. London: Bailliére Tindall.
Scambler, Graham. 1982a. "Illness Behaviour." In *Sociology as Applied to Medicine*, edited by Donald L. Patrick and Graham Scambler, 43–55. Bailliére's Concise Medical Textbooks. London: Bailliére Tindall.
Scambler, Graham. 1982b. '"Deviance, Labelling and Stigma." In *Sociology as Applied to Medicine*, edited by Donald L. Patrick and Graham Scambler, 184–91. Bailliére's Concise Medical Textbooks. London: Bailliére Tindall.
Selye, Hans. 1956. *The Stress of Life: A New Theory of Disease.* New York: McGraw-Hill.
Shem, Samuel. 2010. "Afterword." In *The House of God.* New York: Berkley Books [1978].
Sontag, Susan. 1978. *Illness as Metaphor.* New York: Vintage Books.
Sorokin, Pitirim. 1956. *Fads and Foibles in Modern Sociology and Related Sciences.* Chicago: Henry Regnery Company.
Torrance, George M. 1987a. "Socio-Historical Overview." In *Health and Canadian Society: Sociological Perspectives, Second Edition*, edited by George Torrance, 6–32. Toronto: Fitzhenry and Whiteside.
Torrance, George M. 1987b. 'Hospitals as Health Factories.' In *Health and Canadian Society: Sociological Perspectives, Second Edition*, edited by George Torrance, 479–500. Toronto: Fitzhenry and Whiteside.
Westlake, Aubrey T. 1973. *The Pattern of Health: A Search for a Greater Understanding of the Life Force in Health and Disease.* London: Shambhalla and Routledge and Kegan Paul.
Wolff, B. Berthold, and Sarah Langley. 1977. "Cultural Factors in Response to Pain." In *Culture, Disease, and Healing: Studies in Medical Anthropology*, edited by David Landy, 313–18. New York: Macmillan.

CHAPTER FOUR

'Doctor, Feel Thyself'

The Aura of the Alternative

> Better health care will not depend on some new therapeutic standard, but on the level of willingness and competence to engage in self-care.
>
> —ILLICH (1975, 165)

> The creativity of freedom is precisely what cannot be programmed beforehand. It may seem and irregular, uncertain and circuitous path toward the improvement of the human lot, but there is no other that we can trust.
>
> —BARRETT (1979, 343)

> Theoretically, no limits can be set to the field of consciousness, since it is capable of indefinite extension. Empirically, however, it always finds its limit when it comes up against the *unknown*.
>
> —JUNG (1959, 3, ITALICS IN THE ORIGINAL)

There can be no surprise that in an age where a combination of elite scientific and political dominance is maintained and reproduced by social hierarchy, all those left to the margins of this predominant process will feel some degree of alienation. Movements both reactionary and radical, the former seeking the mythical 'good old days' when their constituents held on to some form of power or at the very least were left alone by those who did, and the latter imagining a future utopia where they would replace the decaying and self-centered elites of our own time, have arisen perennially during our version of highly stratified organic solidarity.

It is the same in the more specific world of medicine, with midwifery being an example of reactionary activity and cybernetic implants an example of that radical. In this chapter, however, we will concentrate on an amalgam of ideas that seeks to both resurrect 'traditional' medicine of a great variety of cultural, mythical and historical sources and yet with an eye to 'holistic' health that lies somehow 'beyond' the limits of current Western ideas of science.

At stake in all of these alternatives to the dominant applied science of allopathic practice is the 'life force'. This concept is itself an amalgam of diverse interests and ideas, including animus, psyche, consciousness, the body-mind, the soul and many others. From within the alternative discourses of homeopathy, all these are labels for either the same thing, or aspects thereof. At once, though, it must be noted that in order to explore the assumptions of alternative health practices, one must at once neither share them nor dismiss them outright. It is correct to say that the history of science is replete with episodes and ideas that for today's standards fall well short on both methodological and epistemological grounds. That said, none of the alternatives to science-based medicine either meets or exceeds these same standards. What can be said is that success rates involving alternative therapies have stayed the course over the decades and are not miniscule. As well, many therapeutic maneuvers, originally accepted only within tight circles marginal to dominant medical discourses have, over the same period, been taken into the institutions of health and health are systems far and wide, as well as becoming more or less fully professionalized in the process. These two facts that on the one hand alternative therapies do work for some persons and that some of these therapies have in turn found themselves ensconced in accepted general practice tell us that homeopathies and their analogs cannot be ignored by any study of medical discourse.

4.1 Homeopathic Histories

But what exactly are the alternatives to the medicine with which most of us are familiar? "… Homeopathy has been the Cinderella of medicine. At no time has it had any general acceptance, and today it has even less than formerly" (Westlake 1973, 174). From the Bach flower remedies to Reich's Orgone accumulator devices, from yoga to aromatherapy, myofascial release to that chiropractic, these therapies and many more bill themselves as specifically 'alternative'. But alternative to what? This is not, after all, a question directed at some epistemological stance or privileged epistemic location. No doubt dominant medical discourses and their attendant institutional hierarchies occupy the vast majority of these kinds of spaces in both our language of healing and health and also, perhaps more importantly, our public budgets and the public trust that goes along with them. No, such a question opens up the possibility of an ontological shift. For alternative therapies conceptualize health quite differently than do the mechanistic models of the applied sciences, where engineering and medicine can be seen as relative intimates.

4.1.1 Historical Moments

The homeopathic language seeks holism. It does not vivisect the body, mind and 'life-force', whatever this last may be composed of. Instead of treating elements or effects, it attempts to treat the whole person. It takes from the idea of life in general certain speciations of what lives, not unlike one of the dominant discourse's ideas of that which threatens life, on the whole: "So the idea of a disease attacking life must be replaced by the much denser notion of *pathological life*. Morbid phenomena are to be understood on the basis of the same text of life, and not as a nosological essence" (Foucault 1973, 153, italics in the original). If the threat to the whole of life is to be regarded as itself a holistic event, it only makes sense to understand that which is threatened or even to be threatened as its own whole. How could only a part of something defend against a whole of something else? How could only a part of something defend the whole of itself? On the surface, these are apt questions. At the same time, even if dominant medicine appears to cut up the body in a million bits and treat each separately, we know, in the end, that the entirety of the body and even aspect of selfhood and 'the mind'—an idea, by the way, not so different in both its vapid timidity and it correspondingly arrogant boldness, than the 'life-force' when compared to hard-nosed nosological practice—is involved in any treatment and especially any potential cure. The anecdotes of cancer victims recovering fully in part through watching marathons of *Monty Python* episodes while in critical care are well known. But the very fact that we tell and retell such stories within the confines of institutional medicine speaks volumes. Even so, it is also clear, holistically speaking, that the cancer would not have been overcome had not there been present as well the usual suite of treatments, however unresponsive the organism may at first have been to them. The presence of the idea of holism is not, in fact, entirely the property of alternative medicine. It does, however, act as an undercurrent to science, and is not as often proffered as either the means or the end to which science aspires: "Instead, science believed fervently in absolute objectivity and assiduously overlooked the fundamental difficulty that the real vehicle and begetter of all knowledge is the *psyche*, the very thing that science knew the least about" (Jung 1959, 173–4). Of late, consciousness, an updated and more 'scientific' term for the psyche *et al*, has been most gallantly portrayed by evolutionary biology as a kind of gestalt. When complex systems reach a certain level of sophistication, they automatically and of their own accord leap into another level.

Notes become a melody, the brain becomes a mind. These events of 'step-wise' evolution, kindred to Gould's 'punctuated equilibrium', are said to account for the aspects of humanity and other forms of being of which we have but partial or speculative knowledge. This would include, more than anything else, exactly what 'consciousness' is and of what it is composed. With this model, still dominant, we do not have to search for obscure and dubious phenomena such as ghosts in the proverbial machines. This is perhaps the most distinct difference between the two major versions of what constitutes health. The homeopathic idea does not shy away from positing, often in the most extravagantly and ill-evidenced terms, the presence of a force beyond the usual means of accession and over and above the usual standards of evidence. Indeed, part of the aura of the alternative is just that, that it *has* an aura to it and mainstream medicine manifestly does not, nor wishes to. Furthermore, any such aura that is demanded of the clientele for alternative practices and therapies would, if instilled in dominant medicine, detract from the aura of the doctor and the specialist, and thus be subversive to the awe that the patient needs to feel as part of her therapeutic program. This awe begets a kind of wide-eyed trust, but the eyes are opened by a kind of fearful or at least, trepidatious respect for authority. The doctor becomes quite easily a filial figure in the eyes of the patient. But if medical personnel are Freudian, alternative therapists are Jungian. Instead of representing the *locus parenti*, they take on the role of siblings or more generalized elders, even friends.

Thus the major interactional tension between the competing discourses of health is often interpersonal. Those of us who require replacement parents seek the institutional version of health and therapy. Those of us more comfortable with a kind of equality, if not in experience, at least in cooperative learning and such efforts to restore the 'balance'—another key word in the rhetoric of alternative medicine—to ourselves and our lives, gravitate to the homeopaths. Some of us do not feel the need to control our own destinies quite as much, perhaps, while at the same time some of us might be said to be more trusting in the science of medical discourse and in its arts of application. It is certainly not a semantic issue, but it is equally certain that this is not a matter for simple subjectivity, no less opinion. On the one side, "What seems to be something irrational is, in the eyes of the scientist, a phenomenon on the frontier of science; this is how phenomena appear on that border where science finds applications to practice" (Gadamer 1996, 3 [1972]). This is precisely the situation of medical science as both practiced and applied. The elements of alternative therapies that are now well ensconced within official medical discourse, as well as being able to apply for state funding or as automatically funded as part of the systemic health care apparatus, were all once deemed 'irrational' in this scientific manner. But how is it that aspects of competing discourses can find their way into that dominant without at first being subject to scientific approval? It is not a matter of coincidence that demand pushes supply along this very frontier. Akin to the advent of psychoanalysis and its startling languages of Oedipus and Electra—two desires that, however bourgeois and limited in cultural region, were already well known under other nomenclature in every family; the filial piety that bled into erotic supplantation of whichever parent was in question and thus that other who was in competition with the child, son or daughter—and at the same time the outlawing of incest in a formal manner (cf. Foucault 1980, 130), the sometimes bizarre evocations and invocations of alternative or homeopathic practice leaves much to the established mindset that is not only unexplained, but downright inexplicable.

At least, this is so at first. Illness 'itself', robbed of its own ontological structures and robed with the strictures of medicine *itself*, could thus be utilized in other manners: "The Romantics invented invalidism as a pretext for leisure, and for dismissing bourgeois obligations in order to live only for one's art. It was a way of retiring from the world without having to take responsibility for the decision …" (Sontag 1978, 32–33). The vague euphemistic rhetoric of the invalid, the emotionally or mentally incapacitated, the languorous and the wretched, all call to mind the equally obscure yet still highly formalized language of the previous age's melancholia. Sontag quotes Schlegel as stating that while health is scientifically interesting, only illness is truly of interest precisely because it belongs to the individual sufferer, and hence confers its annotated pathology upon him or her (ibid, 30). If illness could be relocated and once again made interesting in these ways and others—and once again, it is not a coincidence that the rise of the mass asylum systems, psychoanalysis and its immediate predecessors in Charcot and Binet, the separation of the mentally ill from the criminal, industrialization and urbanization, and perhaps most symbolic of all, the bourgeois marriage, family, and household with all of the accoutrement of 'incestuosity' built right into it from the start all occurred in the wink of a Victorian eye—surely then treatment as well could be reconstructed as of great individuating interest. This was the key to homeopathic victory, or at least, advancement, against that allopathic. *Treat the person who is ill as his or her own person, as an individual.* Tailor very specific treatments and therapies for them and to them, and in some cases, even with them and by them, so that the person who ails maintains his or her interesting state. Indeed, so that the person who suffers can be made to understand suffering as of great personal interest, not unlike Western religiosity, which, in the classes that could not afford the new bourgeois sensibilities, had just 'reawakened' its fervor and force.

The entirety of this alternative structure and its history bears an uncanny resemblance to the tension and division found between the scientific conceptualization and exposition of cosmic nature and "… the nature whose impulse we feel within, with which we can feel ourselves out of alignment and with which we can aspire to be in attunement" (Taylor 1989, 416–7). Note that here again, it is the idea of *balance* that plays a keystone role. What one is to balance remains vague at best. Before it was humors and their associated moods or states of being. In our own time these have been elucidated so finely that no layperson could ever keep track of them, let alone their effects. So there must be some kind of replacement for the more easily grasped frameworks of yesteryear that are also conveniently linked into the symbolic order of a gloss on the visionary, allowing the singularly uninspired and insignificant amongst us to feel not only a balance of forces—some or most of them far greater than he, but he himself is nonetheless greater for their continued and efficacious presence—but the fact that we are part of the cosmos after all. The cosmic nature as revealed by science is far too aloof and infinite for us to grasp on a daily basis. It is where the true 'vision' is. For the rest of us, ill-endowed with the training and status of the cosmologists and their kin, illness, lack of balance, and suffering can continue their role in making our lives more interesting than they actually are. And we, the supplicants and penitents of this personalized introversion of the visionary, can gaze at our navels and behold a universe within.

4.1.2 Contemporary Traces

To be fair, the alternative discourses of balance and holism do not solely recommend the flight from the world as it is nor from the cosmos as it currently understood. These understandings too are not as new as they may be touted. The 'multiplicity of universes' is asserted in Pre-Socratic texts, for example (cf. Gadamer 1998, 88–89). The bursting of the cosmic egg is mindful of the Big Bang. The examples proliferate the more we read. But we also have to bear in mind how much we may be reading into these mythogonical elements. With each interpretation, text is being at once put 'under erasure' without in fact being 'destroyed' in the usual Heideggerean sense. Rather, it is being bracketed. There is more of Hegel than Heidegger in history to this day, which suggests that our desire for romance both past and present is unalleviated by the interest we might also find in romanticizing suffering or the curing of it. Something is being created, however, and whenever that occurs, we are told, something else must at least give way, if not merely to avoid outright destruction and replacement: "But isn't it more difficult to replatonize or rehellenize creationism? Now creationism often belongs to the logical structure of a good many apophatic discourses. In this way, creationism would also be their historic limit [ ] the limit of history and the limit *as* history" (Derrida 1995, 73, italics in the original). Our fetish for the past as nostalgia, certainly as mythical as cosmogony in general but in no profound sense of the term, keeps the historical river unchecked by either data or insight, but ever overflowing its desiring and submissive banks. This too represents a structure of general desire in the lifeworld and one that is repeated writ small in our desire to make our suffering apparent to others and to demand of those others to aid us in recovering from it. It is, in itself intrinsically of interest to all, for any of us could begin our own vision of suffering at any time. We are aware of this, so we play along with this effusive and genuflective discourse of love of self-suffering. It looks like concernful being and circumspection at once, but it remains an ontic validification of the larger and less controlled structures that permeate our consciousness and everyday life as well. This is yet another keystone tin the architecture of alternative therapy: make the individual *responsible* for his suffering. In this way, we become of interest to ourselves—'Why am I feeling this way?' is a common note and query, or the more baleful 'However did I come to end up like this?'—while at the same time being decoyed away from any nominal or incipient interest in the way the world works or is run.

In this, homeopathy shares out the disseminative fluid of its discourses of analysis. Its mode of progress to this regard is responding to the model of allopathic analytics recently invented: "If the disease is to be analyzed, it is because it is itself analysis; and ideological decomposition can only be the repetition in the doctor's consciousness of the decomposition raging in the patient's body" (Foucault 1973, 130). This iterative process of explicating 'what is going on' is taken up obversely by homeopathy, even though it could be said historically and prehistorically that homeopathy itself invented the necessity for repetition, for making external what is at first deemed internal, for turning the interiority of the victim, patient, client, sufferer, inside out for all literate community to observe and understand. In this way one's fellow persons can not only judge what is occurring to the specific person, but have some advance experience of what can or will eventually occur to themselves. We need to *repeat* the suffering of the one in order to generate the community of empathy that binds the social contract.

But dominant medical science cannot manage this repetition without the use of its vast machinery of discourse and technique, the observation of which would stun into mute silence or even an awe bereft of wonder for the vast majority of us. So alternative therapies not only are employed in treating the specific individual person, *not* case, mind you, but more importantly, are *talked* about in the most banal and informal of social circumstance. Only a doctor can speak of medicine, but almost anyone can tell of the process and results of homeopathic genres of experience. Indeed, we are encouraged to do so, because the dominant industry of practical science has all of the market and legal advantages already on its side: "Interestingly, though, doctors in an international context have often moved further towards incorporating alternative medicine into their own repertoire when the legal restrictions on their external competitors have been at their strongest" (Saks 1994, 97). Though Canada had a homeopathic representative on its National Council until 1960 (cf. Torrance 1987, 12), there entered a period where for some decades alternative practices were viewed with increasing suspicion in part because they began to be associated with youth and thus with a variety of social and political movements that tended to be anti-state or anti-authority in general. Medical authority was, under the auspices of these new ideas of the 'counter-culture', no different from that of the police, for instance, and thus should be 'questioned' in the now proverbial manner. All of this new kind of talk, including that which disseminated the experiences of those who participated in, and not 'underwent', alternative therapies eventually had an effect. Our current situation is one in which more and more marginal and outré practices are pushing themselves onto the scene, or back onto it after a lengthy sabbatical, and as stated, many of the once odd-ball ideas such as massage and chiropractic work are well centered in the 'legitimate' spectrum of medicine. Insurance dossiers are perhaps the best evidence of their wider and official acceptance, though it is interesting to note that within the insurance benefits of professional classes and public sector workers there are more likely to be longer lists of alternative therapies such as aromatherapy or hypnosis.

But practices that use different tools and techniques than do those of the dominant model are not the only additional contenders to this latter: "... self-help groups can also be seen as part of a new social movement, resisting the dominance of medicine's instrumental-cognitive rationality ..." (Kelleher, Gabe, and Williams 1994a, xxiv). These kinds of groups, not unlike their predecessors in both the light and shadow of community, the chamber of commerce on the one hand and the militia on the other, for instance, have both the time-honoured role of benevolent societies about them but as well, the even more ancient idea of the 'mysteries'. Though access is hardly exclusive—after all, such groups as these need more market and cannot afford to paint themselves into some arcane corner—nevertheless there is deliberately put forward an aura of those who are 'in the know' about something the remainder of us are not. Such groups are said to 'value experiential knowledge' and to 'see things differently' than institutional medicine (ibid.). But as all knowledge comes from experience, as Hume famously declaimed, so the contention of these alternative social groups has to do with the kinds of experience they are supposedly having as well as suggesting that others join them. Indeed, the first and perhaps the foremost problem any alternative idea faces when confronting the doxa of this or that historical or institutional discourse or ideology is that they themselves come off as ideological due to the apparent lack of scientific credence that they can maintain. By definition, we can expect this kind of tension given that one of the grander claims of alternative health is that science *per se* is either too limited in its epistemological spectrum or that it is simply 'behind the times', as if non-scientific ideas are part of a more intuitively correct and holistically aware human future: "In developing such 'competing rationalities', lay people have found themselves engaged in disagreements with those experts from orthodox epidemiology and public health who insist that the evidence does not support the claims they are making" (ibid: xviii). What is of most ethical risk in these kinds of confrontations is establishing beyond doubt the source of problems that effect communities. In the more narrow case of public health and epidemiology, it is not so much epistemological questions that muddy the waters but vested political interests. Love Canal is now a tired, if still tragic example of industrial cause and effect that vested interests were apt to keep silent about and resent any intrusive investigation. There are hundreds of like cases, but they all share the penchant for using not alternative manners of 'experience' but those scientific in making their claims. So the contentions surrounding public health and alternative medicine are not so much about disagreements over what science is capable of but rather what it is actually being used for, and for whom, and thus, finally, against whom as well.

Whether or not modern institutional medicine has lost the 'human touch' and become reductive or materialistic, or whether through a 'laissez-faire' system of organization and delivery it neglects the patient in other ways (cf. Westlake, op. cit., 26), it is clear, if ironic, that when lives are truly at stake it is to science that all sides come running. Certainly there is industrial and ideological sabotage of the scientific method when its suits such interests as there may be. Given even the sometimes generous laws regarding industrial pollution and other health and environmental hazards with which we live on a daily basis in modern capital, there are still enough punitive stigmata available to the community and to governments to make both private sector organizations, and even some aspects of the state itself—witness the ongoing scandals over casinos and their ill effects—to push certain interests to cover their tracks. Perhaps most effective of all is the potential loss of business and market, consumer or otherwise. Of course, this stick can cut both ways, and rightly so. The recent and highly localized cases of Indiana and Georgia floating legislation that allows businesses to refuse services based on religious or sexual orientation grounds caused a powerful and impressive corporate backlash which included the likes of the Disney Corporation. Indiana had to scrap their efforts to this regard, and it is doubtful any other state will push such anti-constitutional bills through. Note however, that the penumbra of such a back and forth suggests that government itself, that is, the body armed with the constitution or charter or rights, is content to let private concerns play the heroes of freedom and democracy. Whether or not this is a distinctly 'American' manner of working things out remains to be seen.

Either way, there is something worth studying here in reference to the wider notion that we as a society have the tendency to pass the buck when it comes to illustrating our ideals. This, in turn, may be seen to be a response to the denial of those things we fear. Our aspirations are also driven by our anxieties. Alternative medicine offers hope to those who suffer because it recognizes their suffering as something human, something about which we cannot be in any ultimate denial. Political rights or human rights aside for the moment, homeopathy considers, rather oddly, it to be a fundamental human right to experience pain and to communicate about the suffering in a humane context. This, at least, is fundamental to its rhetoric. The idea of overcoming suffering or facing down one's pain is also present, as if some heroic and mythological countenance was part of the overtone infiltrating its generally benign and sunny chorus. Even so, the recognition of pain is something that in general, allopathic medicine is interested in only for the purposes of diagnosis: "Modern cosmopolitan medical civilization denies the need for man's acceptance of pain, sickness and death. Medical civilization is organized to kill pain, to eliminate sickness, and to struggle against death. These are new goals, and goals which have never before been guidelines for social life" (Illich 1975, 90). On the face of it, such goals are clearly children of the enlightenment, with value put on a future-looking universality of a new humanity, perhaps finally overcoming humanity itself through a new form of species evolution. Just because the goals are new and their horizon sometimes far forward of where society actually is at the moment should not put them out of court. But it is sage to remind ourselves of the difference and the distance between such ideals as we may be bringing about gradually and inconsistently, and the many realities of human suffering that still exist and are not even being addressed, or *cannot* be addressed, within the ambit of these optimisms. No doubt this is Illich's main point, but it is obscured by the sense that we must in fact be human only in the face of sickness and death. Rather, it is a problem for both ethics and ontology that we imagine that what makes us most alike, what brings our humanity closest together given cultural and historical differences, are things like suffering, illness, and mortality. These kinds of ideas are manifestly *not* emanating from the enlightenment and indeed hark back to much older forms of social organization and thought. To allow them a back door entry into one's argument is risky, though culture critics of all kinds, from Rousseau to Marx to Freud have all done so, possibly to their detriment as well as to our own. Instead, one might suggest that the more authentic, if grass roots, optimism and enlightenment *ethical* ideals are more squarely made manifest in the hopes of homeopathic doctrines, though their content is itself often contradictory to such ideals. That is, alternative content is pre-industrial while its ideals are not, while the content of allopathic medical discourses is clearly ultra-modern, even if its ideals are a neurotically inclined avoidance of suffering and death and thus it comes off as desperate and faithless. Yet it too uses the same rhetoric when it touts its wares: "The patient comes to feel differently about the world, about himself and other people, and as a consequence he will see things differently" (Barrett 1979, 261). Though talking cures of all stripes were also originally disputed and made the object of a suspicious materialism, there is no insurance policy, public or private, that denies its clientele access to these kinds of services today. The goal of a medically inclined plane is to have all of the subjectivities that once possessed its patients roll off the near end. Seeing differently means letting go of both one's possession and the ideas or states of mind that had possessed one. This sounds more or less like any kind of hortatory spiel, religiously inspired or no. To be cured is to have undergone a conversion experience. Homeopathy brings out the underlying intonation of medical treatment and ideal goals more clearly than does the allopathic or dominant discourses, and it is to this that we are attracted, hoping against hope that there is more than what meets the eye to being ill and, all the more so, to being healthy in return.

4.2 Mainstream Attractions

While the dominant institutional and scientific model of medicine states that it has the greatest weight of experience and evidence at its back regarding the cause, effect, and banishment of disease and like states, its attraction cannot be reduced to our rational acceptance to these statements at face value. For to be ill is almost by definition to have lost at least some of the capacity for rational thought and action, even when the health condition may be a joyous one, such as giving birth. The proverbial chase to the hospital, where one is stopped for speeding and then let loose again with a police escort in tow, is perhaps a romantic folly, but it does point up the fact that no matter the actual state of the body, the state of the mind takes precedence. What we are reacting to is a deviance, a transgression of normalcy, and in doing so, we are not unlike allopathic medicine's response to homeopathy. Two types of rationality are here involved: at first, the response to the ill-evidenced humors of alternative therapies is one of disdain and disbelief, but skepticism gradually enters the scene, allowing for the more civil-mannered suggestion that these practices be examined in the light of experimental evidence, even if such a suggestions is invariably accompanied by a smirking smugness. One of the ways in which homeopathic discourses may be distinguished from their more authoritative competitors is simply by defining them negatively, and the mainstream medicine's reactions to them will help us do just that.

4.2.1 Holistic Bases

This immediate response to any challenge to its authority or trespass into its discursive space reminds us of the same kind of looking askance that we may as individual patients receive from a doctor or other medical professional if we have the nerve, or the gall, to question his or her interpretation of the symptoms we have just listed. After all, we are here to consult with the doctor, not with ourselves. The clinic is a special space, unlike any other that we might regularly or even from time to time be called on to visit. This is why the period of the doctor consulting the patient is sometimes still referred to as a 'visitation', as if the players involved were akin to the spirits of old, and something uncanny and perhaps untoward was occurring. Certainly to be 'visited upon' by an illness, to continue in this archaic tongue, is seen as a malfeasance. Medicine cannot quite shrug off the shroud of subjectivity by which it was birthed and through which it continues to see the world. For the reality that medicine works within is the human or social *lifeworld*, even though it takes as much of the physical sciences, discourse, tools and methods, along with it when it enters this world: "This reality is, of course, dependent on us, in the sense that a condition for its existence is our existence. But once granted that we exist, it is no more a subjective projection than what physics deals with" (Taylor 1989, 59). This is mainstream medicine's greatest challenge, the irksome fact that its reality can never ascend to the relatively pure vistas of physics and like studies of objects utterly alien and anonymous to humanity. We have already seen how the major historical response to this issue is to reduce the human person to his or her component parts and take these as quasars or black holes respectively, depending on how much relative light emanates from or disappears into them. These degrees of illumination mirror our ability to treat the elements not only as the essentialities of living being but indeed, how we can manipulate them into doing what we want. In a word, can we cajole them, by various medical means, into functioning as proper members of a team, a system of organicity whereby the whole is not only maintained but enhanced. Mainstream medicine seeks the whole as well as does holistic therapy, but it *begins with the parts*, whereas homeopathy starts out with a *vision*, and the word is used advisedly, of the whole and what it *could* be and not only what it is at present.

And it is no surprise that in our own day such a vision is more and more attractive, given that the mainstream understanding of the cosmos and all of its inhabitants, no matter how insignificant, is charged as well with its own destructive capabilities. Science has forced us to confront our greatest anxiety, though it, ironically, has also made it possible for the first time in human history. Homeopathy, bracketing for the time being the 'dark arts' of sorcery, does not have to share such a burden. Hardly anyone believes in black magic—though we are much more willing to at least smile at the Hallmark version of what is to be considered some enchanted evening—and this lack of belief in that activities of human beings that balance the alternative ledger books is very convenient for all the rhetorics, ideologies, and even studied discourses that purport to actually be a viable alternative to science and its mainstream. Not only an alternative in the sense of there being presented to us a choice of matters, but an alternative reality, one in which we 'come to see things differently'. The attractiveness of the challengers to the mainstream have an additional card to play: "People who fear science today are chiefly disturbed by the way in which these imperialistic ideologies import irrelevant, inhuman standards into non-scientific aspects of life and lead people to neglect the relevant ones" (Midgely 2004, 21). 'Scientism' is the term that has been invented to characterize these 'ideologies' of which Midgely critiques. It too has a greeting card understanding of science proper, its hallmarks generally being reductionism, behaviorism, and mechanism. It is easy to immediately see why medicine can be construed as dangerously close to scientism. Taking apart the body and examining its elements is reductive in its method, mechanistic in its assumptions, and any subjectivity left over from these operations can be put down to a behavioristic response to pain and change. So much for the person, we might think. The occlusive and overdone 'forces' of homeopathy, distant successors to the shaman's visions of our primordial past, have all of the nuance, but none of the concreteness, of the most awe inspiring cosmic forces known. Yet this too is not a vision that is exclusive to homeopathy. It is rather the state and status of the applied sciences that tends to eschew these grander statements: "Francis Bacon constantly hammers home the point that the traditional sciences have aimed at discovering some satisfying overall order in things, rather than being concerned to see how things function" (Taylor, op. cit., 213). After all, 'cosmos' is order. It is also the whole of things. Cosmology, the reigning regal presence of all the sciences, is the study of the holistic order of things that is presumed to exist. This presumption is reasonable, given that the opposite of cosmos, chaos, has retained much of its original meaning in casual language in a way that cosmos ironically has not. The order of the universe may be implicit, but it too is a reflection of both our desire for an enduring social order and an ordered social world, the one maintaining the social contract, the other reproducing ordinary civil day to day life. *Nothing* else can occur without these two orders, including any study of that cosmic. This may sound oddly conservative, as if Edmund Burke had suddenly poked his head around the theatre curtains and uttered some staid remark. But just as we seek order in everyday life, our discomfort with the unexpected is proof enough of this, we also seek it within our bodies and 'inside' our heads. Cosmos is everywhere, but just so, it must defend itself in all places, perhaps the more so the more intimate.

Not only do the heights of mainstream science share the holistic vision, so too do the stratospheres of philosophy: "Each object in turn is exhibited only as an item within the world, and we have already to be in the world to make the addition. Our Being-in-the-world is a unitary phenomenon and not the total of separate components" (Barrett 1979, 161). Heidegger himself asks why 'authentic being' tends to be sought in 'beings of things in nature' (cf. 1999, 69), and why the dissolution of the everyday world into its component or yet 'primordial' elements should be considered to be more 'real' than the experience which is our own within the day to day. These kinds of questions are now generally seen as part of the movement towards existentialism and away from the so-called 'essentialism' of earlier metaphysics. To its credit, allopathic medicine treads an existentialist path in that, though it may be reductivist, it does not posit some other form of being that is more authentic than the parts it views as being real. These parts are part of the everyday world and as such are sources of the day to day experience of being in that world. It is that being that is either healthy or unhealthy, and not some other form of being, human or otherwise, that is either the paragon or the root of illness and even evil. Homeopathy, on the other hand, tends to resonate with the previous metaphysics of vital forces and wholes greater than the sum of their parts. This would not necessarily have to be taken as different from the modern discursive concept of the *Gestalt* if it were not for the mystical appurtenances that ride along with most of these conceptions. If the mainstream has an attractiveness then it must be taken in an oddly and perhaps experientially, though not logically, contradictory sense; at once it shuns the vague and mysterious while at the same time sticking to the everyday and making its own forces a part thereof. This has the decided advantage of convincing the patient that there should be no *real* mystery to why they feel so poorly, and if there is an apparent one at first, then the 'forces' that are engaged to be with us during this journey are those of the detective. Their purpose is the opposite of those held to be important in homeopathy for they seek the solution to the mystery of cause and effect and not to simply acknowledge that there simply *is* mystery and we must adapt to it in order to recover our good health.

So for allopathic methods and institutional discourses, the mysteries that are encountered are purely bureaucratic and intersubjective. That is, on the one hand, there are rules and on the other people either follow them or they don't. The recognition of this social situatedness of Dasein, however potentially reductive and even flippant, nonetheless helps us to conceive of our experience as in fact quite normal, akin to any other experience of a work-space with people in it who are all trying, more or less, to get the job at hand successfully completed. This is both pat and patent. We want to feel at home in a world that has cast us out through the facticity of being-ill. We know we can feel that way once again, but this is something that takes place *after* one has recovered. To feel the social theatre and the authentic compassion of those around us *before* the recovery occurs is an optimum situation. What we are learning is not only a truth about ourselves cut adrift from the regular run of things, but also how those fellow humans whose purpose it is to restore us to our usual world follow in fact the same courses and regulations that the world to which we long to return does as well. This is also a marked attraction, for some, of mainstream medicine as opposed to that alternative: "It is a question, in the absence of any previous structure, of a domain in which truth teaches itself, and, in exactly the same way, offers itself the gaze of both the experienced observer and the naïve apprentice" (Foucault 1973, 68). Like the interns and students which are likely to be present during our course of treatment, we too apprentice to both a system of discourses and agencies but also to the newness of the experience. Though mainstream medicine likens this experience to normal life, it cannot be entirely identified with it. There remains the mystery of the machines around us, for instance, or the pensive faces of the staff intent on dispatching this or that duty before it is 'too late' for once again, this or that to occur or to have occurred. But all of this 'mystery' is a sham, because it precisely belongs to the mundane world and the key authenticity of its presence as simply a figment and function of technique and technicality is that it reminds us that our mundanity is both complex and diverse, that is, potentially of great interest to us as human beings in the world. In this, it rests its case that the truth of things remains in this self-same world.

This is a crucial point in the construction of dominant medical discourses. It cannot be overstated how medicine of this kind plays this experiential card against all alternatives to it time and again. Instead of consulting the priest or shaman because one has a sore throat, institutional medicine arrests the possibility of melodrama or even malingering by its technical trusses. Its entire being as part of the ontic facility of healthiness and hygiene is that the patient is not allowed to *imagine* anything about her condition. It is what it is, and nothing more. By contrast, the human imagination is a vital aspect of the mode of being that has been overshadowed by the presentiment of its coming demise. It is this form of illness that alternative therapies treat in its essence. And 'essence' is still a relevant term here, unlike in allopathy, for the subjectivity of being-ill is the foremost experience that is treatable, and thus treated, in homeopathy. Mainstream medicine cannot allow itself this tack given that its clientele are those who live within the mechanism of caged capital and its allusive recreations alike. Its discourse has the authority it does for us chiefly on the basis that it can restore us to our function within that world as rapidly as possible: "Part of the reason for this is the dominance of the disease-diagnostic model of health and the dependence of the population upon a business-oriented medical system" (Harding 1987, 552). Alternative therapies cost money too, of course, so it is not a question of when, upon entering into the viscous and sometimes apparently at first vacuous space of homeopathic processes we regress into the barter system or some other 'primitive' economy. Hardly, as we are attracted to alternative precisely by the idea of consumer choice. We are aware of the commodity character of these treatments, no matter if they once hailed from some arcane cultural or even mythical source. The shaman and aromatherapist must eat too, and one cannot consume the symbolic life alone. Alternative medicine has its normalizing functions as well. It has to have them, otherwise it might risk being truly unrecognizable to the modern consumer market. If this occurs, indeed, the treatments would fail simply due to their being unable to get off the ground. The famous real life experience of Conan-Doyle, and the one that led him to create in turn the most famous of modern fictional characters, underscores all attempts to attract a clientele interested in what one has to offer, whether it be ophthalmology or philosophy. Gadamer reminds us that dialogue is only authentic when it takes place as does a 'normal conversation'. Because of this sometimes stringent standard of conduct—and though it feels quite 'natural' to accede to it when it is actually occurring; when one tries to make it occur it fails to do so more often than not—but also because this conduct is specifically 'everyday' in character, alternative therapies have to strive against their own historical and methodological grains in order to achieve a wider and more viable market share: "In our everyday lives we fall into discussions which are sustained by everyone involved rather than led by one person in particular. And this is how it should be even for the special form of dialogue that takes place between doctor and patient" (op. cit., 137 [1989]). The masks that adhere to the more mystical attributes of alternative therapies must somehow either be shed, or if the scene cannot be breeched in this way, ameliorated before and after the treatment occurs, or risk giving over to the 'other world' metaphysics in its entirety. The occurrence of this liminality too soon during the apprenticeship of the patient—kindred to any conversion experience undergone in cult worship of the classical variety or sectarian in our own day—will tend to sabotage the success of the treatment itself. Belief in the process, in this case, that one does better than to see a 'mere' doctor of general medicine for one's ills, is key. In this, mainstream medicine stops its advances, because its morality, like its methods and its interactions, must remain as well mundane.

4.2.2 Moral Bases

Not so alternative medicine's. Even if the faith-based aspect of healing in homeopathy cannot be proclaimed immediately after one darkens its already somewhat shadowy doors, it has to be kept at one's side, in reserve but at the ready. If it is the case that "The objective world of natural science can only function as a symbol for the moral order, [ ] it can do so precisely because one has first an idea of law itself, which is immediately evident in the moral imperative" (Lingis 1989, 42). This Kantian idealism precludes the sense that there could be anything other than some form of law for the mind. Reason would balk, not at the unlawful, which is to be taken here as both immoral and illegal, but at the lawless, which would be amoral, that is, without conscience. And the social contract, what undertakes and births our common humanity for enlightenment thinking, precludes the sense that one could exist as a human being without a conscience. Not only this, but without conscience proper that is, once again, the sense one has that one is part of something greater than oneself and that indeed one's selfhood is defined by this membership and not at all by one's being a self must be accepted. So it is a small step from this logic to that of homeopathy. Even though allopathy can claim a greater discursive and metaphysical kinship with the enlightenment sciences and their philosophical backdrops, it is the alternative world of holistic health that can claim the larger share of moral kinship. The fact that we share both the moral conscience and the experience of being healthy or otherwise underscores our shared and universal humanity, the very idea about which the enlightenment sought to first give us an autonomous sense.

Thus a nineteenth century idea such as 'healthy-mindedness', which James famously notes as a category of faith, is understandable along these lines: one's moral health is commanded by one's conscience. One's moral hygiene is dictated by one's actions and their reception by the specific community into which one was born. But more widely, and more ultimately, one's actions reflect upon the state of being human in general, and thus, once out in the world, could be judged by any other human being. A healthy mind is always aware of this wider potential evaluation and also maintains a corresponding awareness that one's thoughts are not as free as the casual saying has it. For what one thinks is inevitably reflected in one's actions, and hence the 'categorical' quality of the various definitions given by Kant regarding moral imperatives. Thought and action, *as* perceived in the world, belong to the same ontological category because both can be 'shared' *as* an experience by others, though somewhat vicariously unless one places oneself in the others' shoes. This act is only possible due to the 'as-if' quality of human perception and imagination. Though we have already spoken of the shared ability to work out projects of action and its saliency regarding the processes of treatment and recovery, the subjectivity of such projects is a path towards their becoming objectively shared in the world. Everyone can see when we are either sick or healthy, or even 'out of sorts', a kind of half-way house between such normative poles. The will of the subject can become an observable project in the world because "… shared experience points to the autonomy of the object, its independence, and its refusal to be reduced to the status of a possession" (Natanson 1970, 111). Like thought being both free relative to 'unfreedom' but not free relative to whatever action may stem from it, the will, whether to good health or to seek care or even to note discomfort and confront it rather than dismiss it, becomes objectifiable through the projection of its efforts into the world. When this occurs, "Experience may be shared without changing the object being experienced into a private content of consciousness" (ibid). In a word, once 'out', one's subjectivity cannot retreat into itself. And we are constantly 'outing' ourselves in every way imaginable. It is because illness cannot be hidden as it advances within us and uses us as a vehicle of its advance upon the world, that we are beholden to the shared moral conscience of the enlightenment for both subjective guidance and objective aid. Allopathic medicine assumes this relationship tacitly and makes technique the manner in which moral obligation is played out in the object realm. It is more convenient to universalize one's humanity through mechanism due to the immediate sensation that one can be placed as an object with other things that have always been objects. To 'objectify' a human being is not so much to adore her in a certain possessive or desiring way as it is to make her feel that her subjectivity had never been noted in the first place.

This mechanistic 'voyeurism' is precisely the issue that homeopathic medicine seeks to avoid. It does so, in part, by taking the moral imperative to be loyal to one's community and to heed one's objectifying conscience as a non-technical call to concernful arms. In short, it places a value upon the experience of being ill, rather than trying to conquer it by technical virtuosity. For holistic care, the event of being ill or healthy is not a technical affair at all, but a gestalt of the psyche or the 'spirit': "But the psychic phenomenon cannot be grasped in its totality by the intellect, for it consists not only of *meaning* but also of *value*" (Jung 1959, 27, italics the text's). The valuation of being sick occurs first to the individual experiencing the issue. But even here, we have somewhere in the back of our minds the ability to imagine that others must have felt the same way. No project of action tending towards recovery could proceed if we did not immediately accept the article of faith that one could not possibly be the first human being ever to feel this or that way. Even the lovelorn adolescent does not maintain such a stance when pressed. So following upon the enlightenment sense that we are already more than individuals and our humanity comes specifically out of the sharing of community and the awareness of law and morality as universally binding and objectifying, sociologists can then define something like 'illness behavior' as part of the sick role "… as the way in which symptoms are perceived, evaluated, and acted upon by the person who recognizes some pain …" (Scambler 1982, 47). Since it might matter very much how we act when such perceptions occur to our consciousness, our evaluation of them takes on a kind of ontological primacy, prompting philosophers to yet another somewhat trite generalization that suggests value has a form of being all its own. That our ability to evaluate rests primarily on the cultural assumptions with which we have grown and lived amongst, the idea that we are as individuals somehow *responsible*, if not to blame, remains key to this day. Bu the origins of *this* idea are not so objective as the enlightenment imagined: "Both the myth of TB and the current myth about cancer propose that one is responsible for one's disease" (Sontag 1978, 46). It is homeopathy, however, that carries the notion of responsibility directly into the objectivity of the moral realm. Here, it is not machines and technologies that are objects to reckon with, but the manner in which we object to our own incapacitation. To the degree we do so as persons defines in stark terms the character of our own morality. For mainstream medicine, morality remains in the subjective space. The decision to seek care and to ask questions is our only burden of conscience. Once accomplished, we are already judged by the wider community, including its health care personnel and apparatus, as a moral being, that is, one who has effected his or her moral duty toward and within the social contract. Homeopathy thus attracts those who are more aware of, or perhaps more paranoid about, their conscience and how it is perceived in the world.

Either way, the narrative of one's imagined project of action 'in order to' get better must take place. In the mainstream, it takes its place amongst the subjectivity of the 'case' and leads to an initial diagnosis. Lab tests further this first assay into something much more objective and scientifically valid along probability lines. In alternative medicine, this narrative takes a place of self-evaluative significance. For it is, after all, the self which is at stake and the reason why one is sick is not merely technical, in the same way as the 'phenomenon of the psyche' are not merely intellectual. Yet in both discursive spaces, the one reductive and dismissive, the other hyperventilating in its moralizing, "… a whole hermeneutics of the pathological fact, based on modulated, coloured experience is required …" (Foucault 1973, 14). This is so because "The patient is the rediscovered portrait of the disease; he is the disease itself …" (ibid, 15). Recalling that in modern medicine the disease has no essence 'in itself', its thingness can be proclaimed only through its manifestation as an intrusiveness into the interior of the corpuscular formations that make up the human body, the painting metaphor is more easily comprehended. If we add to this the historical fact that a disease *never* was an essence in alternative or pre-modern medicine, we can now grasp the sense that its persona is liquid, shadowy, and ever dynamic. It requires a host. Its 'half-life' in the mainstream is short and it 'presence' in the alternative seeks this host. The language of both echoes eerily with that of the incubus. Though the sciences of the occult have been shed in the discourses of natural science and dimmed to the point of obliqueness in the rhetoric of holistic health, their presence, an actuating historical resonance more than a *remanant*, still provides the murkiness that is necessary for a self-diagnosis to take place and, more to the point, to be listened to.

And this reportage is of course received in different ways. For the mainstream, it is a gross compass, providing the direction that a real science might take to get to the truth of things more quickly. For the alternative it is more like a confessional. If the goal of holistic health is a conversion experience that remakes the self in a new form, then one's own shadows, implicit by the fact that the shadow of disease has been visited upon us through at least some of our own doing—in general, as we have seen, most of this responsibility is 'on us', as it were, if we have sought out alternative medicine at all—and it is these shadows of the self that are somehow at the root of things. So on the one hand, the truth of things can be exposed by a simple relation of representation—the painting metaphor is always in the genre of a still-life realism; it is still of life and the effects of the disease are acknowledged as real even if the subjectivity of the potential causes is debatable—and on the other, the root of things is plumbed by a converted self-understanding that recognizes one's own role in the mode of being unhealthy and thus pledges to change, just as in the ordeal of the post-confessional habitus.

But most importantly, and providing the student of forms of medicine with his actual existential cause, is the difference between the attitudes toward the threat that illness itself presents. In the mainstream, doctors are trained to ignore this as much as possible: "You can't function if you think of things like that (death and dying). Everything you see sort of gets in there and turns about in your mind and you aren't productive …" (quoted in Haas and Shaffir 1987, 406). From interns to experienced physicians and specialists, the refrain is the same: "But here again in this busy practice there was little or no time to think about health. I was far too busy dealing with disease in its manifold forms" (Westlake 1973, 2). The irony of this business of producing health while consuming illness is not lost on the foremost minds of the mainstream discourses: "It was indeed very stressful to spend all my adult life in the laboratory, working on stress; it was perhaps even more stressful to express my thoughts in the form of this book" (Selye 1956, 281). At the same time, there must be some kind of outlet for those on the forefront of medicine in their own time: "But well do I know that not to express all this would have been much more stressful still" (ibid). A Hobson's choice awaits all who enter the dominant institutional languages and practices of modern medicine. Its general 'stress', ironies and hypocrisies are so well known as well as of great general interest that writers like Shem, himself an intern turned novelist can detail them in exacting and rather pedantic narratives and still sell millions of copies. This is so because all of us are affected by the training of our health specialists. It is to us that they dedicate their work and even their lives, though we do not feel that dedication in the same compassionate sense that we might feel the love of an intimate. To do this would break the system entirely. We do not, in fact, expect such intimacy or authenticity from mainstream medicine, and this is a final irony about its enduring attractiveness.

4.2.3 Opening Onto …

But it is also an impetus for us to seek alternatives to it whenever we find that it has somehow failed us. So a further attraction of the mainstream is that it opens itself onto the space of its competition and inevitably lets some of its market escape onto this expanse. Because the spatiality of modern medicine had turned inward, transforming what had been the Augustinian interiority of Man into a simple interior which then could be decorated as one liked, but also inhabited by illness as happenstance had it, the outer space of health could then be invested by alternative medicine. As well, the conceptualization of disease classes and categories had fundamentally been altered by the new presence of an inner space within which they could not so much manifest themselves, but through the medical gaze and analytic operations and tests, be *made* manifest: "Disease is perceived fundamentally in a space of projection without depth, of coincidence without development. There is only one plane and one moment" (Foucault 1973, 6). Though a history of cases is still possible, a genealogy of types of subjects who could contract this or that and why, no history of a 'disease entity' has any meaning. It simply *is present*. And though this kind of declamation rings with the murmur of *Geist*, as well as *Geistlichkeit*, such a resonance is passed over like the residue of a medical test and the residuum of faith itself. But the very presence of such a residue is precisely one of the openings onto the alternative that we may desire to follow if all of the tests and operations, pills and placebos have little effect for us. For we ourselves *do* have a history, and it is we who must, in the end reckon with as well as be reckoned by it.

Coming to this conclusion, we must confront another challenge. If we have been at first attracted by the mainstream and its successes and then distracted by its failures, we move into this expansive but ill-defined space nominally aware that it does contain risks. All of a sudden we are responsible for understanding what is going on and we must do so without the help of the techniques of the mainstream specialists and their machines: "As soon as we enter the phase of interpretation, we find ourselves in a region of shadows and all sorts of fantasmas and spooks about which nothing certain can be stated, and still less can be proved" (Sorokin, op. cit., 88). Not that any hermeneutics of the self is bereft of phantasm. They are, however, usually of the sort defined by Schutz as daydreams constructing projects of action in possible future worlds. But when it comes to our health, our imagination is only conscious of the memory of what it was like to feel healthy rather than unhealthy, as we now feel. We hope it is but a passing thing, but we cannot 'prove' this. If the mainstream contains within its weft its own potential undoing—no treatment is guaranteed to be a success or provide a complete cure, and what is more, we already know this upon entering the closed and highly articulated spaces of the dominant medical discourse—it also contains as part of its own history the fact that its own practitioners have also regularly stepped out onto this plane of the otherness of thought and being: "But does not the path of science include many precarious emergency bridges over which we have all been willing to pass provided they would help us forward on our road?" (Lösch 1967, 100). Kuhn's epistemic genealogy is so well evidenced that it is now widely accepted that science proceeds by making such leaps of faith kindred with those of the subject who feels his case has been slighted in some way. Not that we necessarily assign any fault to the practice of modern medicine as it is. The holistic practitioners may do this for us as part of their sales pitch, but it is not of the utmost to pay any attention to it. What we need to know is what *we* can do to save ourselves. If it is the case that in science and in art alike "... the precept itself, that the study of all phenomena should always begin with the simplest forms and pass to those which are more and more complex, is not to be taken as a universal rule" (Sorokin, op. cit., 228), then our assay into the 'opened up space of the private' must be ready to confront within our own being other beings with some degree of advanced sophistication. That is, what ails us is to be now thought of as *a* complex, rather than as merely relatively complex.

This form of being can only be 'encountered' and not confronted as in the case of how disease is understood in mainstream medicine. This is because, within the alternative realm, illness is as well an aspect of self, whatever else it may have been before it 'encountered' us and provoked in us the objection to our ongoing subjectivity. What we are now to be seeking through our egress from the dominant discourses is a kind of disclosure rather than an exposure: "Significance can only be understood on the basis of the disclosedness which is found in it and from out of which *what is being* encountered signifies itself through a pointing within the other things we encounter and in this way presses forth into its there" (Heidegger 1999, 73, italics in the original). The 'thereness' of any object-being is both spatially relative and perhaps also relevant to all other objects and their hinterlands. Things 'point' to other things in a specifically pointed manner. They are not entirely of themselves even if they are perceived as being by themselves. Disease is a thing of thing kind, whereby it points itself up as an object within the space wherein is encountered other objects—objects that 'should' be there, such as functioning organs or vessels etc.—as well as pointing up the fact of its presence as an objection to the health of the space into which it has 'pressed forth' or, from our perspective, intruded. Thus it is disclosed. Disease in the mainstream utters its disclosure thoroughly by means of its objective status, but in the alternative realm, it is its objection to our ongoing healthiness and even existence that pronounces its perhaps more full disclosure of itself.; 'of itself', precisely because it is now a part of ourselves.

So our understanding of ill-health in advance of its appearance is negotiated on the one hand by the presence of objects other to the self in the world and the various objections these objects or more regularly, other persons, make to our presence in that same world. Heidegger continues: "This being-ready-to-hand, being-at-our-disposal, constitutes its *availability in advance*" (ibid, 75, italics in the original text). Today, much of our advance knowledge of anything that we have yet to experience of ourselves is presented through media of various kinds. Indeed, we seek experience vicariously and sometimes voyeuristically through these channels. Knowledge in this realm is of course more like information, and we participate in media on generally a 'need to know' basis. The more mainstream media we consume in this manner, the less likely we are to engage in alternative forms of life, medicine included: “The influence of the mass media and mass education contributed to lay acceptance of medical knowledge and to the decline of alternative belief systems and practices” (Torrance 1987, 24). Like all forms of ‘folk’ belief worldwide, medicine based on worldviews that were ‘enchanted’ by magical means and beings have not only been sidelined by media and education in our modern period. These two factors or vectors are rather epiphenomenal to the globalization of industrial strength capital and its technical accoutrement. Media and education may influence or even culturally transform peoples but it does not tend to wipe them entirely off the face of the earth. So it was with homeopathic medicine. The counterculture of the 1960s and 1970s created a market for a hybrid set of alternative ideas regarding medical care and even what concepts of health and well-being might be debated. In large part, the existence of alternative health care in Western systems today is due to demographics. Equally, the persistence of medicine as a hard-nosed applied science amalgam of chemistry and biology with some physics thrown in the mix through the machinery of techniques used is also due to the fact that the post-war demographic was so large that many of its members simply by statistic would continue to be attracted to find employment within the mainstream venues. This is certainly also true today, perhaps even more so, where young health care workers find themselves employed in the technical and scientific apparatus all day and then spend part of the evening participating in some different kind of arcane sphere, a sweat-lodge ritual or deep tissue massage. Pragmatic and sensible nurse by day, romantic and sensual body-sage by night.

Whatever may be the case, it is clear that the mainstream has had to adjust what it considers to be its strongest suit regarding holding on to the majority of the health care market and thus also its funding in the face of growing competition on its margins and perhaps also a developing sense amongst its clientele that there might be other ways in which to think about health and its maintenance.

4.3 Alternative Mindsets

Let us then examine how homeopathic medicine and its close relatives have managed their side of the marketing equation as well as their conceptualizations of what health is and how it is to be sought and reproduced.

4.3.1 General Holism

One of its chief principles underlying the suasion it can exert upon the layperson is that it does not make hard and fast distinctions between emotion and intellect:

"Thought and feeling are not opponents, any more than shape and size. They are complementary aspects which appear on both sides of any argument" (Midgely 2004, 9). In spite of the drive to objectify human character in all of its guises, the sensate of emotion remains uncannily part of the equation. It cannot be ignored though it has been successfully reduced, as we have seen, to both statistics and behaviors alike. Yet neither the mainstream *nor* the alternative science of medicine have made emotion their primary basis for treatment and definitions of health. Yes, one is asked 'how one feels' in both venues and by both kinds of practitioners, but given that this is seen as part of the subjective narrative of first run diagnostics in scientific medicine, does it really fare any differently in holism? Not really. The question of explaining what is 'wrong' with me ultimately hinges not on how I cognitively or experientially 'feel' about it or what kinds of discomfort I am physiologically feeling, but rather on forces that are not deemed to be objective, though they are, as stated, different in nature than those to which science attributes health and disease. No, how one 'feels' is equally irrelevant in both systems. It is just that we are a little more aware by what follows our contribution to the diagnosis in the mainstream that our feelings and the reports thereof don't count for that much. At the same time, alternative medicine unduly hyperbolizes our feelings and statements about them as part of its therapy. The placebo effect, however much it contributes to the successful drug trial, underscores alternative therapy in a much more patent manner. The sound question "How can we ever know that humans can be explained by any scientific theory *until* we actually explain how they live their lives in its terms …" (Taylor 1989, 58, italics in the original), is not itself obviated by its narrowed use in alternative practice as leverage for doubting the validity of science in general. The desire to press on with the 'until' part of the question, however, is lost.

In fact, 'explaining' illness or health for that matter depend more specifically on *not* pressing on with such epistemically oriented questions which, in the realm of public health and hygiene, most often take the form of epidemiological ones. We are not to be taken in by policy statements when we enter into the mindset of the alternative. We are first and at once individuals who suffer, and though our feelings represent a refractory image of what is 'actually' going on—in this there is no difference between homeopathy and allopathy; the fact that this latter term when used by homeopaths could take on the intonation of a pejorative is also a clue to where we are meant to stand upon entering the alternative domain—they are still 'true' or within the truth in a way that conventional medicine does not tend to recognize. The introduction to our persons to the idea that we ourselves could speak the truth of something without being a scientist or some other kind of philosophical specialist is to be taken as revelatory. It leads directly to our feeling of being converted. If we can speak the truth, perhaps we can also be led by this voice into the space of truth. This is a crucial idea in preparing oneself for treatment to indeed to accept the idea that one is sick in the first place. This is so because "The sick person is no longer simply identical with the person he or she was before. For the sick individual 'falls out' of things, has already fallen out of their normal place in life" (Gadamer 1996, 42 [1967]). Kindred to the general existential *Verfallen* of the human condition, and ethically charged with the ambuscade that all forms of fallenness confront us with, sickness at once repeals the duties of the day while at the same time reveals what remains at its close. Alternative medicine claims thus to be reordering one's life experience in order not only to feel better but to better understand the gravity of the issue that appears to be only 'at hand'. That is, its 'at-handedness' seems to strike one as only an object in the realm of possible objects, as when our general practitioner assuages us by saying that we could have 'picked up this bug anywhere'. This attempt at reordering also acts as a form of leverage to our confidence in the process to come because we are still oriented to the 'former life of health' though we know we are in absence of it or from it (cf. ibid). Homeopathy, through pointing out the distinction between the absence of health and the presence of illness, can now prepare us to accept ourselves as the concurrent vehicle for a mild case of enantiodromia: "Union of opposites is equivalent to unconsciousness, so far as human logic goes, for consciousness presupposes a differentiation into subject and object and a relation between them" (Jung 1959, 193). The idea of the 'other', quite specifically identified with something, rather than the abstraction of otherness, is key to mainstream medicine. The latter is indeed the counter-position of homeopathic medicine. Science seeks the other and thence to make it part of our differentiating consciousness, while alternative practices seek to negotiate with 'otherness' without attempting to possess it, which is in any case regarded as an impossibility.

Yet an abstraction is as convenient as a thing. Consider this well-known critique, emanating from a humanist, feminist and literary critic, and yet taking as a given the sense that explanation is and must be scientific when it comes to health: "Theories that disease are caused by mental states and can be cured by will power are always an index of how much is not understood about the physical terrain of the disease" (Sontag 1978, 54). Further, just because health not merely impinges upon existence but in a broad sense defines it, the abstraction of health as a non-thing-in-itself cannot be presupposed to be more than what can contain it, that is, the body. Any successive 'mental states' must therefore also be contents of this same corpus, and cannot somehow be taken outside of it in order to act as a 'causal' agency, disembodied and bereft of any rational consciousness. For what rationality would cause a disease condition that threatened its own existence? The union of opposites which is said to lie in our unconscious and also demonstrate the model of the collective unconscious in history and myth is neither prior to nor somehow transcendent of consciousness in the allopathic model. Even in humanist philosophy, the 'hermeneutic' of this relation admits to the co-incidence, the simultaneity of any unconscious process and a consciousness that is perceiving or in dialogue with it. Dreams are an easy example: produced by the unconscious they nevertheless are received by an aspect of consciousness even while we are asleep, and all the more so, though usually in a half-recalled form, upon awakening, though most dreams are not in fact processed in this waking manner. Similarly with waking perception proper, where we are not so much recollecting 'events' or images that hail from elsewhere or the past, but are fully present in the 'wide-awake' world of the everyday. It must be even more transparent that such perceptions could not be in any fundamental opposition to each other, their unity a function of the desire for the unconscious life to be reborn in the waking world. So "… we should not, of course, come to a stop with the opposition between the relativity of sense perceptions and the absoluteness 'thinking'. Sensory perception is in a certain sense already conscious perception" (Gadamer 1998, 106). Yet a common understanding of the process by which consciousness comes to know itself as part of the world does not immediately assume its prior integration. This Cartesian viewpoint dominates mainstream medical practice, but it is also of great interest to note that it is not its opposite that commands the therapeutic intellect of alternative medicine, but rather an oddly populated inversion thereof. First: "Consciousness, suspended outside the world, has to begin by examining itself. When it does, it is surprised to find out that it is almost nothing" (Barrett 1979, 131). Indeed, Barrett suggests that if we wish to speak of what consciousness is, we must speak of it in terms of what *objects* we are conscious of. Phenomenologically so reduced, consciousness ends up being a focal point for relationships, which is merely a more technical way of describing what Gadamer above is implying. Consciousness is here characterized by its 'intentionality', which should be taken in its more Latin sense of a 'tending towards' or 'pointing to' (ibid). No problem so far. We are already and always aware, even in a dreaming sleep, that we are one thing amongst other things in the world. Some of these things have as their form of being a consciousness, developed and sophisticated to a certain degree. Even plants and viruses may be so included to a point. Instinct seems also to fit this model, as it certainly 'points' animals in their proper directions in order to maintain their survivability and over time, evolve. But, we must ask at this juncture, to what is intentionality pointing? Is it merely other objects taken in themselves as singular instances or 'events' in phenomenological space? Or is it to some kind of idea, abstract and aloof to the very world we are supposed to be already integrated within? It appears on the face of it to be both, but while the first is, as we have stated, the lynchpin of the epistemological privilege accorded to the applied science of medicine, descending as it does from scientific 'method' in general and thus having an enormous inertia which *as well* is phenomenologically reckoned with as an event in the world—it is *this* fact rather than the facts about which and through which objects are discovered and described, disease identified and defeated that betrays any hope alternative medicine may hold regarding competing on the same level as allopathy—it is yet more influential than what it appears to be. For the abstractions desired and approached by homeopathic medicine are also objects in this phenomenological sense. They both object to our existence as objects, like or unlike, depending on one's relative perspective—for instance, the cosmological makes all objects relating to human consciousness the same thing, more or less—and they are manifestly seen as *not* us. They stand over against us, and whether or not they offer the enantiodromian *Pharmakon* to us as either cure or poison, they possess their very-ownness in the same way that my death is 'in every case mine'. Part of their apperceptive inertia lies in the belief we maintain that their existence continues after our demise. The cancer that finally struck down my mother, for instance, still exists, though not within that specific host. Diseases too are abstractions, but because they act in a manner that the definitions of causality inherited from modern science can logically apprehend, they are seen as a different class of objects than are the 'forces' which inhabit the 'terrain' of the alternative health discourses.

4.3.2 Examples

Or do they? If it is reasonable to suggest "… that the growth of alternative medicine is a product of the disillusionment many people feel with the dehumanizing effects of 'scientific' medicine …" (Kelleher, Gabe, and Williams 1994a, xv), is it the case that reduction *per se* makes us feel less than human or is it the idea that an object, foreign and threatening, has invaded our space, a space which we feel to be as objectively my own as my death and a lot less abstract at that? Homeopathy may be attracting clientele more on a basis such as this: that we feel more comfortable about engaging with an abstract force that is seen as only impinging upon us. That is, its main body or the majority of its being rests *outside* of our bodies and beings. It does not exist by virtue of our existence, unlike regularly identified disease pathogens or even conditions. The 'environment' that conditions certain states of ill health must also include our bodies. Not that in mainstream medicine the body as such can balance or even always counteract the disease, at least without outside help. But the forces involved in allopathy can also be reduced. Indeed, the reduction of the person to a body or its elements is not at all one-sided. *Everything* is so reduced in the applied sciences. So, speaking once again in more phenomenological terms, what we begin to understand is that any object is objectionable in its presence along these lines as well; it must be reduced, parsed out, even 'deconstructed' to its essential elements, none of which alone bear any recognizable semblance to the reality of their 'force' in the world and within our body. The chief difference between the mainstream conventions of medicine and their alternative counterparts now appears to be this and only this: in alternative medicine, abstraction is reduced through its interaction within the being of the person who is ill, and in conventional and dominant discursive medicine, abstractions are reduced prior to their interaction with the body. We enter into a pre-reduced phenomenologically inclined plane of existence when we seek the clinic. For alternative health practitioners, we are already within such a space and thus need to be raised out of it.

The mindset that will allow us egress from our pre-reduced state involves self-care as much as external suasion: "… even greater and more widespread emphasis was placed on self-help in health care and health was usually seen as the achievement of an appropriate equilibrium, involving both mind and body" (Saks 1994, 87). Note that the third eye of the Western conception of being has dropped off. Even in alternative realms the market could not bear the inclusion,—or is it intrusion?—of the 'spirit'. If one is already so far down that road one might do better joining a sectarian church. With two variables to focus upon, the balancing act required for true health becomes at once simpler and more complex. The first due to the idea, transplanted from allopathic medicine, that the mind is a Gestalt of a part of the body. Yes, it still belongs to bodily function, but not in any base sense. As Sagan famously noted, if we had to consciously control all of our bodily functions we would likely starve to death in short order. Proprioceptive processes aside, it is at least clear that 'mind', however unempirical a thing, is the center for the agency of both self-care and the adjudicator of what is healthy and what is not. The complexity of a dualistic balance appears when one has already committed to raising oneself out of the reductive state of affairs that mainstream medicine has foisted upon us. Mind becomes rather more than something that can be 'mapped onto the brain' as some neuroscience discussions have it, but the question regarding why it is or can become so is begged. With the sidelining or even loss of the idea of spirit, we are left grasping for some other concept that will endow mind with the faculty it needs to raise itself out of the horizontal axis of mind and body and allow it to act as the holder of the scales. What balance can be measured without this third position overlooking the corporeal plane? This is the ontological challenge that is faced by any discourse which claims that conventional modern medicine is 'missing' something. 'What, exactly?', would be the first reply.

The first clue comes from medicine itself: "Death is disease made possible in life" (Foucault 1973, 156). This displaces the deontology of death. It brings it into our own purview, that of the living and still to live. It suggests that how we can approximate our own demise rests more than in analogy or even the metaphor of sleep, the 'brother of death' from Heraclitus onward. We have already stated that illness reminds us of our ultimate fate. It acts as an augur, and even if the atmosphere which it portrays has an Augean quality about it, we have to be prepared ahead of time to do what we can to clean up our act. Clearly, those who are 'healthy', whatever this may consist of, last longer on average than those who are not. We make this presumption before knowing at all of what health might consist or how to attain it. It is what underlies our ability to care for the self in ontic contexts and more ontologically, 'act' as a concernful being in the world. It has a suasion whose dynamic is persuasion. So, for homeopathic medicine, such a suasion, the tendency of most of us to gravitate in authentic manners toward the vaguest notions of health and healthiness—of late, marketeers geared towards aging baby-boomers has reacted by making 'healthy living' and 'healthy eating' into lucrative commodities—has to act in place of spirit. Alternative medicine replaces spirit with desire, and if this would have no doubt been a sacral offense to the Greeks and those who followed them, nevertheless it is a necessity for us moderns given the new language of being and history that we employ with regard to historical consciousness and our place within history as a purely human construct.

Yet this desire is no base affair. It is even called, in unguarded moments, 'spiritual' by homeopaths. Lest this lose potential market, the idea of spirit too is commuted from its purgatorial sentence, indefinitely hung out to dry in the desert of non-time. Our just desserts in this case allows us to enjoy the rather inane chestnut of 'having one's cake' and eating it as well. But all of this, taken either with a pinch of salt or a 'little sugar for the bird', rests on the assumption that both the dualism of mind and body as well as the larger, more ontological claim surrounding what exactly the world and consciousness are made of are not really dualisms at all: "… there is no hard and fast frontier between matter and spirit. The artificial divisions created by centuries of materialism take as a matter of course until very recently have been abolished" (Westlake 1973, 126). Of course, this too requires a leap of faith, though it lies in the opposite direction of the mainstream, wherein the leap is made that spirit is non-existent and therefore irrelevant to any consideration regarding health or anything else for that matter. This too is a leap, but it is the easier one to make given cultural conditions, as Westlake points out. Nonetheless, such an argument that rests its premise on the idea that if the majority of discourses and also people think something then it must be wrong is hardly very impressive. It is one thing to engage in 'thoughts out of season' and another to propose that truth will be found in the opposite of thought.

Westlake himself cites three of the four Christian gospels with regard to Jesus being ignored or seen as a charlatan in his hometown environs and amongst those who are not socially marginal (cf. ibid 102ff). This is taken as a kind of model for truth. Those who are too close to the subject cannot see the forest for the trees. What is required is not only faith, it appears, but also distance. In the case of messianic work, social distance is the key kind of objectivity that allows people to believe in something new and different. These are strictly mundane sociological observations. No history of religious ideas is without them. But the sacred science of medicine has within it the germs of a religion as well. Homeopathy exploits this aspect that has been inherited by medicine through its connection with the occult sciences of the medieval period and even before. Doctors might well also be alchemists. Conventional medicine plays down its sacred quality and, as we will see in the concluding chapter, points to ritual rather than to miracle as the secret of its successes. If "Lack of *conscious* faith makes no difference to the healing taking place" (ibid, 103, italics the text's; cf. also Jung, op. cit., 157ff where alchemy is characterized as a psychical process ahead of whatever chemical transformations occur), then allopathic medicine could well be relying upon the same kind of thing that homeopathic medicine uses as a rhetorical tactic to induce self-care. But 'faith' in modern medicine seems misplaced or at least misdirected. The official discourse of conventional care states baldly that all success rests on scientific knowledge, evidence, and method, and therefore, like spirit, faith is irrelevant. It is manifestly *not* a matter of faith to seek and receive medical care in modernity, we are told. Yet irrepressibly it remains so. Like disappointment, faith is something that allopathic medicine has as a part of its own being, but in turn it is something that regularly betrays it. For when one's disappointment affects one's faith, one is galvanized in a more radical manner to seek a 'second opinion'. Note that when this common-place phrase is used it is never being used to refer to homeopathic practitioners. Confirmation of a diagnosis made within conventional boundaries will come only from within those self-same lines. It may be affirmed, disputed, or even negated, but whatever the judgement, it too can be trusted precisely because it hails from the same discursive territory. One can agree to disagree, in other words, if one shares a common language. And only if one does, it seems, because as soon as we step outside of conventional medicine and move toward those forms alternative to it, we place ourselves outside of any judgement at all. In this, we are all like messianic figures, or at least their disciples. We care not what society thinks of us, doctors and all, and are willing to strike out on our own, fishermen and taxpayers, now collecting the soul of humankind as refracted in our own being, a being which like its destiny, is in every case my own.

This dynamic, which homeopathy relies on for its very existence, is ontologically prior to any decision or action we may make with regard to logistical or monetary costs. Like leaving our families and jobs to follow the savior, leaving the clinic behind for the retreat, the hospital for the wilderness, such a 'leap' was actually already built into the very fabric of the institutional text. Its official discourse attempts to prompt one to either dismiss its loose threads or ignore them, but like the stories people tell about their lives, for each its own official records of what happened and what 'certainly did not', "... you have to discover which are the spheres of maximum objectivity and which, on the other hand, are the sensitive and vulnerable areas, most favourable to fantasies ..." (Peneff 1990, 43). Failing to do so places the investigator in the hands of an altered state of affairs. This too may be desired, however, as each of us is subject to both the subjection that history pronounces upon us and the objection that others announce in our presence; the first is of course aloof to any single subjective stance, but the second seeks out precisely this singularity. This dynamic of our semi-conscious relationship to culture and history is played out in the tension between conventional and alternative medicine, the former acting in the role of history—authoritative, empirical, discursive—and the second the subaltern role of the subject—experiential, sensing, anecdotal. The passage between the two is well-documented, but it always takes the form of life-story-telling and personal mythology. Westlake himself tells us that he was told he 'had the power to heal' and thus he proceeded to seek out those who believed in this power as a cosmic fact (op. cit., 62). These 'seventh sons of seventh sons' appeared to abound when one actually took the time to seek them out, and the majority of them were not in fact males. And autohagiography or myth is hardly the only space wherein these ideas occur. Psychiatry is also a favorite abode within which those who practice healing also must believe that they have the power to do so, though this is not generally assumed to be akin to the power of the visionary or even the artist through which some transcendental force is made manifest, and the person is merely a 'vehicle' or a channeller for this force. Shem relates near the end of his famous novel how medical interns are turned towards psychiatry by the idea that they themselves are the tools for healing (1978, 322–3). The alienation that interns feel, the major theme of the book in terms of the subjectivity of its plot development, is something that we have already seen has effected enough patients to make them cross over the epistemological divide in order to heal themselves. This 'feeling', that we are not doing what we need to do, not 'living right', as the archaic expression has it, regains its once lost or moribund impetus when we begin to feel that no one 'really cares' about our state of health or mind. But health care personnel of all stripes and statuses also feel this to a great degree. After all, they are constantly immersed in the settings that have an alienating quality about them. Even the most mundane tasks can effect not only performance of duties but the general sensibility that one is actually doing anything worthwhile. Speaking the rationalized spaces of instrument tray preparation, Torrance remarks, "Here, too, despite the nursing backgrounds of the staff, it was easy to lose sight of the wider mission of the hospital and to develop a sense of isolation and alienation" (1987, 493). Indeed, tools of even the most outlandish kind and about which the broadest claims have been made seemed to be bereft of therapeutic ken when considered as standalone techniques. Westlake relates that even Reich's notorious Orgone accumulator failed him, but worked wonders when used as a 'psychological technique' (op. cit., 43). Yet the handheld version of the Orgone mechanism, which apparently 'shot' doses at close range on the affected parts of patients had also excellent results (ibid, 44), suggesting that the human interplay and even human touch and handling had a great deal to do with its psychosomatic successes, whatever else may have been going on.

Human intimacy is believed to have a healing force that almost anyone can both heal and be healed with. Here, the elements of both the least scientific of the conventional discourses and the most verifiable of those unconventional meet. It is so well-evidenced that human community, even of the professional and yet further, sterile, kind, exerts a broad-band suasion over any of us who have fallen ill. 'Fallen' should be taken in the existential sense, as one has fallen out of the specific human ambit wherein one finds a home. Intimacy includes that sexual or erotic, but it is more the sensuality of being-with that is of the healing variety. 'Sex therapy' aside, that the sensual is included within the domain of general sexuality as a discourse is a clue to how we both desire and actually need this kind of close human community. Any touch, short of caress, that one is subject to as a patient is welcome in some way. Even the firm handling of our dropsy forms, depending upon on our condition at the time, allows us not only to feel cared for, but though an object or in an objectified state, we will still be handled with some care and attentiveness. This is the other side to the discursive analysis of power relations cleaving to sexuality proper; that we can be objectified in a manner that 'feels good' for us. This irony is testament to the vast utility of sexuality as a psychosomatic form: "Sexuality is not the most intractable element in power relations, but rather one of those endowed with the greatest instrumentality: useful for the greatest number of maneuvers ..." (Foucault 1980, 103). Is it a surprise then, that the 'nurse' figure has been so highly sexualized in Western popular culture. There are male nurses, of course, but they are still met with some suspicion. Their sexuality is ill-defined and indeed, we might well see them attached to the space of disease rather than to that of health. But the Florence Nightingale—and such a surname could only propel the fable of the sensual and caring angel of health, her sweet and sophisticated song *enough* for the desiring senses—apical ancestress of modern nursing could only be an augur of health. The nurse combines the physical energy that the job actually demands with the femininity that our culture associates with rejuvenescence. Youth harnesses both to itself; strength and love. Only the schoolgirl is more fetishized as a sexual object and only because she is slightly taboo with regard to relative age and social position but more importantly, because she has not the concernful and maternal demeanour of the nurse. The schoolgirl cannot nurture, only tempt.

4.3.3 Holistic Summaries

To combine effectively the idea of nurturing and sensuality while avoiding the sense that one is being led on in any ulterior manner is the key to the gradual but growing success of homeopathic practices. It has long been noted that in the human realm, science is limited by its object realm. That is, humans do not have the same kind of being as do other things in the world or in nature, and thus science itself is seen to be limited in the amount it can glean from their study. For decades, from Mill and Dilthey onward, the reason for this limitation was assumed to be the problem of simple mimicry; the human sciences desired to base their future success on the demonstrated triumph of the natural sciences, but of course they did not measure up to these latter in their results: "Another reason for the failure lies in the very nature of the slavish imitation of physical science by psychosocial scholars" (Sorokin 1956, 175). Not merely at the level of discourse, then, but also in the training and expectations, the methods and publications of the students involved in aping the sciences of nature contributed directly to the folly to which humanists of all kinds called attention. Aside from reductionism, which is also a charge still regularly leveled at the behavioral sciences and those hybrid disciplines such as cognitive science, there is the claim that whatever consciousness is made up of, it itself is not made but always rather in the making. Once again, we are confronted with the aspiration of homeopathic medicine to the 'whole' of things, in which one finds the truth. The 'life force' which serves as the objectifying principle and the replacement for 'spirit' in alternative therapies is the *only* manner in which the holistic balance that disease has altered can be regained: "It is very evident that with this power we are dealing with something which heals the *whole* man …" (Westlake 1973, 107, italics in the original). This healing is not subjective. It is, in the final analysis, not even about returning this or that patient to personhood or the curing of disease, but of the revelation that unites opposites and resolves tensions amongst competing cosmological claims: "Sooner or later nuclear physics and the psychology of the unconscious will draw closer together as both of them, independently of one another and from opposite directions, push forward into transcendental territory …" (Jung 1959, 261). Jung states that the 'analogy with physics is not a digression', and that the physical sciences also seek to unite enantiodromian phenomena. Since all of science is a human endeavor, it is argued that its results should not only be favourable to the psyche of humankind but also that its methods be fully participant in the *Mitsein* that living beings have with their own histories.

These are grand goals. Part of the rhetorical force that emanates from alternative health practices is that their ultimate purpose retains the missionary zeal of former days. When rationalized institutions unveil 'mission statements' there may be applause and genuflection of various kinds, but never awe. No matter its content, such institutional missions have only the power to surprise and impress. Haas and Shaffir relate how one Canadian university's medical program departs radically from the usual training procedures, including no formal exams (cf. 1987, 400ff). But these practices, however enlightened, remain in the space of both the ontic and can possess only technical or logistical means. Homeopathy from the start states baldly that one's health is a matter of little consequence if we cannot ourselves be redefined in terms of existential experiences, much like Jung's statements regarding the experiential character of knowledge relating to the collective unconscious, such as the shadow archetype or syzygy (cf. op. cit., 33–34). In fact these ideas cannot be related conceptually or reported on discursively, but affirms that "Wherever my methods were really applied the facts I give have been confirmed" (ibid, 33). Needless to say, models such as Jung's, working as it does within the assumptions of cosmological holism, are a challenge for conventional discourses to fathom, though we know full well about the power of symbols in social and political life: "This was why Jung proposed that psychology should enlarge itself to deal adequately with these wider territories. Since his day, however, academic psychologists have systematically resisted such suggestions, seeking instead to construct their discipline so as to look more like a physical science" (Midgely 2004, 42). Such a macro point of view has its corresponding micro action. At the level of discourse the producers of culture—and science is obviously as much a product of our culture as is our art—are generally as resistant to innovation as is the society culture for which they produce. But though this is a hoary chestnut, it cannot be taken entirely at face value. Nietzsche, Gide, Sapir and The Sex Pistols, to set up a wide band of cultural rebels, were not merely innovators in the general sense. They were critics, some much more sophisticated than others, needless to say, but nevertheless their original marginality and then their subsequent and ironic fame came not from the fact that they produced something new, but that it was somehow threatening to what was already there. This is the case in a profound way with a figure like Jung. But to simply state that Jung's ideas are resisted is only half the story here. At the level of social interaction there occurs all of the actual and actuating resistance that lends itself to defending the discursive pickets with regard to who and what has the authority to make claims about and suggest treatments for disease. In the clinical space, patients are encouraged to 'participate', but only to a point: "… the optimal outcome would be that patients could use their knowledge as a basis for asking non-threatening and intelligent questions, and to work with providers as partners towards the common goal of improved health outcomes" (Frankel, Speechley, and Wade 1996, 194). Indeed, with regard to institutions and formal processes of education in general, 'intelligent' is almost to be equated with 'non-threatening'. Those on the margins who *do* threaten are the first to be branded with the label of unintelligent, whether in philosophy or popular music. Remuneration, first in terms of status points, gilt awards, and the absence of guilt, and then in terms of lifetime earnings and benefits, those who conform to any system of standards and knowledge will be the most successful. This is so well known that instead of the cynicism one might expect it to breed, we have instead seen a massive rise in the level of pragmatism amongst students of all stripes and inclinations, including those in the health care field who have in fact always been at the forefront of such practicality. Those now vintage 'Boys In White' remain the archetypical ethnographic exemplars of this reaction.

But there is a cost to overt pragmatism: "The physician as 'crude pragmatist' tends to try things out in an overly optimistic manner [ ] Hence, there is the considerable literature in the medical journals on the dubious use or overuse of particular interventions" (Evans 1987, 627). Innovators are sometimes drawn into the pragmatic atmosphere as well. Jung himself is a notorious example of this, with his use of corporal correction on a patient recently celebrated in a popular feature film. Such an 'intervention' would have been deemed commonplace enough in his time, though his mentor, Freud, was very critical of it on ethical grounds. Today, of course, such 'therapies' only occur in the even more marginal spaces of professional discipline, only amongst adults—unless one includes the yet more dubious and indeed criminal use of physical coercion in the 'boot camps' a few desperate and irresponsible Americans send their teenagers to in order to make them 'healthy' again—and generally advertised as part of the sexual theatre of the internet. Freud's concern that punishment of any kind was a displaced and therefore risky eroticism is well taken here and remains in our day an important critical viewpoint. Nations that have outlawed such forms of 'discipline' have done so partly on his grounds. It is no surprise that the United States lags sorely behind in this area, given the Puritanical and sexually repressed background of much of its cultural immigration, right from the beginning of European contact. This is but one example of intervening with the most convenient and simplest method and then checking results over time. From authoritarian parents to Bruno Bettelheim, it is safe to say that the presence of unthought drives an aspect of these kinds of reactions to what is judged to be indiscipline amongst youth and perhaps some adults as well. What is clear is that just as intelligence is equated with conformity, maturity with the defense of norms, so is health equated with both of these in addition to disciplined self-care and the ability to question only in support of recognized and conventional authorities.

So cynicism, rampant enough in training and for a time, the chief competitor to pragmatism, is gradually brought under control by sentiment and rationalization (cf. Shem's many dialogues concerning this transition, for example 1978, 148ff and the bald opening statement regarding the difference between sex and love on page 4). The outcome of this kind of self-discipline, after the goal of learning self-discipline itself is attained, is called professionalism: "Doctors are assumed to be persons who can transcend the pressures, emotional or otherwise, of life-and-death situations and act competently and coolly, yet they must do so in the face of the most provocative of human feelings" (Haas and Shaffir 1987, 406). No doubt this takes its toll in burn out issues over time. Doctors with whom I spoke said this was the greatest threat to their careers longevity but also to their sense of self. Not unlike combat veterans, physicians and other staffers are, if not constantly at least consistently interacting with fellow humans in crisis. The melodramas of entertainment fiction hyperbolize these scenes for plot purposes, but there is nonetheless a grain of truth in them. In the setting of his popular novel, Shem uses the grind rather than the crisis to propel his story, and the reactions of readers who are themselves doctors is well-documented, focusing on the 'realism' of Shem's portrayal. For it is the grind rather than the out and out crisis that wears one down. Indeed, one of the more cynical desires that develops amongst those undergoing this grind is the hope that a crisis will suddenly develop, once again, not at all unlike soldiers in war-time where most of their day is spent *waiting* to kill or die rather than actually doing it.

If it is correct to state that "The bond that attaches us to the life outside ourselves is the same bond that hold us to our own" (Barrett 1979, 320), then the suffering of others will 'get to' us given enough time. It is more than the case of 'what comes around goes around' or, in an older guise, 'one reaps what one sows'. For it must also confront the problem of truth in itself: "Physicians can no more prove the worth of their art to themselves than they can to others" (Gadamer 1996, 33 [1967]). Fate and art stand alongside one another, Gadamer maintains, hence the Greek sentiment that 'Tyche loves Techne'. Any defense of any kind of healing whatsoever, conventional or alternative, can only rest its case in how the person healed feels about his or her healing, and whether or not they can recall the difference between health and sickness as a mode of being in the world as well as the demonstration of an ethics.

4.4 Critical Actions

If life is for the living, then an intellectual life could be construed as the most unhealthy form of living. It surpasses what is lived through its focus on what is not alive. Yet it remains our major source of critiques in all its forms. This Socratic penchant runs like an amber thread through the tapestry of Western consciousness, and indeed, pre-dating Plato by some few generations, may be said to be the first authentic moment of *thought* in our culture. Before this existed myth alone.

Not that primordial symbolic systems are manifestations of 'unthought'—*this* form of life, sometimes anti-intellectual but also and more importantly anti-living in its conservative and conformitarian tendencies is peculiarly associated with our own modern society—but rather they participate in a source of thinking that places thought squarely in an imagination dominated by the unconscious. Though we have not completely forsaken this source—and mythologists, especially of the Jungian variety, warn us against doing so—it is certainly muted in our day.

4.4.1 Delusions

But the real danger is not so much the utter ignorance of the symbolic life, for it surfaces in our psyche in any case and we must ultimately confront it with our deaths, but our general indifference to it as a form of explanation for aspects of the human condition: "What is preposterous is the suggestion that we ought to disregard altogether the terms that can figure in the non-explanatory contexts of living for the purposes of our explanatory theory" (Taylor 1989, 58). Given that, as Taylor is wont to suggest, we judge other's actions within the ambit of what we also judge to be the best case. The overlap of a culture's values, however metaphysically inclined or no, do impinge upon our subjectivity as it relates to how and even how often we must deal with 'the others'. When we are suffering, whatever the health condition contains as both its source, vector, manifestation and diagnosis, its moral force, as we have stated, carries us into the arms of precisely the others by whom we are judged. The 'best case' for us as a subject is to 'get better quickly'. This is not always possible in reality, and ultimately it is impossible. But the symbolic language, though deteriorated into sentiment and the etiquette of get well cards and bouquets of condolences, resonates in both our aspirations and our anxieties. Illness brings both of these human passions to the fore. It is one thing to reduce both disease and the person to a confluence of symptomatologies, but it is quite another to claim that what is going on, either subjectively or socially, is also merely a function of technique and technicality. This form of reduction frames the class of delusions that we will briefly investigate with regard to how the alternative discourses of health and illness attempt to critique those conventional along these same lines.

If it is somewhat abstract to be concerned about the place of metaphysics in modern life, however much the self may be sourced in them, there is another level of life where the living self must confront the problem of an objectivity apparently bereft, not of metaphysics, values or symbols, but precisely of the stuff that makes up human selfhood. More than this, such an objectifying stance seems to pick and choose which aspects of the human condition are to be deemed relevant and 'operational': "What is really worrying at present is the impression many people have that the revulsion is somehow more scientific than the affection or respect" (Midgely 2004, 148). Similarly, whether it is our relationship with animal life or the wider nature that contains both this and our unique form of being, the 'mastery over beings' that technology in general allows for also increase the distance between form of Being and thus contributes to our ignorance of the ontological in particular (cf. Barrett 1979, xx). Technology looks like 'the pure servant of freedom', but the question we must ask of it—this is both an ethical and a phenomenological question—is how much does it affect our understanding of human freedom vis-à-vis our confrontation with finitude? We have already discussed how futurist oriented technology and perhaps also technocracy avoid the question of mortality and seek to overcome the very need for asking it. Death is reacted to by revulsion, and it is this revulsion, shared with our enduring, and purely symbolic, sense that we *cannot* be kindred to animal life, that impels and compels our headlong flight from it. This fleeing in the face of human freedom is a leitmotif of existentialist analytics, but within the arena of health and illness it is much less abstract. Here, people can actually feel its suasion, the push and pull of whether or not I am going to sicken and die. The existentialist argument fails to move precisely because it never moves in the direction of how life is actually lived. People manifestly do *not* walk around worrying about their own deaths. Finances, family, jobs and to a certain extent, health, are what occupy most people's minds in the day to day. If these concerns are ontic and thus ethically inauthentic it is not disparaging to suggest they consist of reality nonetheless. Their instrumental quality is the mirage, and it is a delusion in fact to imagine that they are somehow wanting in their awareness of freedom. No, freedom, if not to be found directly within their embrace, is 'served' by the concernful, or 'circumspective' being with which we approach them. The 'demands of the day' are our true ethical duty, as Goethe stated.

'Deontic facticity' could describe the class of events that are both mundane and concernfully circumspect with regard to ontology yet without being otiose. Health and illness fall into this category of phenomena. Their expression is one of the day to day, but their expressiveness is one of finitude. It is quintessentially human to partake in both at one, and the ontic realm cannot simply and neatly be cast as a discretely defined division distancing itself irrevocably from the ontological. There is a third kind of grounding for Dasein in the world. This is why medicine is the 'sacred science', and why circumspection seeks to both avoid and confront the ipssissimosity of finitude. Here we are not interested in the 'cause' of disease, but in the source of illness. We are not moved by the therapies that may return us to health, but by the return itself. *This* is what must be understood: "The notion that a disease can be explained by a variety of causes is precisely characteristic of thinking about disease whose causation is *not* understood" (Sontag 1978, 60, italics in the original). Shem speaks to this when the protagonist's mentor states that it is the iatrogenic relationship that is the real cause of illness, the 'cure is the disease'. (cf. Shem 1978, 183–4). The doctor's own illness is what is, in effect, transferred to the patient. Just as Nietzsche artfully noted that we cannot escape seeking a 'doer for every deed', medical discourse of the conventional variety makes it its true study to parse out the doers at the most miniscule level. Homeopathy does not neglect this bit of 'moralic acid', but it pins its perpetrators high in an overcast sky.

4.4.2 Explications

Like the abstraction of being concerned with the place of metaphysics in modern life, alternative medicine abstracts the causality of illness itself, thus allowing the person to overlook its effects, as if one were having an out-of-body experience. The question that animates all who enter either the conventional clinic or the studio of the alternative is 'what is happening *to me*?', and never so much simply '*what* is happening?' The latter question is the one the physician asks and follows through on. It is the scientific question and however nominated to the forefront by revulsion—in most cases this kind of emotional reaction is not to be considered 'scientific' and must be at least professionally disguised, as we have seen above—it must be treated systematically and probabilistically. The iatrogenetic relationship that occurs is one in which the patient loses sight of his or her ownmost owning of what ails them. But just here the doctor is assuming he is doing me a favor by 'taking over', just as the nurse may later on take over for the doctor, and finally, we receive ourselves as a return on our investment in the institutional process of treatment and cure. But this aspect of circumspective facticity has its 're-ontic' uptake in the separation between what is afflicting us and our affliction. This is why health care appears to be strictly ontic, and thus inauthentic existentially, to the analyst: "Ultimately, both disturbance and the overcoming of disturbance belong together. This fact is constitutive of life itself. And it is this which places a critical limit on the concept of treatment" (Gadamer 1996, 136 [1989]). Given that "… more and more people are killed by disease-producers which cannot be eliminated by the methods of classic medicine" (Selye 1956, 275), and that these sources include those taken as 'the cure' for disease, overcoming ailment, however psychologically connoted or no, remains part of my ownmost capability, and thus it never enters fully into the ontic realm. It itself is overfull with the deontic facticity of living on in the face of that which *does not feel like a life worth living*. It is our ethical pronouncement upon this form of life that links it back inextricably with the authenticity of ontology. It is the manner in which beings reconnect themselves with their Being. It is both ownmost and utmost.

So it is *not* in fact the confrontation with death itself and alone that is crucial to an ontological prescription for good health. Rather, it is our realization that illness destroys our quality of life *as lived*, that is, a confrontation with life that must be reckoned with and whose understanding must become an intimate form of self-understanding: "Thus, in this sense, there is only one disease. [ ] and no disease can be cured unless the balance is restored" (Westlake 1973, 118). In the existential sense, non-existence is merely the outcome of inexistence. Generally, and 'historically', one would favour the term 'inexistence' to refer to something that has not yet occurred or a form of being not yet been, as in the God concept when viewed from pre-agrarian symbolic systems. But just here, where existence meets its match while still living, inexistence appears as the death concept, and not 'drive', not yet extant. For death has its own form of being that we refer to as not-being rather than non-being, which, once again, is the existential equivalent of something historically or cultural inexistent or non-existent, depending on whether or not a specific form that might be imagined by a sole mind in isolation ever takes root in a society or leaves a trace for those to come. *Disease therefore is the inexistence of death.*

This relationship which permeates human consciousness does so by virtue of our modern and 'progressive' or evolutionary understanding of culture, if not the species *per se*: "… consciousness as the acting center precedes consciousness as the cognitive center, in the same way ritual precedes myth, or magic ceremonial and ethical action precede the scientific view of the world and anthropological knowledge" (Neumann 1970, 126 [1949]). The most salient characteristic of this relationship of precedence and gradual objectifying of the world and of the self is that the more densely imbricated the dynamic between what is conscious and what is unconscious in culture and in the person the less one can separate act and thought by observation alone, especially because, in this sense, all observation is self-observation: "Between the conscious and the unconscious there is a kind of 'uncertainty relationship', because the observer is inseparable from the observed and always disturbs it by the act of observation" (Jung 1959, 226). The unconscious however, cannot be said to be typically 'inexistent'. It exists, if as an objective shadow, a form of para-being which is neither fully observable in any epistemological sense nor fully culpable in that ethical. The 'devil', then, cannot be said to have 'made us do it'. Yet illness *can* be spoken of in this manner. 'It' makes us do all kinds of things we would not otherwise do, feel, or think. Illness afflicts both the conscious and the unconscious at once. The content and messages of our dream-language alters when we are seriously ill. The level of anxiety and the number of warnings reach ever new heights unless or until we recover. After the fact of the objective disease, we must then also recover our subjective equanimity. This process, which is often viewed as secondary by conventional medicine, can take far longer than the initial ridding of the physical illness. That alternative medicine both favors and thus concentrates upon this second phase of recovery also remarks upon it as being qualitatively different in viewpoint from 'allopathy'. At the same time, it is equally clear that homeopathic remedies from the beginning concentrate on the recovery of the 'whole' person, as we have already seen, and thus allow themselves the appropriate scope and indeed vagueness to work successfully for many simply because of the lack of definition of what is 'actually' going on. In other words, the observer effect of which Jung speaks is an active and necessary dynamic within alternative health regimes. That which is to be sidelined or even expunged, treated as non-existent, in mainstream medical processes and treatments is something to be used as the most important tool in those alternative. It is regarded as once extant and thus existent, but regressed into inexistence by an illness which is itself death inexistent. Phenomenologically, it is through this dynamic that we become aware of our own existence and that it is suffering from an indigency of inexistence on two fronts, that of both life and death. Here, life acts as the crucible of death, the womb for the tomb, as it were. In doing so, in hosting the pre-natality of what is always to be still-born—and, if one overcomes the illness and recovers, that which is to be *still* born and also that which cannot ultimately be stilled as an existential qualifier—life itself must retreat into an inexistence of its own. Disease may thus be defined existentially as *the presence of two forms of inexistence*, one of life and the other of death. When we experience the discomfort, suffering and pain of being ill, both unconsciously and consciously, it is our balance of consciousness as a whole that is not so much imbalanced, as homeopathy patently has it, but placed on another set of scales entirely: "In our normal dealings with things, we disregard this dimension of experience and focus on the things experienced" (Taylor 1989, 130). Neither aspect of consciousness as living can be experienced now as simply a thing. It is, rather, a thing removed or transformed. It is not itself transformed by disease *per se*, but by our experience of being placed in a state of existential evaluation. We may not have the shudder of the premonition of death, one folkloric expression being 'someone just walked over your grave'. What we do experience is the absence of the life that we thought our ownmost and that could not be taken away from us. Yet we live on. It is this paradox that for the time being disables normative experience and transfers our focus from 'things experienced' to experience *as* a thing.

And once within the envelope of inexistent existing we quickly become aware that this may over time become a do or die situation. Just as doctors cannot cure 'things' by themselves—as Gadamer states, 'it is nature that they help to victory' (1996, 89 [1987])—we also act within precise limits, of late constructed even more by the presence of illness and its effects. To help 'nature' recover its balance or yet its existence, we first must respond to the question, 'what is our nature?' To do this requires of us not merely a new self-understanding not limited by what we have mourned as suddenly absent or gradually deteriorating, but also an objective glancing into the heart of the matter: what is it that we desire of ourselves to be?, what is our mode of being whose expression is life? The worldliness of this being, its being-there, its being-with, and its concernful circumspection all contribute to this new agency, at first but a memory called to arms. Even if we incorrectly pursue the dream that equates recovery with replication rather than resurrection, this misunderstanding of selfhood as Dasein soon passes. Indeed, our realization that we cannot return to such a state places this idea squarely within the same plot as the sense that we cannot lie in-state. In this, we recapitulate as subjects within the form of subjection known as illness the manner in which medicine must function with regard to an objective nature: "It is this which characterizes the unique position of medicine within human science as a whole" (ibid). At the personal level, this is the process that characterizes growth and the gradual maturity of our consciousness. Shem notes acerbically through the voice of the protagonist's spouse that interns perform the exact opposite relation in order to escape the confrontation with objective death and dying (1978, 283–4). In his novel, this figure acts as the conscience to the hero's consciousness precisely because, in denying the day to day dynamic of health care and what it means to those who lie this side or that side of its curative capabilities and limitations, the hero's subjectivity is forced into inexistence. In order to treat those who must die and those one cannot save, one must kill one's own self first.

This is not, in the final analysis, a form of subjectivity to be narrated and made the object of high romance and hero-quest. Its coincidence with the inexistence of death appearing as a gestating form in life—in this, death is never 'alongside' us as are other kinds of objects or forms of being; as Heidegger iterates, it is rather held within the ownmost and utmost possibility of each of us—subsequently surfaces in objective social organizations and their relations with their clientele, the layperson as struck dumb by patient-hood. To recover from this, one must extricate oneself not only from an existential limitation, however long or short term, but also from the sense that the doctor does cure and that his tools are fallible but yet intentionally pure. The ramifications related to this recovery are much larger than medicine alone: "The medicalization of early diagnosis not only hampers and discourages preventative health-care but it also trains the patient-to-be to in the meantime as an acolyte to his doctor. [ ] He turns into a life-long patient" (Illich 1975, 30). Just as neither health nor its return is something 'made' by the doctor and his technological artifice, "The goal of health is not a condition that is clearly definable from within the medical art. For illness is a social state of affairs" (Gadamer 1996, 20 [1967]). And just as the social produces its own problems so we can look to it to recover its general health through other processes which are equally internal to its function and its art.

4.4.3 Solutions?

Such recoveries are objective in the sense that they can be measured as are the variables for indices such as the world quality of life lists. The original idea of the 'social fact' resurfaces in such lists, for it is the *rate* of incidence of this or that illness or illness vector, social context that contributes to risk or outright endangerment, and legal codes which are punitive to victims of crime rather than perpetrators that are compiled. The legalization of prostitution in Australia, for example, was a significant example of 'recovery' that vaulted this country ahead of others very similar to it, such as Canada, in the overall quality of life rankings. Further, policies and programs which highlight a community's ability to engage in mutual and cooperative efforts, health related or otherwise, also seem to be important for these measures: "Only people who have recovered the ability for mutual self-care by the application of contemporary technology will be ready to limit the industrial mode of production in other major areas as well" (Illich 1975, 11). These cannot, of course, be merely cost-cutting compulsions. There is, one might venture to say, a homeopathic balance to be struck within the social body. This kind of characterization verges on a form of fascism, recalling the 'body of the Volk' and other such nonsense. Yet all modern nation states participate in versions of 'neo Nazi' behavior and subsequent social policy. However subtle or camouflaged, the ideas hold within them a Janus; on the one hand, in large mass societies we must indeed think of the whole and put it before special interests. For example, the back-burner but still tepid threat of nuclear annihilation brooks no special interest. But the sense that the individual is suddenly non-responsible for his or her being in the world, that rational organizations and the state can take over every need and every desire is, on the other hand, the very meaning of fascism.

So a 'homeopathy' of society must tread a tight-rope here. There are a myriad of examples of this balancing act in the health arena alone: "If a reduction in services in expensive institutions and those delivered by more expensive professionals does not follow an increase in non-traditional services, then the economic benefits of substitution are unlikely to be realized" (Frankel, Speechley, and Wade 1996, 200). There is the ever-present danger of myth-making that runs alongside, like a shot-gun shadow, any attempt at community making where none ever existed. 'Reduction' in the sense of cutting back may also be read as a form of reductionism; that is, breaking health care down to its elemental subjectivities and then naming it 'preventative'. Where does the knowledge come from that allows individuals to take care of themselves in such a way? We are liable to become libelled for this kind of ruse simply due to the way narrative functions in our society and history: "Often, for instance, a story will pivot on a moment of revelation or truth, and in the talismanic importance attached to 'extraordinary coincidence' and 'pluck' it is possible to discern, concealed as in a memory trace, ideas of destiny and fate, a hidden hand guiding the subject forward" (Samuel and Thompson 1990a, 10). Aside from both the market and the state, two not so hidden hands that impel us, indeed, often compel us toward specifically calculated goals that are not of our own making, the subjectivity of memorialization at the biographical level finds itself fighting a two-front conflict. At once it must defend its 'privacy'—the territory of selfhood in general—and at the same time gain knowledge through much larger and thus more socially 'objective' sources—the authority of institutions and discourses, including most importantly, those health related. We have to become professionalized in a manner not unlike the doctor. We must trade hearing for listening, fixation for raptness, but also seeing for the gaze: "In the clinician's catalogue, the purity of the gaze is bound up with a certain silence that enables him to listen" (Foucault 1973, 107). This silence is 'certain' in at least two ways: it is particular, even peculiar, and this is its 'certainty' in the literary sense. But it is also certain in the veridical sense; it has its sureness of footing, its certainty invested in its ability to hear something that others cannot. Since it is silent, we might assume that it cannot communicate. But silence is its own language, its expressiveness is dominated by what we feel to be most sure about our experience and thus our judgments that follow hardest on their heels: "There at the center of the will—where the decision to live or not to live takes place—we are below the level of articulate reasons and rational persuasion" (Barrett 1979, 315). This is not necessarily a bad thing. Language is used just as much to manipulate as to clarify. A certain silence might behoove us in specific contexts. The observer effect here is one of making things more clear. It stands back and may even become dispassionate. Never to the point of misanthrope, which itself 'articulates' a certain passion, that of *ressentiment* turned inward. I wish to replace *myself* with something or someone else, though I am uncertain as to the precise location of either. It is malicious inexistential envy, so to speak. Hence being silent, by either edict or *ad hoc* demand, could also become the fate of an addict dedicated to following his passions in a disinterested manner. For it this ensuite of the passionate, another shadowy presence which does not follow us but rather leads us on in no particular direction for its moral compass is studiously absent. Following from this, our ability to interpret falls by the wayside, not to be recovered because, in its serpentine and malingering course, there is no 'memory trace' to 'guide' us back out of the labyrinth: "… interpreting is itself a possible and distinctive how of the character of being of facticity. Interpreting is a being which belongs to the being of factical life itself" (Heidegger 1999, 12). To step back from this is to rejoin society, if not community. Society may itself be an aspect of what is 'fallen', but it is also a 'how' of Dasein. The "… definite and average state of understanding …" which characterizes the 'every-one' of the how in which the lifeworld worlds itself is a half-way house for existentialist analytics, to be sure. But it does have the unqualified merit of bringing us out of ourselves. Health depends on this clarification: we cannot be said to know our own health from personal experience alone. Both ideas and facts concerning the meaning of health as well as 'unhealth', come from not only the reductive statistics that are the concern of homeopathic practitioners but those self-same numeric measures that emanate from data that includes 'everyone'. Everyone is therefore no one, but this is not always fatal to the self. After all, the self too is no *one*, it is rather, itself, and just as its death is in every case its own, so too is its life.

It is by virtue of living on in the face of life and not death, as we have seen, that one acquires both the ideas and the facts to buttress one's experiences and feelings. One *does* perform a self-diagnostic before one enters the clinic. One *does* prevent certain risks to health by how one lives prior to receiving the 'wisdom of the doctor'. Sometimes it is, of course, not enough. But it is never found wanting because the 'how' of its being in the world is overly participating in the fallenness of rational onticity. The distractions of 'Das Man' hold within them the clues for human freedom. One of the most salient of these is the realization that forms of life, including that of health, do not reside somewhere other than within the consciousness of selfhood and its extensions and intentions; community, concernfulness, circumspection, for instance. And these extend to the forms of life themselves: "… it is nonsense to believe that the world of ideas is only for the gods and the world of facts is only for mortals" (Gadamer 1998, 58). This statement that hails from Parmenides is sometimes seen as the beginning of the critique of the critical distances that lie between human beings and their respective cultures. The metaphor of transcendence provides a rhetorical force that merely acknowledging cultural difference does not have, unless we go too far and imagine that cultures are fundamentally irreconcilable. 'Keeping it unreal' here has a salutary effect, though it must be admitted immediately that this tactic is rarely positive, and for good reason. The inequalities and inequities, the one factual and the other ideal, the one material and the other ethical, combine to do us the united disservice of finding ourselves without a home in the world and, through the suffering of illness, also finding ourselves absent from the home that we carry around with us no matter where we are. The verve for equality in human relations is something that has been historically revived from primordial humanity. Our version of it is very recent, and within the health care fields, it is homeopathy that attempts to reinsert it as a term in the equation of health.

Though it can be critiqued for its 'talking' cures, the psychiatric margins of behavioristic discourses within conventional health care are also attempts to acknowledge the humaneness of the endeavor which is health: "Dialogue and discussion serve to humanize the fundamentally unequal relationship that prevails between doctor and patient. Such unequal relationships represent one of the most difficult challenges which confront us as human beings" (Gadamer 1996, 112 [1991]). There could well be a 'diagnostics' of such dialogues, an analysis of how the inequality present within the clinical context is transposed to another world via the ascension ascribed to the forces which in their own way 'represent' another fundamental human challenge. But inequality is of this world. It is inequity that confronts us in an onto-theological manner, emanating as it does from our imagination of the other world, that of suasions and forms of being that lie beyond the scientific ambit. That homeopathy maintains the resonance of the symbolic life in modern medicine thus cuts both ways: at once it humanizes and revives the faith necessary for beings whose consciousness is neither prescient nor indefinite but by the same token it can foster a re-mythology of health which is detrimental for both faith and for humanity. Either way, it remains an authentic status of deontic Dasein to cleave to first the one and then the other, for this dynamic pushes us to make a decision that is either forward-looking and hopeful while not losing its critical edge or to regress into nostalgia with its always inauthentic selvedge in hand. In making this decision, we are forced to confront one final limit concerning human consciousness: "One can only study what one has first dreamed about. Science is formed rather on a reverie than on an experiment, and it takes a good many experiments to dispel the mists of the dream" (Bachelard 1964, 22 [1938]).

References

Bachelard, Gaston. 1964. *The Psychoanalysis of Fire.* Boston: Beacon Press [1938].

Barrett, William. 1979. *The Illusion of Technique: A Search for Meaning in a Technological Civilization.* New York: Anchors Books.

Derrida, Jacques. 1995. *On the Name.* Stanford: Stanford University Press [1993].

Evans, Robert G. 1987. "Illusions of Necessity: Evading Responsibility for Choice in Health Care." In *Health and Canadian Society: Sociological Perspectives, Second Edition*, edited by George Torrance, 615–36. Toronto: Fitzhenry and Whiteside.

Foucault, Michel. 1973. *The Birth of the Clinic.* New York: Vintage Books [1963].

Foucault, Michel. 1980. *The History of Sexuality Volume One: Introduction.* New York: Vintage Books [1978].

Frankel, B. Gail, Mark Speechley, and Terrance J. Wade. 1996. *The Sociology of Health and Health Care: A Canadian Perspective.* Toronto: Copp Clark.

Gadamer, Hans-Georg. 1967. "Apologia for the Art of Healing." In *The Enigma of Health: The Art of Healing in a Scientific Age*, 31–44. Stanford: Stanford University Press [1996].

Gadamer, Hans-Georg. 1972. "Theory, Technology, Praxis." In *The Enigma of Health: The Art of Healing in a Scientific Age*, 1–30. Stanford: Stanford University Press [1996].

Gadamer, Hans-Georg. 1987. "Between Nature and Art." In *The Enigma of Health: The Art of Healing in a Scientific Age*, 83–91. Stanford: Stanford University Press [1996].

Gadamer, Hans-Georg. 1989. "Hermeneutics and Psychiatry." In *The Enigma of Health: The Art of Healing in a Scientific Age*, 163–73. Stanford: Stanford University Press [1996].

Gadamer, Hans-Georg. 1991. "On the Enigmatic Character of Health." In *The Enigma of Health: The Art of Healing in a Scientific Age*, 103–116. Stanford: Stanford University Press [1996].

Gadamer, Hans-Georg. 1998. *The Beginning of Philosophy.* New York: Continuum [1996].

Haas, Jack, and William Shaffir. 1987. "Taking on the Role of Doctor." In *Health and Canadian Society: Sociological Perspectives, Second Edition*, edited by George Torrance, 399–421. Toronto: Fitzhenry and Whiteside.

Harding, Jim. 1987. "The Pharmaceutical Industry as a Public-Health Hazard and as an Institution of Social Control." In *Health and Canadian Society: Sociological Perspectives, Second Edition*, edited by George Torrance, 545–67. Toronto: Fitzhenry and Whiteside.

Heidegger, Martin. 1999. *Ontology—The Hermeneutics of Facticity.* Bloomington: Indiana University Press [1988].

Illich, Ivan. 1975. *Medical Nemesis: The Expropriation of Health.* Toronto: McClelland and Stewart.

Jung, Carl G. 1959. *Aion: Researches into the Phenomenology of the Self.* Princeton, NJ: Princeton University Press [1951].

Kelleher, David, Jonathan Gabe, and Gareth Williams. 1994a. "Understanding Medical Dominance in the Modern World." In *Challenging Medicine*, edited by Jonathan Gabe, David Kelleher and Gareth Williams, xi–xxix. London: Routledge.

Lingis, Alphonso. 1989. *Deathbound Subjectivity.* Bloomington: Indiana University Press.

Lösch, August. 1967. *The Economics of Location.* New York: Wiley Science Editions, John Wiley and Sons [1945].

Midgely, Mary. 2004. *The Myths We Live By.* London: Routledge.

Natanson, Maurice. 1970. *The Journeying Self: A Study in Philosophy and Social Role.* Reading, MA: Addison-Wesley Publishing Company.

Neumann, Erich. 1970. *The Origins and History of Consciousness.* Princeton, NJ: Princeton University Press [1949].

Peneff, Jean. 1990. "Myths in Life Stores." In *The Myths We Live By,* edited by Raphael Samuel and Paul Thompson, 36–48. London: Routledge.

Saks, Mike. 1994. "The Alternatives to Medicine." In *Challenging Medicine*, edited by Jonathan Gabe, David Kelleher and Gareth Williams, 84–103. London: Routledge.

Samuel, Raphael, and Paul Thompson, eds. 1990a. *The Myths We Live By.* London: Routledge.

Samuel, Raphael, and Paul Thompson, eds. 1990b. "Introduction." In *The Myths We Live By,* edited by Raphael Samuel and Paul Thompson, 1–22. London: Routledge.

Scambler, Graham. 1982. "Illness Behaviour." In *Sociology as Applied to Medicine*, edited by Donald L. Patrick and Graham Scambler, 43–55. Bailliére's Concise Medical Textbooks. London: Bailliére Tindall.

Selye, Hans. 1956. *The Stress of Life: A New Theory of Disease.* New York: McGraw-Hill.

Shem, Samuel. 1978. *The House of God.* New York: Berkley Books.

Sontag, Susan. 1978. *Illness as Metaphor.* New York: Vintage Books.

Sorokin, Pitirim. 1956. *Fads and Foibles in Modern Sociology and Related Sciences.* Chicago: Henry Regnery Company.

Taylor, Charles. 1989. *Sources of the Self: The Making of Modern Identity.* Cambridge, MA: Harvard University Press.

Torrance, George M. 1987. "Socio-Historical Overview.' In *Health and Canadian Society: Sociological Perspectives, Second Edition*, edited by George Torrance, 6–32. Toronto: Fitzhenry and Whiteside.

Westlake, Aubrey T. 1973. *The Pattern of Health: A Search for a Greater Understanding of the Life Force in Health and Disease.* London: Shambhalla and Routledge and Kegan Paul.

CONCLUSION

Sacred Ritual, Profane Miracle

> The opposition between nature and time, between what is manifested and what announces, has disappeared.
>
> —FOUCAULT (1973, 96)

The experience of health brings us closest to what we imagine is our best nature. Though it is also part of our nature to deteriorate and die, and this is no mere metaphor as it also makes us intimate with the affairs of natural processes, we also see in nature the ability to revive itself with each annual cycle. Alkmaion's definition of humanity is still salient, thus far, to our own: man is the part of nature that has not learned to close the circle and bring back life to himself. Not yet, perhaps. But the renewal that nature affords itself, at least when left to its own devices, rests on a force that is far beyond anything our species can hope to conceive in its current state. The ability of any planetary biosphere to survive cosmic cataclysms—the various primordial extinction events that we are aware of through geo-chronological and paleontological science—itself requires the summoning of cosmic forces. Human beings desire such a power, but so far we are mute to utter any such command. Even the next species, a hybrid of cyber-organic technologies, will not have that kind of ability. 'Nature', even in our most blasé and rational conceptualization of it, is something that truly 'contains multitudes'. It is its diversity that serves as its savior. Making our species more and more alike presents a great risk to its future. The reduction of humanity to a technocratic form might represent the triumph of technology over death, but it also might herald the end of any evolutionary processes that allow history itself to survive its cyclical demise.

All such 'endings' must be taken with this caveat, itself historical; that metaphysics survives as does nature, so far, and that history extends itself into the ahistorical causes that science uncovers. That nature as well may follow along in this same way, 'announcing' itself in a time out of time, by making itself 'manifest' as the arbiter of new forms of life, whatever may be their composition and desire.

We stated at the beginning of this book that science has inherited the drive to immortality that the religious vision created and reproduced for millennia. It is on the verge of making much more real this vision, and we called the combination of our desire to overcome finitude and to have immortality as a part of being-in-the world-as-it-is 'indefinitude'. We also stated that the health sciences are at the forefront of this endeavor, and even those alternative discourses are, as we have seen, salient to our understanding that we can and indeed should desire such things, whatever their actual ethical merit. Just as the concept of the sacred survives mode of production revolutions in human prehistory and history alike, the idea of health, though not the content of what it *means* to be healthy *per se*—is something ancient. If the ultimate health is to become a being with indefinitudinal temporal prospects as opened up by species evolution, rather than one with merely indefinite prospects, then surely it has been evidenced thus far that there must be an aura of the sacred surrounding all the sciences and discourses that shape our understanding of health and illness. So it remains to outline and briefly discuss how modern medicine has attuned this primordial concept to its own score, and how it also can bear witness to its profanation given that one cannot have something holy without the perspective of its absence, without excerpting itself from its sacred circle.

Supposed Science

The problem with the sacred was never that it was unbelievable or that one had to have a specific kind of faith to understand its import. No, the sacred rather presented to humanity a metaphoric model for ideal social relations. It was society elevated into the sphere of belief. Durkheim's simple but brilliant definition of religion, 'society worshipping itself', remains fundamentally true. Therefore it really does matter what kind of society and culture we live in far more than it matters what we believe about other worlds and other possible forms of being. The health sciences address this question at its core: what beliefs are necessary to 'produce' health out of a state of nature—ultimately, what conditions are necessary to create the immortal from the mortal—and thence maintain it? Enlisting the leitmotif of belief from homeopathy through both the placebo effect and the status relations extant between forms of institutional authority and the presence of the doctor or specialist, or even the 'lower' ranks of health care personnel, modern medicine bills itself as the center of the ideal society. It cares for social margins, it is, in most places, publicly funded. Its workers are often unionized and receive long-term benefits of various kinds including those related to their own health, and in social democracies, it is something of a 'sacred cow' that politicians fiddle with at their own risk. Though some of these beliefs come and go as the fashion of the economic climate changes, the sacred quality of health care itself as a system of statuses, discourses, and institutional spaces is clear enough.

But it is not this kind of sacred that a hermeneutical study of health and illness within the arc of modern medicine is directly interested in. Instead, we must focus upon the forms of being that enter these sacralized spaces, for it is these, and the events they sponsor and participate in, that demarcate the interiority of both the body and all that operates upon it as an object of the sacred from what is merely profane. This term, lending to our ears as it does the association with both profanation and profanity—one after all, 'swears' one's allegiance to these systems of discourse and the tax money that keeps them going, and then may well curse at having to pay so much *in* such taxes each year—historically may be taken as the relationship between our efforts to manipulate the forces that surround us, making nature into a part of culture, and hoping that our culture can mimic the power of nature so abundantly expressed everywhere but in the human heart.

Predilection

To do so is the function of all ritual, including those of our own day, those of science. But modern rituals of the external world and cosmos have as their backdrop the primordial ones of inner space: "The reality is the object of his science, and his efforts to deal with it in his cults and rituals were just as successful in controlling and manipulating the inner forces of the unconscious as are modern man's efforts to control and manipulate the forces of the physical world" (Neumann 1970, 220). Such success cannot truly be measured. One can experience 'success' as one experiences a recovery to health. One overcomes limits which are temporary, and not those fundamental. In this, recovery is kindred to learning in general, as one at first must accept certain limits and then decide to go beyond them. In science, this involves a concentration that excludes or suppresses other kinds of thought, including that 'enchanted' or purely symbolic. Of course, we may also speak here of 'repression', a term which carries with it both a pronouncement and a pronoun—it is 'she' who is in denial, for instance, or 'he' is evading something. Yet in a certain profound sense objective thinking, philosophical disquisition, or scientific analysis involves us in a world that is not at all part of the second nature of socialization. As

Schutz famously states, the common-sense world of the everyday knows nothing of real science. Experiential knowing, yes, as well as *ad hoc* experimentation and innovation, but not the methodical exploration, the systematic reduction of variables, the cumulative and generative discourses of science as have been developed in our own time. As such, science is the stuff of both ritual and repression: "There can be no scientific thought without repression. Repression is at the origin concentrated, reflective and abstract thought. Every coherent thought is constructed on a system of sound, clear inhibitions" (Bachelard 1964, 100). The scientific imagination, once harnessed to its method, must cast aside, at the very least, the wider human imagination, awe, wonder, and curiosity that led it to its focused experiment. Yet surely this is a narrow view of what science *means* to the species and what it does in its lifeworld. If wonder must be repressed in the search for the wondrous, awe sidelined in order to once again experience the awesome, raw curiosity suppressed and refined, it also must be true that we never completely abandon the idea that we are not only part of the cosmos we are exploring but also by some evolutionary miracle, the vehicle by which the cosmos can be known. Surely this is the most profound relationship we can have with what is unimaginably distant and anonymous to us: "*The source of our pleasure is the intimacy of this contact with nature*; and it is rewarding to cultivate our acquaintance with her and thus make this communion even more intimate" (Selye 1956, 296, italics in the original).

But it is one thing to become intimate with the otherness which is objective to us, and which may, objectively, call our presence to accounting through the object world. Its objection is thus something that no person, no subjectivity, can argue with. We are all in the same boat when it comes to our relationship with the cosmos, however intimate and pleasurable. This is manifestly *not* the case when it comes to our sciences of ourselves, the human sciences, including the more profound part of the medical arts. It is not our presence that is here being objected to or called into question, but our very *being*. And it is not otherness in the abstract that is being studied by human beings, but *others* like ourselves but also unlike ourselves. These others may, unlike natural objects, both object to us in the most stringent and intimate terms, though these terms are still subjective, but they can also study us as subjectitudinal objects in return. We can be subjected to their gaze. We are subject to their regulations, held within the subjection of their means and modes of being in the ontic life. All of us are held hostage by nuclear weapons, for instance, though we have more or less successfully suppressed this reality over the past generation or so, perhaps to our greater risk. Such a form of subjection takes the guise of the a subjectitude, wherein we are cast as both objects in the object realm, but also those objects that are most objectionable and, due to our muted but nevertheless continuing agency and agencies, always potentially objecting subjects. None of this is relevant in the natural sciences or even in medical research that is about disease entities *per se*. But as soon as we turn to ourselves, epidemiology, public policy health, health care systems, the people who work in them and run them, treatment, therapy, diagnosis and prognosis, the anamnestic character of psychiatric recall, the symbolic forms of homeopathy and their somewhat murky references to past ontology, all of this and more point directly to the subject which is us. Controlling our 'natures' is more pointedly and more poignantly the *meaning* of ritual.

So we cannot simply stop at the fact that rituals exist. We do not pause to admire the historical advent of science as a whole. No, we must clamber on towards the significance that 'even' in our most contemporary knowledge there resides the host of spirit, the soul of the unconscious, and the psyche of human character as a worldly being who also must walk alongside both objects and himself. In the nineteenth century, Mill and Dilthey developed the proper and serious analytics of the study of this strange form of being, and it has been noted many times that the translator of Mill's *System of Logic* used the German word for 'spirit' to denote the human sciences, causing ever since confusion and consternation alike. The *Geisteswissenschaften* has a meaning that in English is 'repressed': "This science is then no longer one which selects human beings themselves as the immediate object of its research. On the contrary, it takes up as its object *the knowledge* of human beings themselves which is mediated by the historical and cultural tradition" (Gadamer 1996, 28 [1972], italics in the original). It has become commonplace to also note that the natural sciences are as well mediated by such traditions that technically and discursively lie outside their objective boundaries. But the introduction of the subjectivity of humanity into the scientific equation, not merely on the side of the observer, as in the 'observer effect', but as the goal of its sciences, means for us that we are now standing inside the circle of any possible knowledge, that knowledge and knowing rest side by side, as do sleeping and dying.

Death and sleep are the objective states of natural science. But getting there means traversing the Stygian boundedness of our lifeworld, and there is always some kind of toll to be paid. We have seen that models from the sciences of pure nature are so powerful, especially in medicine, that we are almost automatically apt to shrug off any other kind of scientific experience as at best, a version of the homeopathy that also should be used with great caution and then only as a possible last resort. This aversion to the human sciences in all their forms—witness the flight from the liberal arts in contemporary universities, though pure research sciences are not doing much better enrollment wise—is certainly partly influenced by general market forces. But does not the market also respond to the sense that where our greatest human influence lies in the world is where the money should follow? Why even make efforts in other arenas, dubious as their history of success has been? "But the ascendancy of these models is one of the great sources of illusion and error in these sciences [ ] In a sense, however, premodern notions of science have also contributed to this over-hasty inference" (Taylor 1989, 58). The inference is that what is good for the goose of nature is good for the gander of 'human nature'. Perhaps the greatest necessary 'repression' of scientific thought is that of the self. The fragmentation that operational science often leads into would surely help along such a sense that meaningfulness, mystery, and the general messiness of human life can be swept under the epistemological rug (cf. Sorokin 1956, 34ff). So the philosophical response to such an historical situation is to, somewhat ironically, maintain it as merely a 'situation', one that can be negotiated and indeed diagnosed, rather than letting it become a situatedness, a mode of Dasein that is fundamental to its historical structure of consciousness. Repression in general may be part of the necessity for living on—one is heedful of Nietzsche's warning concerning those who must recall everything to themselves—but it is not an elemental aspect of what consciousness is. It is, like science, only a tool: "It is our task to point out again and again that our scientific culture owes its proficiency to the vigilant accompaniment of the enlightenment and [ ] to be reminded again and again of the limits that are placed on the knowledge and ability of humanity" (Gadamer 2003, 19 [1998b]). Knowing something and knowing *about* something may be the obverses of a coinage that carries the Janus of epistemology and experience alike. But coinage and currency are also not quite the same. To be contemporary is at one glance to forsake limits for limitations. The idea of a limit strikes the same chord as that of finitude, while limitation is more like something that is at rest for the time being. Science demands the faith that we acknowledge the temporary character of human knowledge, but in the name of its advancement, 'again and again'. Medical science is always at the forefront of this kind of demand, at once old world and almost otherworldly. The desire to overcome ourselves as we are—though our general use of technology is such that we strive to keep what is already ours our own; the privileges of wealth and work, the lack of cooperation and sharing of resources at a global level, etc.—rides shotgun with the goal of remaining just as we are. The contents of what should stay the same and what should change may not consistently overlap, and there still is extant cultural tension internecine to the demand that we both alter and conserve our culture at once. And at once, without delay, we are thrust into the arena of competing and conflicting self-understanding, the majuscule of our ideas regarding health and illness that come home to us within the experience of being something in the world about which we always know too little.

Predictions

Human experience is handy precisely because it can be used to predict the future. It cannot identify what is to come, but it can help us come to terms with that fact. It makes the open book more tolerable to proximally scan. To gaze afar is to lose the scripted melody of what has been and yet to find no sure replacement. This unutterable experience is one of the existential aspects of Dasein and it opens itself onto the space of deontic facticity, including that of the desire for a return to health. The 'magical' quality of these returns is not entirely lost on us, even as we would like also to pretend that the illness never occurred on the first place. Like the advent of precision and system in the sciences, ascending from their occult forebears in a way that Weil and others felt to be a 'degradation'—scientific clarity 'represents a fading of human engagement with the world' (cf. Lilburn 1999, 73–74)—its hallmark of measurable gradations allows itself to attain a different kind of truth: "Science is only true knowledge when it can be proven" (Gadamer 2003, 131 [1994–5]). Such proof, however, does not rest in the older idea of redemption or even a resentment that stakes its claims to favour by warning the relatively inexperienced that 'such shall come to pass', or 'wait and see'. Rather, science proves itself currently and in our own time, as a daily event. Though not quite quotidian—science must be learned as both a method and a discourse, and there was no culture that included science as a worldview in its primary socialization until that of the post-enlightenment West and its globalizing forces—it is nevertheless a mundane event. Science does not ask us to 'believe in future promises' or take its premises to be promissory in any ethical regard (cf. Sorokin, op. cit., 190). The alternate demand that we do not take things on faith and in our own turn make the corresponding demand that things be shown and thence known in the present, is one way of dealing with the always finitudinal challenge of walking ahead blind. But, one moment, science reminds us; 'it is not that we are blind but merely blindfolded'. Knowing and knowledge are in fact the same thing after all, and one will see that when one raises one's eyes to what is immanent. Religion demanded that we lower our eyes. Science demands we do the opposite. The old metaphysics of transcendence often used the convenient metaphor of a magical figure healing the blind. Sight and vision for them was the same thing. For us, we must be content with the contents of what can be *seen* and not those that might be envisaged.

All of this proves to be something of a set-up when it comes to the demands that both health and illness make upon our beings. For health is not something strictly empirical. It cannot be seen to be in its entirety. And seeing is not always enough during the process of therapy and treatment necessary to regain our health and all that follows from it. We need, in other words, both vision and faith to escort us, even if neither have anything material to offer in the present circumstance of working back towards one's imagination of what it meant to be healthy. Some of the stress that we experience during illness and recovery can be put down to our emotions, but another aspect of such stress is more empirically verifiable in clinical statements regarding pain thresholds and levels of shock. These measure insert a token of validity into the experience of stress without stating that everything else a person feels is necessarily invalid. Our invalidism is of two minds: we know we have been socially invalidated by illness but hopefully in an equal way, social re-validated by our suffering and our willingness to participate in conventional medical efforts. We are invalids without being invalid. Our recovery rate may well be affected by our levels of stress, whether these are purely subjective or whether they can be measured or both. It is certainly true to also say that "… the hypothesis that distress can lower immunological responsiveness [ ] is hardly the same—or constitutes evidence for—the view that emotions cause diseases, much less for the belief that specific emotions can produce specific diseases" (Sontag 1978, 52–53). At the same time, however, traditional cultural practices often do recognize empirical relationships in the world. The fact that they are covered over in symbolic rhetoric and forms of magic does not obviate their practicality in the locales in which they are practiced or even ritualized. Medicine's ritual theater is based on these older forms. All of us, even in the modern West, take as a given the idea that a crucial aspect of health is education, and all learning flows from these earlier historical social formations wherein symbology contained the rubrics to be learned and their maintenance was accomplished through guises of rhetorical force and flavour (cf. Khare 1977, 249ff for examples).

This being said, culture of the contemporary variety has also its rhetorical flourishes and ritual purifications. Those marginal to the centers of cultural production whereby such languages and symbolic forms are cast into the world as are nets into an unsuspecting liquid can expect to be enmeshed. Heidegger's sense of this term includes the idea of being 'ensnared', which puts the net into a rather different light. One of the most transparent examples of this problem—why, in a vast, wealthy and diverse society, do we need everyone on the same page all the time regarding capital, democracy, and education?—is the medication of social groups that we imagine are most liable to fly off on a tangent from the culture-circle the rest of us are content to rest within: "From a social-pharmacological perspective, the fundamental question to be answered is why mood- and behaviour-altering drugs are increasingly being prescribed to different social groupings in significantly different amounts" (Harding 1987, 550). Surely this kind of event concerns our ability to predict such moods, behaviors, and subsequent forms of being that may be expected to emanate from them. Predictability is thus the goal, and not merely prediction. A 'prediction', taken literally, could include anything at all. This is manifestly *not* what we are after. We desire conformity. We want this from others chiefly because we have been forced to accept our own. Resentment is indeed a factor here. Accepting conformity as part of health flies in the face of much of the individuating rhetoric and ideology of the enlightenment and the romantic reaction to the enlightenment both. Yet the order of society in general is something we also desire. Such a conflicting existentiality—though both forms of being might be thought of as inauthentic due to their concernfulness directed at 'only' ontic grounds of reality—is the root of both legal and illegal use of narcotics and other drug genres. Hallucinogenic experiences allow one to imagine that one's world is more to one's taste. They make otherwise dull people interesting, if only to themselves. But the dullness in question is to be considered part of the uniform of the conformitarian. One pretends that through a substance one can both escape the confines of the material world while also bidding farewell to the limits of one's worldview. But this is quite clearly a mirage, a turning away from the world as it is and ourselves in it. If there is one outstanding challenge to health in today's society, it is the health of the 'social body' and the illnesses we suffer together that make people turn away in these manners. On top of this, given that "… many licit and illicit drugs have common active ingredients and effects", (ibid), it is not surprising that what we are actually seeing and experiencing is an intense *competition* between institutionally sanctioned and thereby conventional forms of substances and their underground alternatives. The level of cynicism involved on both sides should not be underestimated, and this outlook on human life is patently unhealthy.

Protection

How then can one address both the issue of ill-health at a societal level and yet secure the interest of that self-same society in correcting it? The idea that elite vested interests can be manipulated or that they even exist in an organized way has its sociological limits. There is a model historically in place that sheds some light on the problem, and that is the relationship nascent science had with its cultural forebears. These too had vested interest to protect, and the new knowledge was certainly seen as sometimes and somehow threatening. Drug addiction is a non-threatening response to a society wherein opportunities and sacrifices are unequal and often unjust. 'Experimenting' with drugs is surely an abuse of the term, for no validity, measurement, or replicability applies. Within the ambit of scientific discourse, the pre-existing state of affairs both in the cosmos and in the lifeworld was one of relative ignorance, and thus "… a worldview that did not yet have this or that knowledge and therefore suffered under the misapprehensions that have since been overcome" (Gadamer 2003, 82 [1935]) could not, by definition, be of relevance itself for current scientific investigation. Ethno-history and archaeology aside, the pursuit of cosmic truth could only look ahead. Not even lingering alongside itself for overlong, this kind of study is the hallmark of our age alone. This understanding of history, wherein one could find antecedent and precedent alike, but never insight relative to the knowledge and especially the know-how of one's own day, sabotaged any attempt at authentic historical consciousness. Indeed, looking always ahead in this technical manner could be seen itself as a version of denial or avoidance behavior of some kind, kindred with the 'suppression' that science itself was said to require for thought to become focused on a technical task or an objective problem.

It makes sense, however, to distinguish this new form of knowing by which medicine and the ideas of health and illness were thrust into the lifeworld from the consciousness dominated by myth, itself an expression of what was mostly unconscious in a culture. It also made sense back when it was actually occurring. The birth of the 'logos', so-called, heralded both the 'first idea', the beginning of thinking as we know it in the Western tradition, and the advent of what was conscious. It is still regarded, somewhat ironically, as a kind of mythic event of its own: "This outburst of light in ancient Greece that led to philosophy and from philosophy into science need not ever have happened to the human race at all. Humankind would have gone on in some fashion or other as it had done for millennia before" (Barrett 1979, 206). We understand this 'beforehand' as one in which our ancestors existed in a kind of darkness. This relative ignorance, characterized in Plato by the cave-dwellers and their disbelief and even dangerous stigmata heaped upon the one who walks outside and grasps reality as it is, is both disdained and feared. The so-called 'culture wars' in the United States, the residue of which linger even today, is often seen as a contemporary by-product of the original conflict between myth and science that occurred in the Attic and Aegean diaspora some 2.5 millennia ago. Medicine is sometimes front and center within the culture wars. Witness the reaction against certain medical procedures, most especially abortion and access thereto, and other forms of research such as that involving stem cells. Modern magic and 'magical thinking' appear to be like oil and water.

But this is too rapid a realization of the facts of these cases. We do not exactly know what occurred in Classical Greece to upend the dominance of mythic thought and replace it with logic, logos, and experiment. What we know of the present is also incomplete, though much more detailed with regard to specific moments or cases. A more sociologically interesting viewpoint is one that takes into account the kinds of social groups involved in being marginalized by science as a whole. It is true to say, as did Sagan, that we tend to accept the products of science, that is, our vaunted and precious technological commodities, while rejecting its methods. Plenty of creationists drive cars. But this apparent hypocrisy alludes more directly to the sense that what knowledge is about is the invention and construction of new things and not new ideas. Philosophy's job over the time elapsed between Heraclitus and his fellows and ourselves concerned the world of ideas, and ideas could always be ignored. But science works in the real world and does not rest with ideas alone. Its products cannot be denied, and thus it itself cannot be ignored. If the doorways into these new discourses are blocked by *social* impedimenta such as inequality of opportunity along structural lines, those that fall outside these specifically social boundaries will feel resentment against not only the lack of opportunity but also what itself has been denied to them. In a classic example of *ressentiment*, these newly marginalized groups—though they are also descendants of the already marginal religious communities that settled the United States in the colonial periods—coalesce and attempt to gain political and legal traction based on their outsider status in a nation that formally acknowledges equal access to all constitutional rights and privileges. For about a quarter of a century beginning around 1980 these groups had varying degrees of success, especially early on in this recent if brief period. Eventually, however, their lack of numbers caught up with them. It is difficult to take on a dominant society with only about 15 percent of the population consistently on your side. The point remains that medical technique and technology was cast in the role of villain not due to its effects but more with respect to its social position in the dominant and conventional centers of authority and education. It was a symbol of 'secular' thinking. The old saw about not necessarily doing something just because one could do something was often trotted out as an apparent historical insight. More than any other applied or practical discourse, medicine became the poster-child of what was to be demonized, its position from within the religious oriented franchise akin to that of heavy metal in popular music. 'Abortion doctors' were gunned down, clinics attacked, stem cell research curtailed, much to the delight of European and Japanese universities. In some local political regions, animals appeared to have more rights than some people, especially children.

Ironically, this last aspect of the reaction to social marginality—in the United States, uniquely self-conscious about the expression of one's individuated worldview, especially those having to do with, or at least hanging their ideological hats on, religion or faith-based beliefs—the protection of animals as non-responsible chattel was originally part of the scientific redefinition of nature and thus our responsibility thereto which ultimately culminated in the environmentalist movements, something the religious factor had, up until very recently ignored: "Darwin himself responded positively to this change. It seemed to him obvious that the new ideas implied a strong and significant continuum between human nature and the nature of other creatures. Scientific method therefore called for an end of all prejudice against a serious, dispassionate comparison between their psychologies" (Midgely 2004, 140). Although, as we have already seen, stigmatizing metaphor had come to dominate the folk culture vocabulary regarding animal life and even the more alien and wider natural forces that surround us, animals could also demonstrate the best human qualities better than did human beings themselves; loyalty, obedience, respect for authority, consistency in behavior, all of these also happen to be, not at all coincidentally, the kind of attitudes that religiously influenced people of all stripes adore and strive to instill in their own children and perhaps also in their spouses etc. However disingenuous all of this may be, it is clearly the marginal culture's manner of expressing what in science, and specifically, in medical sickness, are also necessary features. The difference lies in their notion of what constitutes valid authority. In the symbolic forms of folk culture, such authority ultimately descends from a god, as when children are told that they must follow the 'teachings of the lord' which apparently can include being submissive to assault. In the applied sciences, the same authority descends from previous experimental research experience emanating from the natural sciences themselves. In these discourses, a similar separation of the operating mode of discovery of these authorities and their use in the human world occurs. For the anti-science person, though he accepts scientific products without so much as a blink, the distance between action and the source of morality guiding such action is the different form of being accorded to a divinity. For the scientist who is not also a religious person, the distance necessary for there to be imagined a non-human source of authority is accomplished by the presence of discourse itself. The fact that any human or group of humans would discover the same thing through the scientific method is enough to assure the objectivity of the case.

Yet it is not objectivity alone that is of the greatest import, but rather the distance created by placing authority apart from human action so it then can direct the latter and be appealed to as a kind of third party. In this, religion and science share a metaphysics in the same way that nature and Godhead are conceptions that share an historical ontology. Even so, just as the religious man cannot live by bread alone, humanity more generally does not live by science alone. There is more: "If no scientist can live by methodology alone, neither can science survive without it. The tension created by what seems to be an unnatural strain between role and person is intensified when we move from the natural to the social sciences" (Natanson 1970, 71). The medical sciences are arguably the most intense forum animated by such tensions. If not the crucible for the metaphysical conflict—usually, cultural roles and values in general harbor such an historical tension—medical science is where the tension is displayed. The enduring practice of allowing priests or ministers into palliative wards after science has 'done all it can', or more personally, and proverbially, the doctor's own admission of his limitations, is testament to the reality of having to agree to disagree over the meaning of life and death. More aptly, we may find ourselves desiring both forms of life at once, and indeed, it is not yet certain if human beings can choose between them in any final manner. Just what constitutes the supplement to 'bread alone' is ambiguous, though we are aware that it involves some kind of faith. Medicine has, as we have seen earlier, staked a claim to this faith, most importantly, to all those who seek its care or recovery through its therapies. At the same time, in taking in the sick it reveals its limits regarding their healing. In order to avoid facing up to this tension, and for the protection of its own authorities, the very purpose of science in its applied settings is altered in a dangerous manner: "… contrary to the meaning of science, one dares to claim the prerogative of never having to know anything in a fundamental manner" (Heidegger 1999, 85). In part, the ambiguities created when this or that disease vector encounters an individuated host, both socially and at the chemical or physiological level, makes any essentializing irrelevant. But what the phenomenologist is calling our attention to is not so much the idea that something elemental is being overlooked in methodological terms. It is more the sense that treatment reveals nothing about being in the world. It attempts to avoid the confrontation with itself by making simple recovery its utmost point. It reduces the experience of illness to a broken lamp. Not a hammer, as in Heidegger's own examples, wherein we realize the specifically objective being of the tool in the absence of its ability to actually do what it was designed for—the existentiality of the human equivalent might include the atheist, as in Nietzsche's 'ugliest man', whose inability to esteem anything includes himself—but a source of light that must be relit only for the purpose of regaining the objective knowledge of one's surroundings rather than one's place and perspective. In this way we use the *lux aeterna* as a mere flashlight.

For medicine, as a scion of research science proper, there is an incessant demand upon its original values to move aside in the face of the desire for health and well-being. One never desires illness to befall oneself. But the philosophical contribution of illness to the living is thereby lost. The discursive 'curse' runs its way back into the being of science as a whole: "Science never creates values but requires a value-creating power in the service of which one could believe in itself. The scientist believes in truth and does so in a way that he makes of his life the sacrificial animal of his faith" (Lingis 1989, 66–67). Contempt cannot be respect, even though when turned against the self it provides a rather predestinative vulgar Protestantism a self-assured stoicism that *looks* like a form of self-respect—something that still resonates particularly amongst the remaining Anabaptists and their run-offs in North America—as well as being particularly paternalistic in the way it treats others. It is masculinity emasculated. The tools of medicine are broken from the beginning. They never had what the hammer did before it wore itself out being what it was in the world of objects and in the hand of its master. Because the body of the other, not to mention her mind is never truly within the mastery of the doctor, his prosthetics must take on a value-creating mechanism of their own. Since objects cannot 'believe' in themselves, it falls to the patient to develop a misplaced faith in them. This is accomplished not only by the marketing of technology as a panacea but as well by the doctor's own efforts to buttress his authority by citing techniques and instruments as but extensions of his will to power. The morality of the prosthesis floats ambiguously above the corpus of the patient, not only depersonalizing but reassuring that one's place is not inside oneself but inside the gendered dynamics of emasculation. A time-honoured male fear wherein women are the villains and as such are dangerous to male sexuality, prompts the paternalistic conventions of medical art to auto-emasculate, transferring their desires into their instruments and wielding them as the sadist wields the 'implement' of juvenile 'correction'. After all, one is to correct the problem of illness, the body is broken, and the mind altered by its experience of pain. Just as the bifurcation of gender in bourgeois society rested not only on a convenient division of labour but also on the fear of women as public figures (cf. Martin 1994, 216ff), the problem of the public/private distinction breaking down in social contexts such as the clinic and the hospital—'professionalism' is thus all the more the incessant rallying cry herein, another example of Heidegger's plaintiff regarding 'never' knowing what underlies these tensions and striving to avoid such knowledge—presents medical care with one of its most intense tensions.

Furthermore, there is a tension extant between the doing of science for its own sake, of even for the sake of the extension of certain therapies, and the practice of science as accomplished. Knowledge as it might be and as it has been are always in a tension that also avoids the phenomenological backdrop. To protect against this more 'epistemological' frontier collapsing, to defend its honour as partner in care, is to be loyal to the studied ignorance of all things 'theoretical'. It is almost as if theory and hypothesis become the same thing. This is most felt in the medical spaces where a form of research must be accomplished in order to find out what is going on with this or that specific patient complaint: "The laboratories, therefore, exhibit dual trends: one the one hand, they are the cutting edge where exciting new technologies are introduced into routine use in patient care; on the other, the rationalization of work moves in the opposite direction" (Torrance 1987, 497). Between the divisions present through the gender, method, epistemic function, and discursive being of medical care there still remains the person as patient. She has, not of her own accord, become the otherwise missing crucible responsible for casting a novel amalgam of all these sites of surrounding life. It is as if the hinterlands of existence had suddenly appeared at one's front step, intent on rusticating within our homes, our beds. Our temporary resting in the beds of the hospitals and clinics but affirms this swap. We have become the living vehicle of all that supports life when it comes face to face with its own limitations. In doing so, the idea that the recovery of one's previous existence as a simple living form, the hammer before its use heralded its demise, is not merely a naivety but is itself the most profound form of self-contempt.

Sacralizing the Profane

If the rituals of medicine are to be taken as what truly matters—miracles are rare and can be used as positive media in the same way as are national and regional lottery winners; a kind of profanation of the conventions and of one's own expectations—there must be a way in which medical discourse and its institutions make good on such a premise.

Patient

The premise as promise is one such way: "… what occurred was the restructuring, in a precise historical context, of the theme of 'medicine in liberty' …" (Foucault 1973, 69). The truth that was embodied in the patient, that is, the facticality of illness as manifest in a host that does not succumb to disease *per se* but becomes part of the problem, was to "… define its own institutional and scientific structures" (ibid). Medicine, more than other applied sciences and far more than those of nature 'proper' appears to give the subject the first deal in inscribing the overleaf of its own discourses. Akin to Bachelard's 'phenomenotechnique', where natural objects such as landforms and laboratory data can take on symbolic qualities due to their proximity to myth creating tropes—they are either within the category of the source of certain kinds of myth, often cosmogonical, such as mountains, or they emanate from other objects which have both threatening and messianic qualities to them, such as machines—the human body, the corpus read as a corpuscularity, takes on the symbolic function of being something other to itself. It contains no longer multitudes of recognizably human, though diverse and even bizarre, features, but instead has taken into itself the means of its own annihilation.

Therefore, the objectifying stance that carries both the clinical gaze and the distanciated discourse of diagnosis parries the beseeching glance of the patient. The paternalism of the *gaze*—it may be directed to the nakedness of the patient or her sister, the nudity of oil painting, for instance, but it is *virtually* the same thing—thrust back into the endangered corpus its leveraged limb, limning from the subject a representation. Anatomically, not unlike the pleasureful use of pre-photographic representation—though it is sage to note that the very first Fox-Talbot gelatin print was inevitably of a nude female—we are now in possession of the thing threatened and, somewhere beneath its folds, kindred to the prize of hymen, the illness that must be struck from her being. In this, all patients are 'female'. In patient-hood, we give over our care to a technique of caring, we trade concern for consternation. Our own gaze is focused as never before through the instrumentation of medicine. Here, all sharps have the same purpose. We are transfixed by them before ever they actually penetrate our bodies. They have the ability to call rapt attention to themselves because, unlike the unseen illness, their presence is at once transparently threatening yet can be called to arms in our defense. Illness forces us to give up our own ability to gaze at ourselves. Is it any wonder that the most symbolically heavy illnesses remove our ability to procreate and to bear children as well as to enjoy the bodies of others? But there is an odd consolation to all of this: "Those who had lost the exclusive privilege of worrying over their sexuality henceforth have the privilege of experiencing more than others the thing that prohibited it and of possessing the method which made it possible to remove the repression" (Foucault 1980, 130). Psychoanalysis is the symbolic form of medicine that attempts to reiterate both the miniscule cosmogonies of biographical illness vectors—'tell me about your father'—as well as to install the patient within some kind of landscape wherein he can come home to himself. Medicine exposes its reliance on the metaphoric languages of pre-modernity most obviously when it has to deal with illnesses or disease categories that do not conform to the gaze. Indeed, the very gaze of the clinic must be altered in order to penetrate these suddenly hermeneutic veils. Its process bears then a recklessly intimate intimacy with that of both homeopathic treatments but all the more so and with all the more risk, magic itself: "The application of remedies, effective or not, is by no means the only way of mediating between man and his disease. Magic, or healing through the impact of ceremonial, is certainly one among several important functions medicine has served. Magic works because the intent of patient and magician coincide" (Illich 1975, 52). Once again it is the patient's role, not to cure himself alone, but to provide for the ambient discourse both the subject matter to be worked upon but also the very subjectivity that is transformed into an object. Magical rituals are the basis upon which the most contemporary scientific medicine can occur. The key is not so much the facticality of socially sanctioned apparatus in the object realm—the sorcerer's sleights of hand or the machinery of our own age in which there is also an invisibility; 'how did this machine *know* that my blood contains this or that'?—but the purpose of being a being who is sick. This deontic facticity of which we have spoken earlier is the center of what centers our being in state, lying in wait for its own demise, playing close to the edge of its own abyss and carrying its own weight to the brink of a form of para-being which 'is in every case my own'. It is this that reminds others whose role it is to maintain the social contract through whatever forms and formulations may be necessary, health being perhaps its supreme exemplar, that they must act. They act not precisely on our own behalf but on behalf of the social body from which we have strayed. Illness by itself cannot force us out, but the danger of us giving up ourselves to the illness, giving in to it, must be arrested and turned back on itself. This is the function all shamans and doctors ultimately perform.

And I, as the being who testifies at first to my complaint and then admits to my reaction to it, must submit to the others that they are still in the right of things. In this, every medical diagnosis is kindred with the magical trial: "Through the defendant, witchcraft and ideas associated with it cease to exist as a diffuse complex of poorly formulated sentiments and representations and become embodied in experience. The defendant, who serves as a witness, gives the group the satisfaction of truth" (Lévi-Strauss 1977, 448). It is but a short step from playing the role of perpetrator to that of victim. It is the relative or absolute invisibility of the illness or its contrived vectors that binds them together, much as the master and slave are bound by their mutual needs. Such roles can be reversed of course, either through ritual or revolution, but the essence of the social relationship lies in its ability to unmask the unasked: "The place of the sick man is understood in this kind of culture to be a magico-religious one. Prescribed actions must be performed in order to restore the sick man to the favor of the human witch or nonhuman spirits. The diseased man is a victim of powerful and secret forces" (Sigerist 1977, 390). We have already seen that the moral career of the patient contains the threat of social dissolution. Even in our most mundane interpretation of such a medically centered apocalypse, that of a plague that ends our species tenure on this world, the forces at work are 'powerful' by virtue of their being 'secret'. Medicine is always at its forefront when it is working to expose the secrets of this or that disease. It is always marketing itself by virtue of the potential cures it can offer in the nearest future possible, that for AIDS or cancer etc. Miracle must be made mundane, even profane, for just like in primordial social organizations from which all of us have both descended *and* ascended, it is ritual and not miracle that restores, cures, and recreates the balance of the human condition.

If it is part of this condition to contain that which conflicts with itself—witness the usual order of disease vectors in pre-modern cultures; ritual impurity due to happenstance, the intrusion of material objects, other humans maleficent actions or intents or yet our own spirits being intrinsically accursed in some manner (cf. Khare 1977, 243ff), and none of these vectors has truly altered its structural implications, only the kind of content that may be admitted to them—then it must be admitted that its discourses doubly *contain* such a conflict as well. They contain it in the more immediate sense of stopping it from spreading; their quarantine is in effect as soon as we decide to take ourselves to the clinic even under our own locomotion. But they also contain it in this other, more ambiguous sense: from magic to medicine the trope of the *Pharmakon* is always in play. The cure and the poison rest side by side, even within the same potion or prescription, as in morphine. The *Pharmakon* has been famously interpreted by Derrida as being the embrasure of erasure. It puts itself out of action, always and already, differing and deferring its abilities along a chain of existential signifiers. This is not so much an aside but a phenomenological description of its symbolic content. It is never content to just be the thing that we desire the most, but must always remind us, the 'users' of its pharmacopeia, for instance, that our desires are linked to our knowledge of personal finitude.

In our own time, we have managed this volatile mixture of presence and absence through making the prescription something that can cure and kill the responsibility of a number of people, and not just the one who takes the medicine. More than this, drugs are a lucrative commodity, one of the most sought after and profitable business ventures that we know. It bears its uncanniness into the commodity market precisely because it continues to be the bearer of both life and death at once. *Its* 'rationalization' contains doubly the sense that it does not *have* to kill us, there is no need for us to die in this way, as well as it being *only* a pill, after all, for how could one render an existential erasure of logocentric consciousness 'over the counter'?: "Not only material objects such as pharmaceuticals and prosthetic devices but also the entire range of health services become commodities to be bought and sold. Commodification encourages both the sick and well to become avid consumers of the nebulous product known as health" (Freund and McGuire 1999, 211). Not only are outsiders, laypersons and those who are not truly ill, bystanders and collateral workers whose employment indirectly relates to health care systems affected by this process, personnel intimately involved with the direction and dispensation of this vague product—better, production or reproduction since health is not an object *per se* but a way of seeing in its relationship to capital, rather than a mode of being, though in homeopathy, the 'existentialized' version of what it means to be healthy is also bought and sold—are as well part of the consumptive efforts. In particular, the amount of technological miracle is costed out and adjusted for year to year or even month to month depending upon ease of access. The proverbial stories of those who must leave the political region in which they have automatic access to most health care and travel to a place where they can access more specialized or crisis care is too well known to be repeated here. Part of the way medicine mutes its potential miracles is to simply deny access to them. Some of this denial is disguised under budgetary items, and such operations or treatments are debated by institutions or even the wider society alike focusing upon "... how it should draw the line on access to these glamorous but terribly expensive interventions. [Meanwhile] The level of waste in the existing system continues, carefully screened from view" (Evans 1987, 628).

The focus upon the patient as not only the object of medical science but also its subject matter also has the ironic effect of decoying attention away from health as a product in itself. Instead, the individual person as patient is returned to health and this person now becomes the product of successful medical interventions. Or not. For a significant percentage of treatments ultimately fail, depending upon the condition of the original input. It is certainly a slice of well-meaning to have the sense that 'the patient is the world', as Shem notes with enthusiasm in his 2010 afterword, as well as stating flatly that in the case of the United States, a universally public system is the only answer to the ill-health of the system itself (cf. 2010, 378ff, written precisely at the time when this issue became very much public in that country). This *is* something to note: iatrogenesis effects its own sources, and not merely those who enter into some kind of contractuality with it. It is not only and necessarily an output function of a mismanaged or overcompensatory desire. It is rather the sum of all of its parts in a system where each part is more than the sum of the whole. For each element of medical care takes on a larger than life presence when it is our own health and even life that has become its center. The patient remains the fulcrum of care but his consciousness is decentered by the manner in which care is to be carried out. We are so desperate for this or that treatment though we are often dimly aware of its rate of success, positive or middling or as desperate as we, that the remainder of what health care represents in wider terms is lost on us. Even the idea that emergency services must take in and take on more critical cases than ourselves becomes bereft of conscience, as is witnessed each night in any emergency ward where patients with more mild complaints complain more about being shunted back in the queue. It is the consciousness altering effect of illness that makes the ritual of health care appear to be more magical than the actual cures, and thus the caring for the sick that *can* be cured is the most sacred of health personnel tasks. The less sick can wait, and the sickest can go to the wall.

Doctor

To be fair, any rationalized system must care for its wards in this manner. Those with the highest probability of pulling through 'on their own', or relatively uncared for, are left to the side for the moment. Practical science is, if anything, practical in the casual sense of the term, however impractical its costs and management organizations and policies may appear to be. This practicality, the greatest utility for the greatest number the greatest amount of the time, summarized in one version of utilitarianism as an ethics, is almost primordial to our species. Our ancestors were of the same mentality in drawing the line between ritual and miracle. Miracles were for those whose life in reality had no traction over their consciousness. For whatever reason, these few and rare potential individuals disdained the society current to their time. Indeed, it was this kind of person that most often became a medical specialist himself, and considered this spiritual transformation in the epoch of transformational metaphysics to be the answer to his quandary of being 'unfit' for the usual social order: "Even though this order is different from the kind we impose, the connection between our conscious order and the magical order of early man can be proved at all pints" (Neumann 1970, 126). One of these points is assuredly the presence of medical specialists in our own day. The traditional shamanic devices have disappeared, such as sleight of hand, cheeking, smoke and ashes, hallucinogens and the like. But their modern counterparts appear in abundance; technologies of all kinds, potions and pills, etc. And what *has* remained intact is the manipulation of the physical body in order to produce mental effects as well as the language of the diagnosis, the idea that something is amiss. For we are still dealing with two people; one has the problem, the other, perhaps, the solution. Medicine is yet regarded as magical by many. As many more people experience the ritual of medical care rather than its rare miracle, it is thus the ritual that gains the most favorable magical characterizations. Each ritual maneuver becomes in its own way some small miracle by which we are cured. A timely but commonplace operation for a hernia, for instance, makes the world of difference to us and our day to day lives. We are also aware, though we have never studied the history of the clinic or its operations, that at one point a hernia procedure could simply not be accomplished. Then, later on, closer to the time of our own specific case, it was done with difficulty for both doctor and patient, and was not always successful. And then it was successful, and so on. Each little ritual, however mundane today, has a pedigree in which it, the farther back one peers, becomes more and more like a miracle. Ritual is, in a word, *the end result of the demythology of miracle.*

This is quite different than medicine as a science whose subject and object is humanity and yet whose epistemology is decidedly not human science aping its progenitors, the natural sciences. Here, the problem is "… the misleading effect of deliberate imitation of another science, and the dangerous false reassurance that can be derived from thinking that mere surface imitation makes one's methods scientific …" (Midgely 2004, 145). The potential epistemological subterfuges that can occur because of this misled mimicry of method is hardly the only danger here. The figure of the doctor, not as a knight errant of epistemology but as a messianic personage cloaks his actual abilities in magical garb. Though naked as the emperor whose mantle he has mimicked or even inherited given our disdain for politicians of all stripes, the doctor's own nakedness is warmed by the brightest sun possible; the glow of the eyes of his patients: "The sudden emergence of the doctor as saviour, culture-hero and miracle worker was not due to the proven efficacy of new techniques but to the need for a magical ritual that would lend credibility to a pursuit at which a political revolution failed" (Illich 1975, 111). Given that politics is intrinsically a matter of ideological druthers, a hero that transcended all politics and indeed, seemingly all culture as well was an instant attraction. All of us, no matter what are political opinions, could get sick and thus would need to be saved by the doctor. In our own day, rationalization processes have converted latent messianism into professionalism. Doctors were for a long while the 'ultimate professionals' in a society where every one of us desired professionalization'. (cf. Kelleher, Gabe, and Williams 1994a, xii). This sensibility continues to be a major force amongst new immigrant groups to the West. Countless young students are told by their parents to become health professionals, especially doctors, because of the prestige associated with the trade. This rather old world sensibility is being reinvigorated by migration. Add to this the idea that the person in charge of the ritual gets the most out of it: "Like all other major rituals of industrial society, medicine in practice takes the form of a game. The chief function of the physician becomes that of an umpire. He is the agent or representative of the social body, with the duty to make sure that everyone plays the game according to the rules" (Illich, op. cit., 147). Hence the stigmata levied against homeopathic discourse and practice. Indeed, it is mainly the former that is disdained. I have interviewed or overheard many doctors simply but gently dismissing the actual practice of alternative medicine by 'well, it can't do any harm', or 'if it makes you feel better about it, go ahead', and the like. Kindred with many vitamins or mineral supplements, many doctors today, though they are discursively convinced that these aids do little or nothing, are content to go along with the placebo effect. After all, it is that very effect that is responsible for some of their own successes (cf. the dialogue in Williams et al. 1994, 183ff where the doctor admits to related issues when pressed).

But the most important aspect of professionalization when it concerns a cohort based group of persons is that they are able to circle the wagons when one member of their group is threatened. Lawyers, professors, civil servants, military officers and sometimes business leaders all join doctors in their respective circles. Fortunately for lay-people of all stripes, the professions themselves don't always get along with one another. The conflict between doctors and lawyers in the nineteenth century is well known. Shem notes that the sense his protagonist has relatively early on in *House of God* that the interns were 'becoming doctors' by not taking advantage of each other's errors and incompetencies was strong (c. 1978, 126ff). This sense is not so much constructed consciously, though in times of crisis it manifests itself in calculations, some of which appear from the outside to be bereft of all conscience, but rather created at a semi-conscious level. In this, it bears a distant kindred with other forms of more profound creation. Though professionalization has become a major fetish in all rational organizations—and it is striking to note the lack of professionalism in the apprentice; it is much more noticeable than any absence of technical competence, for instance—though numerous attempts have been made over the decades to codify the rules of engagement regarding one's profession (these change over time usually from being strict to more permissive; for example, personal relationships with students being off-limits entirely for professors to suggesting that their grading be done by some other faculty member). Such codes fail, in practice, to bring out both the nuances of how the ideas themselves came to be the general sensibility within professional groups of all kinds, as well as the actual behavior of professionals, very often it is here that they come across as patently *unprofessional*, when challenged or threatened. Like more general ideas of creativity, still tinged with the romantic sensibility of the anti-enlightenment and thus also somehow 'anti-rational', the ability to be consistent as well as sincere at all times is often the most difficult challenge. This is so because there are in fact no universally agreed upon means for maintaining professionalism against all comers and within all social contexts: "Genuine creation is precisely that for which we can give no prescribed technique or recipe; and technique reaches its limits precisely at that point beyond which real creativity is called for …" (Barrett 1979, 22).

Such codes and their interface with reality are not in fact templates, but mimic more profound social relations. Perhaps the most ambitious attempt at codification comes not so much from professional policy manuals as from within the ambit of medical techniques whose goal is to transcend the improvisatory nature of nature itself. The human genome project is an excellent current example of this dynamic. Health can be attained by overcoming any hereditarily transmitted ailments (cf. Westlake's bold predictions regarding this technique, not undreamed of in his time but certainly unattainable by the then current technologies; 1973, 126ff). In spite of the 'Nazi' overtones to this and related projects, not to mention its 'Brave New World' qualities as well, most people are quite content to have their pedigree's 'professionalized' in this manner. Purification, hygiene, cleanliness and health, made unambiguous and certain by efforts like those of the Third Reich remain for us today social goals. And it is the 'body of our current peoples' that will benefit from it, from less tax dollars to less burn-out for health personnel. Ultimately, however, it is the doctor who emerges as both umpire and messiah, for he is the one who has not only cured us but has done so according to rules that all can agree upon.

Institution

Even so, none of this would be possible without doctors being firmly ensconced within institutional spaces such as the clinic or hospital. Within these spaces, what passes for truth has essentialized itself through mere force of habit. Truth is the by-product of ritual, and method, otherwise never 'catching up to truth' as Gadamer has put it, rather becomes it almost in its entirety: "Psychological truths are not metaphysical insights; they are habitual modes of thinking, feeling, and behaving which experience has proved appropriate and useful" (Jung 1959, 27). Kindred with the Greek idea that 'we are what we repeatedly do', the outwardly expressed habitus of ritual not only connects people and their daily tasks in a manner about which we rarely have to be entirely conscious, much less circumspect existentially about, it constructs an appropriate distance between self and other as well as self and object. In medical practice, technique and technician cannot be seen as being too much of the same thing, lest the final vestiges of humanity be withdrawn from the scene of health and health care. More than this, the object of health, recovery from disease or the absence of discomfort, must be kept at a distance from the vector of illness. To essentialize either would be to make too discrete a separation where none in fact exists, given that the body is itself diseased, and perhaps the mind as well. In order to avoid the problem of thinking oneself another kind of being simply because one happens to be ill, disease must be given its own fluid frame, its own ability to come into existence in the manner that is most supportive of its vanquishing: "Disease, like the word, is deprived of being, but like the word, it is endowed with a configuration" (Foucault 1973, 119). As such, it can 'fit in' with the rest of the apparatus of the clinic. Those others who bear the badge of office and to whom we have entrusted perhaps even our lives are not only to be seen as the masters of ritual but through this and by it, also the ritual masters of disease 'itself'. But this 'selfhood' is no longer itself, but part of us, so the magic in any medical ritual, primordial, ancient or modern, is to once again make separate that which has made itself, also by a form of darker magic, the same. The great principle of magic has to do with the idea that 'once two things are brought together, they remain connected.' It is this elemental idea regarding what magic is in essence that must be overcome by the novel magic of medicine. This means, as we have seen earlier, the overcoming of the idea of essence.

Doing this means transferring the symbology of magic into an opened up space in which all can participate. It is not so much to demythologize magic but to make its practice as public and reductive as possible. It is still the case that only the doctor *et al*, magical practitioners all, can practice it for the general benefit. But no longer must the patient as layperson be in the dark as to what the doctor is trying to do, though the technical language of the means may remain an obstinate 'mystery'. Alongside this there is a growing sense, evolving into a sensibility, that almost anyone *could* become a doctor if he or she put the necessary amount of effort into it. Magic is demystified without being demythologized: "White coats, antiseptic environments, ambulances and insurance came to serve magical and symbolic functions influencing health. The impact of symbols, myths and rituals on health-levels is distinct from the effect of the same procedures in merely technical terms" (Illich 1975, 53). Except that there is no real difference, socially, between technique and ritual in the modern medical context. One might make a distinction between the tools and the acts, but even here such a difference is slight. The mere sight of medical technology has a reassuring effect. It constructs its own ambience. Sometimes, of course, such an atmosphere is too acerbic, suggesting alienation. It is not surprising that we also use the term 'clinical' to refer to an environment or even a personality that is disinterested in the extreme. One could follow the suggestion detailed in the previous chapter and turn one's back on the whole thing. But even commentators such as Westlake ultimately disagree with the idea that we can travel back in time to some inevitably imaginary anachronism. If the 'spirit' is cast adrift in modernity, there should be no barrier in place to reconstruct our own distinctive *Zeitgeist* rather than retreat to traditional forms: "We should not in fact try to revive this sort of spiritual healing, as is being done by many and various religious bodies, but seek to find what is appropriate to these modern times" (op. cit., 75). Unless, of course, our very alienation and anonymity count as what is 'appropriate'. Even so, *no* institutional grace hailing from any historical period, is bereft of alienation. The fact of the larger other, non-generalized and yet impersonal, populated by living beings who must come and go and whose influence can only last so long in the memories of others who to pass on, should not be lost on us. Illich concurs: "You can count what the friars collect, you can look at the temples they build, you can take part in the liturgies they indulge in, but you can only guess what the traffic in amnesties for purgatory does to the soul after death" (op. cit., 68). The 'spirit' is not necessarily effectively cared for, or even conjured, simply by talking about it anymore than not talking about it. It is either present or it is not. In our neo-Kantian fashion, modern rationalized organizations have opted to treat the question as moot. The boundary of graceful activity to this regard is only transgressed when we begin to endow the institutions themselves with some kind of spiritual life. This can quickly become a fatal error. Indeed, those who temporarily inhabit medical spaces such as clinics and hospitals have the tendency to fall into patterns much more ancient than those that might be deemed 'appropriate' for our own day: "Relationships between different categories of staff tend to be hierarchical and authoritarian, the unquestioning obedience of the lower ranks being justified on the grounds of the emergency nature of most medical tasks" (Morgan 1982, 75). Unions and more democratic contractual agreements and policies have ameliorated this situation to a certain extent, and it is not truly correct to say that 'most' medical tasks are of a critical tone in any case. Yet the institution must give the appearance of order, and without much demur, tasks of all character need still be accomplished in a timely manner. Perhaps the most obvious change regarding the hierarchical nature of the hospital is the language surrounding how many hours and what shifts lower ranking employees can be asked to work. There is mandatory overtime in most union shops, but along with the increased wages associated with these shifts, they are also limited in their periodicity, especially if they include overnight hours. In private institutions, the resemblance to the church as the archetypical institutional model is more transparent: "The gaudy care is financed, like the liturgies of old, by taxes, gifts and sacrifices" (Illich, op. cit., 51). There is a limited argument to be made that, given our acceptance of the wider hierarchy and sometimes authoritarian society in which all of us dwell, that those who can afford expensive and specialized care should be able to opt for a user-pay system, such as the various national park services have used for some time, or, more basically, the idea of the toll road. How far to implement such a system is always the problem. Ethical pitfalls abound if such an idea is over-extended at the cost of the remainder of the population who has available to it only more modest means and yet may well suffer from the same sort of ailments that the privileged could look after more rapidly simply due to the disparity in access to material and technical resources as well as specialized personnel. Generally, it has been beyond alteration in policy, if not quite beyond question, that all must pay for the same system and ride in the same boat regarding delays, shortages, or even the odd absence of specific care in this or that region. In large countries with diverse populations, such a system is incredibly costly, needless to say, and it requires an alert politics that is keen to manifest 'responsible government' to maintain it.

One of the pressures that tends to act against the institution from keeping a democratic line regarding its outputs and services is simply how those who work within it are trained. As the objectification of the person presents a challenge both ethically and empirically the general response has been to enact a variety of distanciation techniques, alongside those techniques that actually emanate from the use of tools or technologies. Once again, institutional 'professionalism' demands that we depersonalize ourselves as well as those we may be caring for. This irony serves to disenchant human relationships in order to keep the magic of technique and technology alive. Not unlike our 'sexting' example above, where young persons and sometimes those older enact intimate performances for one another through the genie of portable technology, medical care, at once intimate and yet anonymous, has long since been able to provide a model for anyone interested in the mere performance of intimacy and authenticity without the actual risk of the real thing. A new kind of symbology is in the making: "Becoming professional, then, involves a symbolic and a psychological transformation. A symbolic distancing and control over constructions of reality is accompanied by a psychological and interpersonal distancing" (Haas and Shaffir 1987, 408). Confined to the hours of work, such a dispassionate stance may aid in certain critical care events. It is not merely a utility to accomplish necessary tasks without sentiment of any kind. Far better to save a life than to express one's condolences instead. Inevitably, however, the distanciatedness of 'being-professional'—this could be seen as the template for all forms of inauthentic being in the purely ontic landscape of policy and bureaucracy—travels afar, into the hinterlands of health care. The most immanent example of this exogamy concerns public health policy and the reaction to certain kinds of events, calculated or happenstance, that affect the health of a wider population who would not otherwise have necessarily consulted the actual institutions and their staff. The response to such professional distanciation has been to create lay or grass-roots versions of epidemiology, though these also have their limits and can test rational thought, as in vaccines and autism, or hydro-electric lines and mental illness. Even so, "in defining as public dangers what might otherwise be perceived as private risks, popular epidemiology poses a direct threat to those who have conventionally been invested with the authority to pronounce on the meaning and significance of public and environmental health problems" (Williams and Popay 1994, 134). Very often, even in the case of accidents rather than insurance fraud or calculated pollution to lower costs or save other monies reserved for more lucrative investment, private sector operations can be relied upon to make light of any health concerns generated by their actions. This is not always the case, but it certainly is something in the public mind as it remains a staple of entertainment fiction from conspiracy and espionage to crime and detective series. Given this, it is not surprising to note that medical institutions are sometimes tarred with the same suspicious brush. This is more likely when public health officials have been persuaded, monetarily or otherwise, to pass over the risk to public health and make health a function of the literal institutional space. That is, those who seek health should do so at the doorstep of the clinic and not the corporation, or, that publicly financed health *care* should be a balance to privately sponsored health *risk*. Not unlike the idea that universities should train workers for corporations so the latter do not have to spend the time and money doing it, one kind of risk generally overlooked is the sense that our society itself maybe unhealthy in a political and an ethical sense: "In a free society, so long as the current prejudice in favour of medicalization prevails, government will be forced to allocate resources according to public demand, even if they do not effectively accomplish what the public desires" (Illich, op. cit., 74). It is an odd situation to begin with when desire and demand do not coincide. But such is the conflict when at once we are attending to the needs of the day—laboring in a potentially risky workspace and eating this or that conventional diet, thence going to the clinic for 'what ails us' and having to do this while taking time away from work and so on—while at the same time wondering about whether or not all of this is somehow related or how it might be so. Furthermore, we are approached, nay, accosted, by those who claim to have figured out just exactly how such things are related and what we can do about it. Then, official and oft officious servants of either the state, the capitalist, or the medical officers interpose and tell us that we have been duped. By whom? When and where, and how often?

One thing is clear: "… we live in the age of institutions and mass society. [ ] What we need to do is build a bridge over the existing divide between the theoretician who knows the general rule and the person involved in practice who wishes to deal with the unique situation of this patient who is need of care" (Gadamer 1996, 94 [1990]). What is not as clear is how far we should go—we, as in, the conglomerate rather than the congery of 'this person' or 'this patient'—in our ability to trust what the person who claims to know the general rule is about. We must not only know these rules but from whence they have come, who states them and why. We need to find out if there are other options, and not only for us, but also to ask of the theorist or the thinker if he or she has developed alternative understandings or why they may not be available. Are the roadblocks to other forms of thought or optional ideas contrived or are they somehow beyond the limits of current human knowledge? How long will they remain so, or could they be judged as permanent in a human history replete with such often premature judgments? The task of philosophy in its widest and most democratic sense, in our day most often remains "… to try to see where technical and technological thinking, with no other principle but itself, must lead us and whether some countervailing mode of thought may not be called for" (Barrett 1979, 230).

Technique fits well within the confines of institutional life. It is understood as neutral, as something that not only may be learned but may be learned by almost anyone. It appears to be the ultimate expression of democratic community, as well as a genuine arbiter for it. One can either do the job or one cannot, adjudicated by the measured and standard pace and premise of technical life and application. Medicine ideally would treat all comers as equally worthy of care respective of complaint. Technique and the technology from which it both emanates and from which that self-same technology is itself constructed would appear to be the best way of delivering this kind of care. Large scale care requires equally large scale spaces to house such mechanisms and the personnel that work with and through them. Institutions of medicine are certainly here to stay, even though out-sourced care for an aging demographic will shunt their focus away from traditional clinical centers and diagnostic arenas.

The most important effect of the presence of such institutions is their ability to make sacred the rituals performed within them. The person becomes the patient through these performances, is treated and indeed even cured by their force. The institutional ambience that lends itself to the creation and maintenance of ritual is part of the scene of sacralization, a scene that no form of medicine, allopathic or homeopathic, can ever afford to completely eschew.

The Miracle of Profanation

Neither the institution nor the doctor can summon the very presence of the divinity that is traditionally associated with being the source of the miraculous. But what medical spaces can do is to perform so few apparent miracles that on the one hand the rarity and genuine character of the miracle is affirmed while at the same time, on the other, the stigmata that may accrue to all those who claim that they can indeed perform miracles is avoided. Miracles in medicine are thus the very opposite of rituals but in an inverted way: a miracle is a profanation of the ritual for it takes itself as a result outside of the due process and known qualities and quantities of medical treatment. It is unexpected though thus not unsuspected. Its presence, sudden and irreversible, lending to the patient all kinds of symbolic content and other-worldly notions that must conflict with modern medical practice and knowledge alike, is anti-heroic. It conflates the purpose of the hospital with that of the church (cf. Illich 1975, 79ff for another version of this conflation). And it allows the patient, now immediately recovered or recovering, to stand in the space that is reserved only for the doctor, the space of both imminence and immanence, the one being where all sense of the 'sudden' should rest, the other being the aura of being-able-to-pronounce health back into the world of the patient. The formula for this space is thus: imminence plus immanence equals eminence.

Suspended of Disbelief

The very status of the doctor and his abilities are radically called into question by the miracle or what is taken for it. Whether or not a 'response' to medically-induced states or judged as coming from the 'body itself', or even nature, as a 'freak' or some other such epithet, it matters not. The standards of medical practice have been transgressed and the status of those who practice it challenged. The interloper is an outsider, and not even a readily identifiable other. It can only be placed inside the vague category of 'force' or process that medical science cannot predict but yet cannot also completely rule out. The miracle is both outsider and outlier, and as such also an insult to the methods of scientific medicine. Though homeopathic discourse more easily accounts for the presence of the unexpected recovery, especially in cases where 'nothing more can be done', it too is wary of too many miracles for the same reason as is conventional practice; their presence creates unreasonably high expectations of their clientele. 'Everyone' has heard the story of 'so and so', and desires the same or similar outcomes for themselves.

More than this, the miraculous seen as something sacred is thus something that one would want to take into themselves. As a profanation it becomes something to be shunned. To alter its evaluation one need not, of course, change its being: "It is naturally not a question of a collective value artificially manufactured or arbitrarily awarded, but of one that is effective and present *per se*, and that makes its effectiveness felt whether the subject is conscious of it or not" (Jung 1959, 44). How miracles are effective, indeed, how they are even acclaimed as being what they are for us, *is* equally and definitively a question of collective value, however 'arbitrary' in the historical or cultural sense. The Jamesian distinction between the possible world of source material or force from which or by which miracles, visions and other signatures of the human imagination as attuned to the infinite and our mundane consciousness with which the conscious mind is mostly attentive and occupied with could be utilized in this arena as well. But it is perhaps simpler to suggest that Jung's 'collective unconscious' and Lévi-Strauss's idea of the grammar of culture are more or less one and the same; the three things necessary for any magic, including miracles, to be 'effective' are thus the shaman's belief in his own techniques as well as the patient's belief in their efficacy, and finally and most importantly, given that this is space from which the beliefs of the other two ultimately can be sourced from, the group's understanding of magical effectiveness. (cf. op. cit., 446) All of this may be but a sham to any outsider, whether anthropologist or psychologist—though Jung's foray into 'primitive' society as a participant in ritual is so well known as to not be detailed yet again—but the power of belief, no less resident and resonant in the cultural spaces of modern medicine, is such that it only needs the insider to work with. The challenge for contemporary medicine or any art and science that claims to be an attempt to work miracles on a daily basis, nay, to make the very concept of the miracle into a mundane object, is to convince those who come to it seeking just this form of the sacred to become converts to the sense that belief actually has nothing to do with what occurs once inside the discourses and techniques of medicine.

To do so means to at first profane the traditional idea of miracle—*they* don't exist, cannot happen, are a figment of overzealous desire, such wishes are understandable given the stakes of life and death, that sort of thing—but this kind of stuffy hard-nosed and even priggish attitude can only take one so far. Especially so when the symbolic quantity of the miraculous is to be at first transferred into the disease and inverted; that is, that which is sudden and unexpected is in fact a villain and not a hero or savior: "The melodramatics of the disease metaphor in modern political discourse assume a punitive notion: of the disease not as a punishment but as a sign of evil, something to be punished" (Sontag 1978, 79). Not unlike a kind of Kierkegaardean anxiety, the *subito* of disease befalls us like an evil thing. Not even an omen, which remains an augur of things yet to come, a shadowy patch along an otherwise everyday horizon, disease is the event itself. It can seem so unlikely to be uncanny. It is a miracle of the dark art of sorcery, an explication that takes us back to primordial social organization and would hardly seem the sort of idea to help us recover from whatever has actually happened to us. This kind of thinking forces us to live within the ambit of the event, but not with the goal of giving us some aspect of existential perspective. The process indeed looks more like a kind of neurosis, a repetitive regression, not unlike the proto-theatrical therapeutics of the first doctors: "The shaman does not limit himself to reproducing or miming certain events. He actually relives them in all their vividness, originality, and violence" (Lévi-Strauss 1977, 452). We ourselves do not 'relive' anything. Our life does in fact go on both in spite of the disease and strangely, because of it. It alerts us to life, as we have already suggested, in a manner nothing else can. And our recovery too has a kindred relationship with the shaman's work: "And since he returns to his normal state at the end of the séance, we may say, borrowing a term from psychoanalysis, that he *abreacts*" (ibid, italics in the original). This is the moment where the actual patient relives the source of the neurotic condition, in order to overcome it. The timing of this abreaction is sometimes as unexpected as was the onset of the disorder or disturbance. Lévi-Strauss refers to the shaman as a 'professional abreactor'. Perhaps much art in many cultures has this purpose as well, abstracted and generalized so that most of the members of the respective culture from which the art works come can understand their purpose and 'use' them to overcome whatever crisis they may be undergoing. The shaman's theater, sleight of hand, and other shadowy trickery as well as his or her rhetoric, smoke and mirrors, fire and brimstone, call and response, could well be seen as an early form of art itself. In the human world, one must generally manufacture one's own miracles.

The medical arts are so named for this reason; to even aid in recovery from the inexistence of death in life is a wondrous achievement. One feels like they have cheated at something, hence the proverbial 'new lease on life', as if a mythical landlord that still bears uncanny personification even in our own rationalized age has reluctantly renewed the agreement 'he' keeps with all humankind. To submit such notions to ridicule is itself to tempt fate. Speaking ill of the already dead is a resonance of some of this as well; the dead received new names upon passing over into the other-world. It is by these that they now must be called, aside from minding what one might say about them. In this, the will to life is revealed yet again, for in that prior life, and thus also being so for all those who yet live on towards their own deaths, names were bestowed and dropped in apophatic fashion. The previous name was itself considered 'dead' as was that form of being, that phase of life. In social contract societies these changes were punctuated in no uncertain terms by rites of passage at which we moderns cringe. There could be no going back, no regression, in social organizations of this type. For ourselves, the very absence of distinct life-phase boundaries creates uncounted problems, including the classic 'neuroses' investigated by psychoanalysis, as well as the enduring belief that something will come 'out of the blue' to save us from ourselves.

This said, it is also clear even for us that changing one's life overnight is a feat that is more suited to disease than cure: "Miracles are not so easy to come by: the mutation that made it possible—and which continues to do so every day—for the patient's 'bed' to become a field of scientific investigation and discourse is not the sudden explosive mixture of old practice and an even older logic …" (Foucault 1973, xv). Rather, the most profound miracle of modernity is the ability to suddenly understand both illness and health as non-magical events sourced in the same world as all other events, that is, the specifically and yet sometimes tacitly *mundane* world. The demystification of the dark miracle of disease is the *true* miracle of modern medicine.

Even so, this event gives forth one that is seen to structurally balance the metaphysical ledger. If miracles 'themselves' are no longer so easy to come by, our desire for them is only seen as increasing with their relative paucity. No doubt the techniques of medicine and their probability rates of success only contribute to our wishful thinking to this regard. Yet once disease as an evil has been vanquished, at least to the medical mind—and part of the reason we seek the doctor's wisdom is because he appears to exist in a state beyond the reach, not of disease *per se*, but of the symbolic quanta the disease carries with it into our consciousness, just as it carries its physical 'selfhood' into our bodies; in this, we have overpopulated the human condition with versions of ourselves, everything has a 'spirit', even, and perhaps especially, that which threatens our own—it is the very techniques and technologies of medical science that now can be imbued with a kind of magical quality. 'Its just a tool' does not satisfy our lust for results. For we know that tools and their use have, in a large degree, as well as with a degree of largesse, 'raised' us above the crowd of animal life that continues to either annoy us or even infect us—pests and pestilence are very much related, and not only etymologically—or inflame us with resentment and jealousy with regard to their apparent 'freedom' from conscious reflection, freedom from the knowledge of their own all the more sudden finitude.

The Suspense of Belief

In the combination of having to face up to this finitude which can only be known in general terms alongside the less potent facticality of our technical achievements and the extension of life in the face of death, we are still prone to desire when we are personally confronted by the threats to life that do not themselves retreat in the face of our technical skills. The metaphor of 'face' is telling: "It can be best understood as the deep-seated need for miracle cures. High-technology medicine is the most solemn element in a ritual celebrating and reinforcing the myth that doctors struggle heroically against death" (Illich 1975, 52). Such a struggle is only the outward manifestation of an interiority that has been darkened by the stain of inexistent death. 'Death walks among us' is the old-fashioned version of this now medicalized state. Its status is one of liminality, therefore it cannot be identified as to its outcomes. Hence the probability rates of success or failure for any medical procedure or health care treatment. We are not merely in the presence of the half-formed death, unable to yet walk but crawling along nevertheless toward us, we are in actual communion with it. This is the 'low' form of what Westlake intones as not only the goal of religion but also of 'life on earth'. Medicine should share this goal. (cf. 1973, 80ff). If we are thought of as a 'vessel', the 'jars of clay' motif so beloved in the Near East and with evangelical Christians in our own society, the *spiritus mundi* has itself abreacted to the presence of the disease and left its hermetic home. Just because we are material beings does not make us only that, it is claimed. We have already seen that it is homeopathy that makes much more mileage of these conceptualizations than does conventional medicine. But the round of life that, like the shaman's trance, does not so much recapitulate but relive, the sphere of being, hermetic in one sense, yes, but in much greater portion hermeneutic, contains all those events that give it its unique if oft unquiet character. This includes disease as well as health, for only in their combination can we gain the perspective necessary regarding why 'on earth' we are alive at all (cf. Jung 1959, 242ff regarding the metaphor of the 'roundness' of being). To recover then, is to experience the miracle of what is also a worldly though not necessarily mundane process. Perhaps the term abnormative would be a better fit; it is sometimes shown to be the case during conventional treatment or alternative therapy alike that one's body or character, one's own 'nature', an idea descended directly from the archaic sense that a divinity has implanted an element of herself in each human being, has taken the problem in hand and dealt with it summarily: "A miracle in acute disease is the operation of normal processes, restoring normality, speeded up until the time element is completely eliminated" (Westlake 1973, 101). Surely only something extramundane could be responsible for such a 'dilation', or someone, if the notion becomes personified, extra-human. The enduring popularity of entertainment fictions based on physics and astronomy use this sensitivity as leverage, given that we are alert to the possibility that we too, as merely human, can extend our abilities through the miraculous technologies of the nearer and farther futures alike. In this, we are never quite in the present, and thus never present to ourselves in the authenticating mode of anxiety that acquits itself not as fear or as obsessive worrying, but as the concernfulness of a being who only overcomes itself in its own death. As such, mortality is not a 'failure', but it is more often perceived as such because of its effect of time dilation. Only in death does time end for us, losing its meaning through the loss of our experience of its 'passage'. To the extent that time 'weighs' on us, we associate this with ill-health. The idea that time can be sped up is more often perceived as a testament to the good life, when we are free and 'having fun', as the casual saying has it. There is enough of this kind of experience still for us to keep up with the speed of medical science, avidly or on an *ad hoc* basis: "We maintain beliefs in drugs, 'wonder cures' and the progress of science even if a particular prescription or visit to a doctor seems ineffective for a particular illness. The wider set of cultural beliefs is not upset by occasional 'failures'" (Patrick and Scambler 1982, 12). Such disappointments have the ironic effect of humanizing the doctor-patient relationship. We know, going into the process that we might not be 'saved' after all. There are limits to the reach of our abilities, and the doctor is no less human than we. At the same time, we also know, perhaps from our own successes petty or profound, that human beings are at least capable of great things. Even if there is a systems failure at the domestic level, from plumbing to one's marriage, we have experienced a rebound. The pipes are fixed, the counselor adjusts our behavior towards our spouse, and all is well again. For social beings, it is our consciousness of the evaluative facticity of relationships that accord health or illness upon them. Their 'deontic' quality rests upon whether or not they push us in the direction of authentic Dasein. Since the world worlds on in its own way without care in the sense that human consciousness attributes to things it is solely our own responsibility to live within its worldly envelope. In this, life and death are exactly the same thing: in each case they are 'in every case my own.' Life may even be seen as the placebo for death. We are alive thanks to the knowledge that we remain ignorant of the timing of our respective demises. We have already cited Gadamer's epigram to this regard, but Heidegger's reality hinges upon the awareness of death as one's own and as one's destiny. We 'run on towards' it like no other form of being known to us.

Yet the placebo metaphor is, even so, a profanation. It works by a form of obscure psychosomatic magic, and is more evident within the body than outside of it. But like all authenticities, it turns the innards of a physical object into an interiority of a form of subjectivity that objects to its own corpus of available materials. This mode of being desires not to be 'alongside itself' but rather 'present to hand' as if it could be both a subject and an object for itself. We desire to make ourselves subject to the forces that heal us, yes, but we also wish to maintain our objection to the idea that we *need* to be healed in the first place. Enter the actual object of the placebo, no longer just a metaphor but a thing which produces, or rather, induces, an effect: "Whether the effectiveness of a placebo is attributed to the doctor's ability to inspire confidence and reduce anxiety, or to the faith and hope experienced by the patient on entry into a general practitioner's surgery or a hospital clinic, it is the social relationship between doctor and patient that engenders this powerful therapeutic effect" (Morgan 1982, 56). Saying this is not saying all that much. It is the surface of a dynamic that more truly finds an abode within the sensibility that one's life is more like another's than we would readily admit under regular circumstances. The doctor becomes *the* Doctor through the relative absence of our living relationship, not with him or her, but with ourselves. For it is our illness that has distanced us from being who we are, who we would generally like to be. No one wants to be ill unless they are so already distanciated from human relationships that this is the only way in which *care* can be conjured. Care, in the existential sense, is not only the keystone of community, it trumps our communalistic needs because it focuses them through the lens of our subjectivity. We may even find ourselves objecting to the care of others in this way, further obviating the pull of community and stretching the basis of the social contract. Since our health is of paramount value, and the health of society often seen as being the supporting cast for it, riding shotgun *alongside* us, but not therefore or thereby being present at hand as other beings like ourselves—more like a forced or even enforced version of present *to* hand, as in things of the object realm—our evaluation of what we now are as both sick and in need of support can never be entirely objective. In their objection, both to altered health and to our altered status, they lose their objectivity. Their facticity overcomes their facticality. In a word, the deontic character of illness is avoided by imagining that our life is more important than that of the other, especially if the other remains healthy while we succumb to this or that ailment, mild or serious. We become our sickness, and we are thus sickened because of this.

And this sickening feeling must be hidden at all costs. Not only is there present the stigmata leveled against those who come across as selfish and without conscience, as we can be when we are stricken in this way, but there is also the immediate sense that we must cooperate with those others because only through this dynamic can we be healed. We must turn our resentment, even our *ressentiment*, depending on whether or not it is our very life that is being threatened by illness, into gratitude and relief. Only the plague equals all comers, and when this approaches us, there is no other left who can be said to heal us *as* an other. Everyone caring about the same thing at once means that no one can care about any one thing. We as a society now suddenly cannot afford to care, and no one is responsible. As long as there are healthy people, it falls to them to heal the sick. The roles can be reversed, or they have already been. Of course this is so, and this gives us impetus to do many things we otherwise might not at all do, like paying school taxes when we ourselves have no children attending, and such like. But, "… in a field as value laden as health care, such perceptions may be extremely important to the providers or funders of care in enabling them to disguise *from themselves* the extent to which the are responsible for particular choices. When the decision is hard, the illusion of necessity may be comforting" (Evans 1987, 617, italics in the original). This sounds much like Nuremberg. And that is not at all 'comforting'.

The placebo metaphor is in fact wide-ranging. It is not contained in a sugar pill, but it certainly sugar-coats the world as it is. A forced choice is no choice at all, and we are very much aware of this. Each of us has had to accede to such a situation. The loss of freedom it entails, however momentary, can be sickening, and it reminds us of nothing other than being physically ill, for this condition too entangles us in a similar loss of our freedoms. For all the discussion of the 'loss of belief' that is accorded to our modern worldview, at least in the West, the faith we have in placebos, semi-conscious in action but still part of our common knowledge base, it is clear that 'unbelief' rusticates in regions that are the least threatening to existence, the least relevant to our self-understanding as living beings who desire to live on. While it is certainly the case that "The other factor which is thought to lead inevitably to unbelief is the spread of science and education. Here the ideological prejudice shows more clearly on the surface. People who hold this usually simply take for granted that religious belief is irrational and unenlightened or unscientific" (Taylor 1989, 310). Indeed, 'maturity' is almost as often used to denote the enlightened society, and it is also certain that almost none of us born into and quite used to the world we know as our own, would trade it for *any* previous period of human tenure on this planet. Even so, certain aspects of the two previous metaphysical world systems must appeal to us, whether they hail from the more primordial 'transformational' or the agrarian-based 'transcendental' varieties. Though we have 'aged', become more mature, the causes of our youth are not entirely lost on us. The youth of our species too, follows this metaphor and allows us to imagine that we are preserving something that is fundamental about ourselves, as if there was but one human nature, however narrowly defined and stripped down in scope. But this is mostly rhetorical, after all. No one actually thinks as did our ancestors, though since we cannot also know how *they* thought, the empiricity of such a question is rather moot. To know our own times is manifestly *not* to be more than a child of them. Gide and others have made that sentiment into a proverb. The ongoing notion that 'today's society' is always in a crisis is more than a media trick to attract readership and viewers. It has its inauthentic dwelling in the exteriority of an ideology that over-values itself; that is, it too serves as a general placebo for avoiding the task of confronting how we live in the day to day, without the notion of crisis present. For it is not crisis *per se* that lends itself to thought—panic often sabotages rational self-understanding at this point and sometimes also points along any process of therapy or healing—but reflection upon the cannily hidden uncanniness of human life as it tends to be lived. Akin to the problems of funding and service in actual health care systems, the wider issue of belief and the suspense it engenders, faux or furious, dilated or dilatory, must overcome the panic of the realization that all 'maturing' brings with it; simply the facticity of getting older combined with the personal experience of aging: "The rhetoric of a 'crisis' of aging is then used to create a spurious impression of inevitability and to screen those choices from relative scrutiny" (Evans 1987, 622). Since aging is in fact inevitable, it is a short step to the perception of it also being a crisis, especially when it brings on the manifestation of dying, however imperceptibly at first. Aging, because it is not what we would ideally do with our lives and since wasting away is also wasting them away in this sense, also may be perceived as a form of deviance. Certainly we have already seen how illness is associated with deviance. Not only that bodily functions may be impaired to the point of not working properly or 'normally', but the way we think subjected to the duress of illness sometimes short-circuits our general and once again, 'normal' rationality. Like an extreme emotion, illness pushes over the normative boundaries of civil behavior *and* thought. 'Uncivil' thinking, like incivility in action, is often observed amongst the aged. We usually put it down to the fact that their quality of life has itself been impaired to the extent that it makes it a grand task to enjoy anything about the day at hand. We 'let things go' in this way because we know that, through no fault of their own, the elderly have had to things let go, give up on much of their former lives and many of the activities that even though they once were able to do and have. Knowing too that it will happen to us eventually, though most often occurring to us in the form of the 'they' and thus inauthentically, is still enough to shrug off the insult or the offensiveness of aged incivility. We must concern ourselves rather with the deviance of those who still matter to society as a whole. Ironically, the forgiving and forgetting of the deviance of the aged is another sign of their irrelevance and even impending doom.

Long ago, Robert Merton understood the relationship between transgression and normative maintenance to be alternative routes to the same goals. Yet further back, it was Durkheim who famously characterized deviance as necessary to a functional society, as it allows the norms to be regularly upheld and even celebrated. We also know "… that disapproving cultural and professional reactions to deviant behaviour can often foster rather than inhibit a continuing commitment to deviance" (Scambler 1982, 188), and that this dynamic occurs in more relationships than simply those between teenagers and their parents. Such adolescent testing of boundaries is associated, also ironically, with the newly emerging maturity of young persons, that is, associated also with simply the aging process. One could view the life-phases as a serial glimpsing of the ultimate deviance which is death. In each, we clamber out of the shell of instilled behavioral and cognitive norms in order to breach their frame. The old self is killed. With each, therefore, there is a rehearsal for the final act which is different in character than the farewells to others we undertake during the life course. We say goodbye to ourselves. That we do it on our own terms is of the greatest importance to us, and hence our revulsion at illnesses that take from us our freedom to immolate ourselves. It is *this* deviance, that death steals from us not our life but our *freedom*, that pushes us to both avoid it and control it at once: "That death is so carefully evaded is linked less to a new anxiety which makes death unbearable for our societies than to the fact that the procedures of power have not ceased to turn way from death" (Foucault 1980, 138). On the frontline of this effort to manipulate the timing of our demise and to ideally censor it from our beings is medical science. Interestingly, part of the draw of homeopathic medicine, as we implied in the previous chapter, is that it performs an existential *volte face* regarding the necessity of dying. Dying is still seen as a 'natural' process, indeed, it becomes part of the 'naturalization of a cultural arbitrary', to borrow Bourdieu and Passeron's famous phrase, because in fact the death of a human being is always and already entirely a cultural event. This is the manner in which alternative therapies and treatments control death and is thus a testament to the fact that these discourses too, though they claim to be sourced in far older and more 'traditional' forms of healing, are in fact as modern as are their conventional competition.

That we focus on the deviance of death also helps us mask the facticality of our efforts to control it, to make its sacred presence as profane as possible –surely death, whether personified or rationalized, remains the ultimate scapegoat, the vehicle upon which all the shadows of humanity can be placed and carried off, crossing the Stygian waters; perhaps this is why 'Death' is the way 'he' is as 'he' has been forced to take on all that humanity finds in itself to be so burdensome—through medical procedures and processes: "Physicians are no longer concerned with the practical art of healing the curable, but with the salvation of mankind from the shackles of illness, impairment, and even the necessity of death" (Illich op. cit., 77). Is the doctor then the living version of the scapegoat of death? If he fails, he is stigmatized to a certain extent, even if medical science itself remains aloof to much criticism. Like bad teachers, poor doctors are remembered and not given recommendation to others. Since the doctor has been set up as the heroic warrior whose cause is the death of death, his life has already been filed away by the rest of us as not only unworthy for any other cause or even activity, but as being worthy only in this existential battle. The doctor is only alive, as it were, by virtue of his role in combatting that which threatens all life. His life is otherwise worth nothing. Hence the incredibly high burn-out rate of hospital doctors and even some clinicians. The social expectations we have regarding the doctor's ability, reflected in their remuneration and their status, the desire many still feel to preen their children to become medical professionals, and the sacredness of health care systems in many nations, all point to the ridiculous dynamic that pretends to involve a specific kind of living being as our favorite to dismount the rider of the pale horse. Akin to having a professional military—whose point it is only to pit the living against the living, at least a more plausible, if still vulgar aspiration—the idea that the vast majority of us simply have to sit back and await the results of fights to the death casts obloquy on our notion of 'civility'. Perhaps this is why deviance is also so enamoured and even adored by those on the sidelines. Norms alone cannot defeat those who are already patently abnormative. Furthermore, "Behind the doctor's back, death remained the great dark threat in which is knowledge and skill were abolished; it was the risk not only of life and disease but of knowledge that questioned them" (Foucault 1973, 146). If by norms alone the villains inhabiting human consciousness could not be eliminated, and a good that stayed good would never triumph over that which was determined to stay evil, then how was it that medicine maintained itself in spite of being given an impossibly unreasonable task as its reason to be?

In Mid Air

Yet the situation is not as mysterious as it first appears. First, it is not so much a situation as a situatedness of being. It an aspect of the authentic existentiality of

Dasein to be concerned about our own finitude and to confront it in a manner that speaks to us of what we are at present in the world as it is. Anxiety is hereby revealed as a positive 'function' of being and also an ippsissimosity to it. It is more than part of an 'identity', as this term is far too hyletic in its politics and overly reliant on structural social variables such as gender or ethnicity. One's existentiality is only disclosed as the world in which one is as one's being must be. There is no being in the 'they' that cannot be understood as what is present at hand in the way objects are perceived. The 'they' is thus an environmental frame. 'What is called thinking' is almost always the received traditions and customs, mores, and folkways of our predecessors. It is unthought while not going so far as to be non-thought, a category which could be reserved for much of popular culture that is overlaid on our more anthropologically definable predilections. As such, any analysis of the discourse that serves us as the repository for life, healing and restoring, curing and rehabilitating, must partake in both the definitions made ostensibly indispensable by the socius—including scapegoating as a facticality; it is only disclosed as a facticity when subjected to a phenomenological lens that attempts to understand the *ethical* implications of human actions and thought—and those made more clear by venturing into a lighted space of worlding, that is, thinking as reflection and involvement, *Phronesis* as a mode of being in the world. For every form of subjection and objection, the Gemini of our thrown projects, then, "… it is not clear what a complete explanation would be, since there are as infinite number of questions that might be asked about it" (Midgely 2004, 52). Not that any single human life has the character of infinitude. We have even suggested throughout this study that what we seek is merely a human version of this, that is, indefinitude, rather than the temporal indefinition within which we currently as a species exist. We are at a loss to express such ambiguities, and thus fall back on remarking upon them. Commentary takes the form of editorial, and few of us are above engaging in at least private homiletics regarding the offensiveness of others. Historically, outward signs of the character of this or that human life were not remarkable in themselves, for the scarlet letters of social stigmata abounded. One could well be suspended by belief, let alone being brought to hang there, in midair, swaying in the not so gentle breezes of one's own cultural suasions.

Such remarking, marking the body so everyone could know what kind of person you in fact were, or executing the miscreant by torturing his or her body publicly, are also quasi-medical devices. They too represent a culture's desire to control death, even though the taking over of death's duties in an 'official' manner, or perhaps better, the making of death a duty rather than a simple happenstance or an inevitability, could reach outlandish proportions, as when a chief would hang a suicide just to put the stamp of office upon the corpse and 'punish' it symbolically. Disease too was interpreted as such a punishment, coming from another form of being or a natural force that had been offended in some way. Since this was the case, there might also be diseases that occur by chance, with no implication of curse or ragged fate. If so, they must be so distinguished by the new sciences of medicine and indeed, generate the first nascent pictures of being healthy meant: "There is no lack of irony in the fact that the scientific expression still used by physicians is Lues Insontium—the plague of the innocent. The stigma that falls upon the syphilitic also extends to the skin diseases generally among large sections of the populace" (Sigerist 1977, 393). Yet this distinction is a crucial one: no science could arise in a culture where all ailments were understood to be either verdicts of a moral judgement or as maleficence caused by witchcraft or sorcery. The very origin of illness had to be redefined, and the idea that one could be innocent of the traditional or customary sources of disease and yet bear the marks of something very similar to it was revolutionary. These kinds of distinctions also remarked upon the novel differences between doctor and priest, and began the separation between the arts of the shaman and that of the physician. In primordial times, all of this was found in one social role-player. At issue was, in the final analysis, the health of the spirit, and hence all discomfort fell under the purview of the shaman or 'witch-doctor', to use the colonialist but not entirely inappropriate nomenclature. Such an expression today not only smacks of 'primitivism' but is logically something that cannot make sense. Not only are these distinct roles—their coexistence was the subject of sometimes intense conflict, much of it gender based, when one considers the witch hunts and trials of the later renaissance and colonial periods—the 'witch' as a recognizable role in contemporary society has been so marginalized as to be non-existent. Aside from social inversion rituals like All Hallows Eve, or anachronistic recreational groups, being a witch today could only be regarded by the vast majority of us to be something that might be a feature of a certain kind of mental illness. Even here, the exertion of control over a potential source of illness and death includes satire, ridicule, and other forms of humor that bear the mark of ancient stigmata. Is it also ironic that it is in children's literature and entertainment that the character of the witch might still appear? Or that there are here also posited 'good' witches, such as those of the North and South in L. Frank Baum. No doubt this reflected the general American effort to get over the carnage and tension of the Civil War, another expression that is kindred with 'witch doctor' in our modern mindset, for how can any war, by definition, be 'civil'? Both North and South were good and had the joint task of administering goodness over the ideal realm expressed in the landscape into which Dorothy and her dog are projected. But the new tension of the latter years of the nineteenth century was clearly between the East, urban, industrialized and 'civilized' and the West, uncivil in the extreme, rural, and proverbially lawless. Hence the characterization of the witches hailing from *these* two directions as 'wicked'. The fact that Dorothy's family home lands on one of them extinguishing her life is a clear reference to settlement being one of the chief vectors of civilization. A farm house, no less, and when water 'melts' the other wicked witch later on, we are to interpret this as simply irrigating the land, also a marker of the advent of civilization and thus civility. This minor assay into literary interpretation is not as tangential as it appears to be. It has its immediate analogues in water and bed rest in the most commonplace of all medical treatments. 'Get plenty of rest and drink plenty of liquids' is perhaps the most obvious and remarked upon advice from any clinician, so much so that it is a very rare layperson or a child who does not know it themselves and thus has no real need of seeking its affirmation in an official or formal manner. There is, in the majority of minor cases of illness, no need at all to be 'off to see the Wizard'.

But there is a further distinction to be made on the historical road that leads this time to the cities of glass and concrete that glisten across the landscape of our own dream worlds. Just as the doctor and the witch come to be separated in terms of role and moral aspect, so too must the doctor distance himself from much closer cousins. The doctor practices and is interested in, if not humanity 'itself', then at least in this or that particular case of human being, the patient or client, the subject whose object is afflicted and is thus causing, objectively, a problem for his subjectivity: "There are, then, good reasons why doctors do not see their profession as equivalent either to that of the scientist or researcher, or to that of a mere technician [ ] Part of what a doctor does closely resembles an art, and is something which cannot be conveyed through theoretical instruction" (Gadamer 1996, 163 [1989]). The art of healing has also an irony imbedded within it, for it brings the doctor back into contact with his early ancestor, the shaman. In fact, even if we have parsed the methodological aspects of these two roles their moral bonds remain much more intact. It is through the almost 'aesthetic' ambience of healing—and does not one feel similar in recovery as one might when in the presence of a work of art, an aesthetic object; and is not, somewhat proverbially and still rather dubiously with regard to sexism, the human body in its youth and freshness considered one of the ultimate aesthetic objects?—that the doctor meets his long lost ancestor and has to come to relative terms with him. We hold the doctor to this because we suspect that his modern relative, the scientist, is inherently incapable of such an encounter: "A scientist observer who had never experienced joy or sorrow, love or hatred, religious or aesthetic bliss, justice or injustice, creative or dull moments, certitude or doubt, can never obtain even the remotest knowledge of these living, feeling, wishing, emotional, and thoughtful states" (Sorokin 1956, 159–60). The hand alone 'cannot touch the part that's dead' (cf. Shem 1978, 211ff). There must be, in other words, a presence of the still alive, and still to be living, for the doctor to act at all. This is not the case with either other kinds of scientific researchers or technicians of any kind. Other students of life even may skirt the issue of the living, by poring over texts, for instance, or engaging only in the world of ideas. It is a symptom of our scientifically idealized culture that we have given over to a specifically formal and rationally discursive sense of truth many other aspects of the mode of being authentic both in the world and 'beyond' it. This concatenation and thence concentration of such a suite of ideals only makes the doctor's task more difficult: "The other values we think of as scientific are intellectual virtues such as honesty, disinterestedness, thoroughness, imaginative enterprise, a devotion to truth. Those virtues are indeed scientific, but they are so in the older and wider sense of that word which is not restricted to physical science" (Midgely 2004, 11). The same values may be present in all human endeavors, for in each a kind of truth is sought. Even in the most petty of circumstances, and certainly in those most profound, we seek to know 'what occurred'; whether it might be spying on our children motivated by jealousy or gazing through the orbital telescope searching for new worlds motivated by a deep curiosity concerning the existence of life.

No doubt curiosity alone cannot guide us to the truth of things in all cases. Reich's notorious and still partially unexplained experiments with Orgone energy and radiation sickness are a case in point (cf. Westlake 1973, 56ff). When the cosmos opens itself up to us, our being opens itself onto it. It is the graceful version of Nietzsche's abyss. Westlake quotes Reich who wrote at the time: "We all felt we had gone through some awful, deadly dangerous experience which we could not yet fully grasp, which had thrown us into some great depth, a hitherto well-hidden domain of cosmic functioning ..." (from April of 1950). Profound emotion does not, of course, always correlate with profound discovery. We humans do replay old tapes, recite aging scripts, and sometimes simply go through the motions. The theatrical aspect of social life cannot stop; the show, as it were, must go on no matter the state of the beings who are scheduled to perform. Medical professionals with whom I spoke agreed to a person that this sensibility, originally made famous by the entertainment business, was like a mantra to them in their daily rounds. The depths of life were quite normative for them, dying and death, sorrow and the sudden of all things made abruptly clear, from lab results to diagnoses to prognoses. This kind of work life might be said to dull the most human of senses, or quite literally replace sensitivity with sensibility, as one begins to sense that one might not be able to afford to be too concerned about the others in one's care. But in so far as the doctor and his coterie of skilled assistants continue to practice a form of science, they do so in respect to the truth of things. And the disclosure of truth in the ambit of human life and death is always going to necessitate an opening of oneself, however slight: "According to this, the meaning that the natural phenomena bear is no longer defined by the order of nature in itself or by the Ideas which they embody. It is defined by the effect of the phenomena on us, in the reactions they awaken" (Taylor 1989, 299). When Reich and his associates experienced trauma, they each did so in a specific manner accorded in correlation with the specific weaknesses or illnesses they were suffering from, or had suffered from in the past. The romantic quality to such experiments, and Reich's is hardly the only example in the history of medicine or science more generally, is something which must give us pause. At the same time, just because results are unexpected and even bizarre, our devotion to truth must always trump our loyalty to whatever may be the current and even fashionable discourses of our own time. Like the artists who have reminded us that though we are children of our own time and always must be so, the trick remains to not be a slave to this time in addition to being its scion. The same goes for science. In profaning all that is strange to us, we are exhibiting an undue and unnecessary allegiance to the social structures and norms that inasmuch as they provide for us the accepted truth of things they also must do so at the expense of knowing truth anew.

Summa Iatrogenica?

Just as the doctor must discover something new in relation to a particular person become patient, and this person must also be opened up by the newness of her experience, medicine as a discourse retains its hermeneutic value. We have stated that illness is a mode of 'deontic facticity', an aspect of the ontic world which brings it within range of both authenticity and ontology. It does so only because it discloses itself both subjectively, as a form of objection to our continued existence, and objectively, as a form of subjection to the discourses of the clinic and to practical science. It remains to discuss how this dual disclosure influences both our understanding of what medical science is in today's world and how it can provide an ongoing source of self-understanding by virtue of the intimacy, even intrusiveness, of its operations and therapies.

Outcomes

Does medicine, in the longer view, offer us an opportunity for a self-understanding that extends beyond the self-absorbed experience of finding out what is the matter with me and then trying to overcome it? This is a question that is focused on relatively singular experiences, but it is one that is but an aspect of the same query writ large and addressing the historical condition in which we find both ourselves and thus our illness and health alike: "We must ask whether the present world situation does not present us with specifically human responsibilities, and whether modern science with its ethos of achievement, which has brought these responsibilities to a crucial point, is not forcing western culture towards a critical self-examination?" (Gadamer 1996, 71 [1986]). Whenever we are ourselves forced to interrogate something about our own lives, we are resonating with this wider question. It can be as, or even more, uncomfortable as the physical malady itself. Indeed, part of the deontology of disease in modern discourse has occurred precisely because of the rise of the very notion of subjectivity that underlies modern politics, aesthetics, and ethics combined. Though we can disdain it as the sole font of 'oceanic' experience, as did Nietzsche and Freud, we nevertheless cannot avoid existing within its epistemological ambit. It is one of the 'entanglements' of which Heidegger speaks so seriously in *Being and Time*, but its very mesh is a clue to the sense that there is another kind of world beyond that we might still grasp, for who is entangled who is not also outside this other world? How can one even speak of an inside without also immediately beckoning the outer frontiers of existence? Illness takes the outside world away from us. We are forced to confront and thence to reckon with our interiors, the real source of being-entangled. Its deonticity is deliberately provocative. One can, of course, ignore illness for many years depending on its character, and one equally can be quite ill and not even know it until very late in the game, sometimes very much too late. Ultimately, however, illness cannot be so denied, in the same way the manner in which we live in the world as a species is brought home to us from time to time. We must face down our selfishness and give up some of our self-interest in order not merely to keep the general peace, but to have a future. The ignorance regarding our own specific ends is more than compensated for by the hyper-calculated means we have at our disposal for ending humankind as a whole. They are not at all unrelated.

The dream of overcoming human finitude begins in the microcosm of a simple farewell. All things come to end, sometimes pleasantly and with the bittersweet taste of something that we would not have missed but that we also know that we shall miss, and sometimes with greater discomforts brought on by knowing that our part in the affair was not up to either social standards or yet the ideals by which our culture has constructed both institutions and ethics alike. However far we fall from general social graces, illness provides us with the opportunity to take stock of the times we have caused pain for others. Not that we do so in the way someone catches a cold from some other person, but how we view the world, our staunch and stalwart opinions, our sense of propriety and predestination, is also catching, sometimes forcibly. To be healthy means far more than the absence of physical illness or infectious disease. It is, at first and most imminently, to avoid being the source of malady and malaise in the world around us, To do so, life and thought must remain intimate with one another, and medicine is in fact a reasonable model to take regarding this kind of intimacy: "… it is right to emphasize the primacy of living, But wrong to suggest that philosophy is an adjunct added on to life, when in fact it should be a vital activity we carry on to clarify our way among the tangled affairs of the everyday" (Barrett 1979, 73). Medicine deals in the everyday but to do so, it must also take part in exercises which are philosophical in character. We have already commented upon the importance of dialogue and interpretation, but concernful being, the care of authenticity, and the rigor of method and epistemology, logic and rationality all come into play at many junctures along the way of healing. If the clinic is today rationalized to the point of stretching its human relationships almost beyond recognition, this has more to do with the external pressures of politics and demographics than with the core values of medical science. To utter this at this late point in a critical analysis of medicine is not to abruptly opt out of any critique. Ideals that emanate from the search for the truth of things cannot be confused with utility. Rationality is not necessarily instrumental. Homeopathic discourses often confuse the two of these, as often as does conventional medicine dismiss the emotional aspect of healing and therapy. The more each competing viewpoint solidifies its position against the other the less insight we can expect from either of them: "No simple rule for the application of theory to practice should be expected, since that is more than science is able to give. There art and venture begin" (Lösch 1967, 138). In fact, "… science must carry on a kind of demythologization of itself and indeed by its very own means: critical information and methodical discipline" (Gadamer 1996, 7 [1972]). The arena of health care is the very place to enact such a self-reflection. Far more so than engineering, with which we opened this study by way of a brief comparison, the humanity of medical discourse can never be avoided. The exterior spaces that we construct for ourselves, beautiful and profound as some of them are, cannot truly be compared to the interiority of consciousness. Even the body's interior is a moving microcosm of evolutionary forces both at work and working themselves out with each intake of breath. They too are theory applied in the most sophisticated sense of the idea. The model for medical success is held within our own beings, corpus mitigated and sometimes overseen by *corps d'esprit*. The body improvises while utilizing time-tested means. Its weakness is our own; when it comes to rely on methods that had always worked but can no longer do so in the face of a new challenge. Perhaps we are still too wedded to our physical forms to understand fully this issue. The body is kindred with the institution. Its parts come and go, and it is said that every seven years or so all cells are replaced so that we are, in a sense, a completely different 'model', like a new line of automobile that looks very much the same but in fact has had all its parts redesigned and substituted. Or, at least, we may feel that we have been given a new lease on life and have, somewhat vicariously and with none of the long-term perenniality of the wider nature, been given a glimpse of what it might be like to live forever. Institutions are also a human way of expressing this same desire. But like the body, if they cannot adapt adeptly and adopt something new in the face of what is equally new, they suffer the malaise of ensuing irrelevance and thus decay. Evans speaks of the 'efflorescence of the health care system' as being part of this problem, simply because in its expansion it has not maintained the necessary diversity to confront a changing human condition (cf. 1987, 633ff). Illich too never tires of reminding us that the over-production of health care does not in any way guarantee a greater health. Further, "The depersonalization of diagnosis and therapy has turned malpractice from an ethical into a technical problem" (1975, 25). There are also ethical questions, as well as those concerning technical competence, about the 'missionizing' of certain therapies, especially those on the alternative side of supply. This is an older question than it would seem to be at first glance: "The experiences of the sick person represent the least important aspect of the system, except for the fact that a patient successfully treated by a shaman is in an especially good position to become a shaman in his own right, as we see today in the case of psychoanalysis" (Lévi-Strauss 1977, 451). Amusement aside—and, indeed, there have been more than a few feature films whose plots make much of this translocution of roles, following perhaps the equally venerable 'apprentice becomes master' trope—to bring such an ascension back into the ambit of ethics is to widen the search for meaning far beyond that of the medical sphere. Healing then takes on, ironically, an older definition, and includes, in our mass societies where politics cannot be said to reliably represent either a people's or much less a person's needs and views, 'speaking up', which is said by Shem in his 2010 afterword to be essential for our 'survival as human beings' (op. cit., 377). The matriculation process in any institution often serves to silence critical voices. One becomes, quite proverbially, 'part of the system'. Even tenure is not a form of freedom in this regard. Veteran professionals are expected to be all the more loyal. A word from the elders is enough to make or break the neophyte, and this relationship is almost as old as is society itself. Interns of all types in health care have as many ethical doubts as their peers in other systems of practice, with the exception perhaps of business where one's doubts are introspective and have to do with the idea of relative competence, or politics, where such doubts are extrospective and concern one's ability to play the game. The most successful institutions wherein training occurs extinguish as many of these kinds of doubts, ethical, technical, intellectual and political or ideological, well before any 'on the job' work begins. We may well say that the 'health' of any system depends on its *lack* of healthy self-reflection.

Divides

But this is something one can say precisely of a *system*, whether of thought or practice, theory or application. And all systems, no matter how seemingly self-contained, do reference outside sources for their most technical operations. These may be found in history and epistemology, language and logic: "The most austere operationist communicates not operations but a prior concept, for operational symbolizing depends upon prior ideas of entities and relations that are symbolized" (Alport in Sorokin, 1956, 34). One version of such an analytic involves the exposition of structural social variables. There have been a multitude of such studies as applied to the contexts of health care over the past few decades and all of them point to 'prior' concepts in their results. Stock phrases such as "… a strong association between gender, type of occupation, work setting and level of autonomy" is revealed through these analyses (Butterick et al. 1994, 85). As insightful as such studies are, they themselves also point to another and farther hinterland of 'symbolizing', such as "… the social and physical reproduction of the working class on a daily and generational level is left to the ingenuity of the workers themselves" (Gimenez 1994, 299). Needless to say, all health care personnel of whatever remuneration and social status must at the end of the day fall back upon a language that does not expressly represent their position or role in the labor force. Doctors proverbially play golf and often, even stereotypically, abuse substances, mostly licit. Nurses and other staffers smoke and over-eat. In the field, I was consistently on guard against not seeing anything *but* these events, and nevertheless I still observed them regularly. If training and status-role divided health care workers, their vices united them.

More than this, there was also observed an undue homologic effect between the care prescribed for others and self-care. One asked, and was asked, if, for instance, "… tranquillizers [are] to be accepted as adequate solutions to social stresses?" (Cooperstock and Lennard 1987, 329). One reminded, and was reminded, that "These are clearly moral and ethical issues that transcend the bounds of the expertise of the medical profession …" (ibid) But even if this is patently correct, the fact remained that it was almost solely the medical professionals' responsibility to grapple with these kinds of issues and others like them, and thence to assign therapies and evaluate their ensuing results. None of this had ever an ethical overtone to it, but rather at most, an undertone. Or, perhaps it would be more precise to say that a moral overtone was present and an ethical undertone absent. Kindred with the placebo effect, moralizing amongst medicos is only a slightly less stereotypical phenomena than substance abuse. The both of them have a similar intent and effect: one is relieved of self-examination through the study of others, recused from self-understanding by, potentially, bringing to another some new enlightenment, and allowed to engage in projection; the vice of the self is certainly present in the other—it still takes one to know one, even in this highly technical and rationalized sense—but it is made into a presence. The shadow of one's own selfhood is deferred by observing its differed form as attached to another person.

Yet in health care systems and their significant sets of symbols, it is also correct to state that "… a distinction must be made between individual or personal systems of ethics and those that prescribe the conduct of health care professionals, although the distinction is often blurred" (Frankel, Speechley, and Wade 1999, 205). Sociologists would be more likely to use the rubric of 'professional mores' rather than ethics, which always turns heads in the direction of a more formal philosophy on the one hand, but also, and in a less thoughtful manner, to morality. Ethics, by definition, cannot be enshrined in a code, one of conduct or ideals. Ethics is a manifestation of Phronesis and therefore occurs on the ground and in action. Not that this is to say that when understood and 'applied' only in this sense does ethics finally and for all time entirely free itself from moral principles. The standards of conduct in a rationalized organization, simply more succinct and staccato formulations of those one finds in the wider community, are only circumnavigated by the most adroit and artful ethical movements. Ethics as reflective practice does not really have a place in medicine, and if this sounds tantamount to anarchy, consider that between the goal of healing and that of maintaining its authority, pragmatism pure and simple, without the manifest and ongoing doubt of any authentic ethics, must carry the day. One must do and therefore one cannot dream.

It is left to the patient to summarize the options regarding human experience, much as we just saw it being left to the workers to sort out their sensibilities regarding class position and gendered hierarchies, not to mention how far their salaries might get them each month. In doing so, the person become patient accrues a kind of ethical honor, but also shame: "Fatal illness has always been viewed as a test of moral character, but in the nineteenth century there is a great reluctance to let anybody flunk the test. And the virtuous only become more so as they slide toward death" (Sontag 1978, 40). Today the outward moralizing of the medical facility is muted, as we have seen. Nonetheless, alongside in a present at hand fashion we still observe the patient's ideas of what constitutes the good life, including her health, in tension with the medical discourse's notions of what a good outcome can be in each case. This is another division within the space of the clinic that can only be confronted if the patient becomes herself a health professional and self-medicates, or becomes a corpse, an object to be dissected or analyzed by the coroner as the case may be.

Even the language of those who have recognized this divide tends to further it rather than the opposite: "When all is said and done, we are still profoundly ignorant as to what constitutes a cure in the fundamental sense. We are too prone to judge everything by a physical cure, and overlook the true needs of the soul" (Westlake 1973, 153). What precisely these may be, even assuming such an outlandish 'thing' as a soul or spirit in our own day, are an even greater mystery than how one overlooks the *idea*, reasonable enough in itself, that the human being has needs that resonate beyond the physical realm of mere objects and object relations. Why should we not begin there? Overstating the case is symptomatic of a situation where one aspect of being has been long neglected. Feminism and Marxism, and even Phenomenology in their most trenchant declarations provide easy examples of this pendulum effect with regard to fashionable discourses. We know that the human condition does not rest on 'bread alone', but does this automatically imply any form of transcendence? Modern medicine has opted to steer clear of the question long enough. It is of the moment to address just what the metaphysics of medical science means for *our* culture without, with nostalgia both hypocritical and vacuous, summoning the 'old gods' of another era to give tired witness to their now vintage retirement.

Visions

If we did so, what might we observe? The hubris of pendulum thinking cannot disclose the lighted space of being in the world. For it always runs headlong, not towards death as an *Aufklärung*, but rather into its opposite: "Nemesis is the inevitable punishment for inhuman attempts to be a hero rather than a human being" (Illich 1975, 28). Such attempts litter the supposedly reenchanted landscape of alternative medical practices, as well as the thoroughly disenchanted but still magical décor of conventional medicine. With each disappointment, the presence of nemesis becomes more clear to us, if only personally. We understand that one of the marks of mature being is recognizing in oneself the heroic attempts that might never have been made. It is not that heroism in principle is uncalled for. There are moments aplenty even in our brief existence where it is necessary. It is the *motivation* for bravery that Nemesis questions us about. And there remain conflicting motives behind the kinds of choices we currently are making in society and culture regarding the value of medical care and the purpose thereof. The 'right to die' movement and subsequent legislation is one particularly delicate yet at once simmering announcement of this conflict. Do we really own ourselves, in a polis of citizenry and as ward of the state in the loosest sense? Every ethics presumes that we do, and hence another tension and division is exposed, though not fully disclosed, regarding what kind of vision we may expect from the lenses of health care systems and the governments or other organizations that sponsor them. There must be a division of ethical and intellectual labor struck amongst these often competing sources of sight: Nodding to Weber, Gadamer states unequivocally that "… it is the task not of science but of politics to supervise the application of the know-how made possible by science. It is also conversely the task not of politics but of science to supervise its own needs, investments in time and money, etc. This is, in the final analysis, the function of scientific criticism" (1996, 25 [1972]). Because the potential material value and political advantage is so heady, the products of science are always accorded greater fanfare than its methods. We lust after them with a patent disregard for how they are achieved. The same science understands evolution to be a fact just as much as it has constructed any factual automobile. It is not entirely the fault of politics that science has been reduced, in many cases, to indentured servitude. Medicine too has contributed to this acceptance of science as a specific kind of tool. Science as a tool used for the benefit of material aims alone is but a shadow of its true character and worth. It is perhaps an odd way of expressing such an ideal, but Selye, a medical doctor and biologist, opines that "… *I do not think anyone has ever died of old age yet.* To permit this would be the ideal accomplishment of medical science" (1956, 276), italics in the original). In this sense, 'old age' glances toward indefinitude, the 'eternal' that is relatively stated in the following: "Disease likewise forces us to recognize the place of destiny in our lives. It activates our spiritual sensitivity. It directs our gaze towards the eternal" (Sigerist 1977, 389). What this kind of language has in common is the retreat from hubris. It is a forced taking stock, yes, but still a well-chosen one. Whether or not this indication carries the human condition beyond itself is not so important as its effects in the here and now. Whether or not a cosmology that is scientifically valid can also presume to have some kind of religious significance is equally dubious (cf., Westlake 1973, 59ff), but what medicine has furnished us with, aside from the techniques and technologies of extending the quantity of life and, it must be admitted, also enhancing its quality especially when compared with other historical epochs, is that we are able to gain an insight about the nature of *care* as an aspect of authentic Dasein. We do care to care, at the least, and this is a beginning.

For each of us, as a potentially caring being, we must also accept that facticity of an enactmental complex that includes our deficits; that we, in our caring, care to be cared for and feel strongly that the care we give to others will, in some version of life and consciousness, be made remedial and even reciprocal. But to care simply because we can is perhaps another matter. Such figures abode in our myths, medical or otherwise, but "… reality is less tidy than myth. Time and again real personal experience breaks through, at times negating the myth, taking the story in unexpected directions and finally giving its own substance to every life story" (Burchardt 1990, 249). However exasperating to both historians, scientists, but most especially, ideologues of all stripes and axes, the experience of the lifeworld as it is, within a structural envelope but also without it, provides for human consciousness its mode of operating, its genesis, and a self-understanding that echoes Marx and Engels' famous 'consciousness too is a social product'. If this is so, specifically in our age and thus for ourselves as conscious beings who understand that we have a history but are unsure of what it truly consists, both culturally and personally, we must rely on experience all the more. We come to know, after hard times which often include illness and recovery, interactions with apparently uncaring places of care, ministries of truth who are caught in a lie of policy and process, and all of the farewells this life rehearses with us, that "… the life world takes precedence. It is, after all, the reality which we live, while the scientific world is a reality we conceive …" (Barrett 1979, 139). Within its ambit, we find two contrasting modes of being: one can be aptly denoted as its 'grasp', the other, its 'embrace'. Not only does reality both grasp and embrace us at once, we exert the same in return. Grasping demeans both ourselves and the world in which we must live with others, while embracing is a sign of both fondness and gentleness, along with the respect that the world of others and the lifeworld itself needs from each of its denizens. It would be sentimental to simply utter 'therefore, choose embrace, so that …', but what one can state is that however real something may be to us, including the suffering that comes with illness and the joy that always attends the experience of health, we do not, in our finitude and our partiality, know the fullest extent of what reality means, for either ourselves and especially for others. We have turned back the pages on many a mystery, but what is mysterious about life remains in the background of all we find puzzling or intriguing about our particular lives. This is a fundamental structure of any curious consciousness, of any sentience that possess the faculties of both reason and wonder. Its continued presence, chased by method and framed by discourse, is likely primordial and as such, both sacred and scientific at once: "In primitive epochs, mystery had 'use-value' and man lived with it, could not avoid it for his life—it was his form of possessing things, even to know—for everything demonic and superstitious is only a label on a sealed bottle. Now, though, when we know so much, mystery has 'scarcity-value'. The more it is repressed, and the more what was once mystery is now in essence knowable or actually becomes known, the more purely is revealed the range and essence of what is inherently mystery" (Simmel 2010, 185 [1918]). Any science that seeks the ultimate mystery and its solution, that of what makes a human life and what does not, that which can be said to underscore the singing architecture of consciousness, found the order of our reason and work the wondrous in front of our very sense of wonder *must*, by definition, inhabit the sacred. Though its policies, processes, treatment and therapies, techniques and technologies often hide this simple facticity from us, or even seek to hide it, this is merely another manifestation of what Simmel has identified as 'inherently' mysterious to us. Neither do we exercise our human faculties in a way that is bereft of mystery, for we do not have the much idealized freedom of being able to know ourselves only as an impartiality of the world: "Such a freedom, such a standing at a distance from the examined object simply does not exist" (Gadamer 1998b, 28).

As long as finitude remains the moment wherein our interiority and our intentionality construe each other as soul-mates, we will conjure the mystery of the soul reimagined through our science. Medical science is not the epitome of this cosmogony, but rather the discourse and practice of the soul ignited by our perennial desire to overtake the soul's own limits, to vivisect and exonerate the spirit by subjecting it to the healing force of all that lies without its freedom.

References

Bachelard, Gaston. 1964 *The Psychoanalysis of Fire.* Boston: Beacon Press [1938].

Barrett, William. 1979. *The Illusion of Technique: A Search for Meaning in a Technological Civilization.* New York: Anchor Books.

Burchardt, Natasha. 1990. "Stepchildren's Memories: Myth, Understanding, and Forgiveness." In *The Myths We Live By*, edited by Raphael Samuel and Paul Thompson, 239–251. London: Routledge.

Butterick, Irene H., E. S. Carpenter, B. J. Kay, and R. S. Simmons. 1994. "Gender Hierarchies in the Health Labor Force." In *Women's Health, Politics, and Power: Essays on Sex/Gender, Medicine and Public Health*, edited by Elizabeth Fee and Nancy Krieger, 79–96. Amityville, NY: Baywood.

Cooperstock, Ruth, and Henry L. Lennard. 1987. "Role Strains and Tranquillizer Use. In *Health and Canadian Society: Sociological Perspectives, Second Edition*, edited by George Torrance, 295–313. Toronto: Fitzhenry and Whiteside.

Evans, Robert G. 1987. "Illusions of Necessity: Evading Responsibility for Choice in Health Care." In *Health and Canadian Society: Sociological Perspectives, Second Edition*, edited by George Torrance, 615–36. Toronto: Fitzhenry and Whiteside.

Foucault, Michel. 1980. *The History of Sexuality Volume One: Introduction.* New York: Vintage Books [1978].

Foucault, Michel. 1973. *The Birth of the Clinic.* New York: Vintage Books [1963].

Frankel, B. Gail, Mark Speechley, and Terrance J. Wade. 1996. *The Sociology of Health and Health Care: A Canadian Perspective.* Toronto: Copp Clark.

Freund, Peter E. S., and Meredith B. McGuire. 1999. *Health, Illness, and the Social Body: A Critical Sociology.* New York: Prentice-Hall.

Gadamer, Hans-Georg. 1935. "Ancient Atomic Theory." In *The Beginning of Knowledge*, 82–101. New York: Continuum [2001].

Gadamer, Hans-Georg. 1972. "Theory, Technology, Praxis." In *The Enigma of Health: The Art of Healing in a Scientific Age*, 1–30. Stanford: Stanford University Press [1996].

Gadamer, Hans-Georg. 1978 "Greek Philosophy and Modern Thought." In *The Beginning of Knowledge*, 119–126. New York: Continuum [2003].

Gadamer, Hans-Georg. 1986. "Bodily Experience and the Limits of Objectification." In *The Enigma of Health: The Art of Healing in a Scientific Age*, 70–82. Stanford: Stanford University Press [1996].

Gadamer, Hans-Georg. 1989. "Hermeneutics and Psychiatry." In *The Enigma of Health: The Art of Healing in a Scientific Age*, 163–73. Stanford: Stanford University Press [1996].

Gadamer, Hans-Georg. 1990. "Philosophy and Practical Medicine." In *The Enigma of Health: The Art of Healing in a Scientific Age*, 92–102. Stanford: Stanford University Press [1996].

Gadamer, Hans-Georg. 1995 "Natural Science and the Concept of Nature." In *The Beginning of Knowledge*, 127–140. New York: Continuum [2003].

Gadamer, Hans-Georg. 1998a. *The Beginning of Philosophy.* New York: Continuum [1996].

Gadamer, Hans-Georg. 1998b. "Author's Preface." In *The Beginning of Knowledge*, 15–19. New York: Continuum [2003].

Gadamer, Hans-Georg. 2003 "Greek Philosophy and Modern Thought." In *The Beginning of Knowledge*, 119–26. New York: Continuum [1978].

Gimenez, Martha E. 1994. "The Feminization of Poverty: Myth or Reality?" In *Women's Health, Politics, and Power: Essays on Sex/Gender, Medicine and Public Health*, edited by Elizabeth Fee and Nancy Krieger, 287–306. Amityville, NY: Baywood.

Haas, Jack, and William Shaffir. 1987. "Taking on the Role of Doctor." In *Health and Canadian Society: Sociological Perspectives, Second Edition*, edited by George Torrance, 399–421. Toronto: Fitzhenry and Whiteside

Harding, Jim. 1987. "The Pharmaceutical Industry as a Public-Health Hazard and as an Institution of Social Control." In *Health and Canadian Society: Sociological Perspectives, Second Edition*, edited by George Torrance, 545–67. Toronto: Fitzhenry and Whiteside.

Heidegger, Martin. 1999. *Ontology—The Hermeneutics of Facticity.* Bloomington: Indiana University Press [1988].

Illich, Ivan. 1975. *Medical Nemesis: The Expropriation of Health.* Toronto: McClelland and Stewart.

Jung, Carl G. 1951. *Aion: Researches into the Phenomenology of the Self.* Princeton, NJ: Princeton University Press [1959].

Kelleher, David, Jonathan Gabe, and Gareth Williams. 1994a. "Understanding Medical Dominance in the Modern World." In *Challenging Medicine*, edited by Jonathan Gabe, David Kelleher, and Gareth Williams, xi–xxix. London: Routledge.

Kelleher, David, Jonathan Gabe, and Gareth Williams. 1994b. "Epilogue: The Last Days of Doctor Power." In *Challenging Medicine*, edited by Jonathan Gabe, David Kelleher, and Gareth Williams, 183–87. London: Routledge.

Khare, R. S. 1977. "Ritual Purity and Pollution in Relation to Domestic Sanitation." In *Culture, Disease, and Healing: Studies in Medical Anthropology*, edited by David Landy, 242–50. New York: Macmillan.

Lévi-Strauss, Claude. 1977. "The Sorcerer and his Magic." In *Culture, Disease, and Healing: Studies in Medical Anthropology*, edited by David Landy, 445–53. New York: Macmillan.

Lilburn, Tim. 1999. *Living in the World as If It Were Home: Essays.* Dunvegen, Ontario: Cormorant Books.

Lingis, Alphonso. 1989. *Deathbound Subjectivity.* Bloomington, Indiana University Press.

Lösch, August. 1967. *The Economics of Location.* New York: Wiley Science Editions, John Wiley and Sons [1945].

Martin, Emily. 1994. "Medical Metaphors of Women's Bodies: Menstruation and Menopause." In *Women's Health, Politics, and Power: Essays on Sex/Gender, Medicine and Public Health*, edited by Elizabeth Fee and Nancy Krieger, 213–32. Amityville, NY: Baywood.

Midgely, Mary. 2004. *The Myths We Live By.* London: Routledge.

Morgan, Myfanwy. 1982. "The Doctor-Patient Relationship." In *Sociology as Applied to Medicine*, edited by Donald L. Patrick and Graham Scambler, 56–70. Bailliére's Concise Medical Textbooks. London: Bailliére Tindall.

Natanson, Maurice. 1970. *The Journeying Self: A Study in Philosophy and Social Role.* Reading, MA: Addison-Wesley Publishing Company.

Neumann, Erich. 1970. *The Origins and History of Consciousness.* Princeton: Princeton University Press [1949].

Patrick, Donald L., and Graham Scambler, eds. 1982, *Sociology as Applied to Medicine.* Bailliére's Concise Medical Textbooks. London: Bailliére Tindall.

Scambler, Graham. 1982. "Deviance, Labelling and Stigma." In *Sociology as Applied to Medicine,* edited by Donald L. Patrick and Graham Scambler, 184–91. Bailliére's Concise Medical Textbooks. London: Bailliére Tindall.

Selye, Hans. 1956. *The Stress of Life: A New Theory of Disease.* New York: McGraw-Hill.

Shem, Samuel. 1978. *The House of God.* New York: Berkley Books.

Shem, Samuel. 2010. "Afterword." In *The House of God.* New York: Berkley Books.

Sigerist, Henry E. 1977. "The Special Position of the Sick." In *Culture, Disease, and Healing: Studies in Medical Anthropology,* edited by David Landy, 388–93. New York: Macmillan.

Simmel, Georg. 2010. *The View of Life: Four Metaphysical Essays with Journal Aphorisms.* Chicago: The University of Chicago Press [1918].

Sontag, Susan. 1978. *Illness as Metaphor.* New York: Vintage Books.

Sorokin, Pitirim. 1956. *Fads and Foibles in Modern Sociology and Related Sciences.* Chicago: Henry Regnery Company.

Taylor, Charles. 1989. *Sources of the Self: The Making of Modern Identity.* Cambridge, MA: Harvard University Press.

Torrance, George M. 1987. "Hospitals as Health Factories." In *Health and Canadian Society: Sociological Perspectives, Second Edition,* edited by George Torrance, 479–500. Toronto: Fitzhenry and Whiteside.

Westlake, Aubrey T. 1973. *The Pattern of Health: A Search for a Greater Understanding of the Life Force in Health and Disease.* London: Shambhalla and Routledge and Kegan Paul.

Williams, Gareth, and Jennie Popay. 1994. "Lay Knowledge and the Privilege of Experience." In *Challenging Medicine,* edited by Jonathan Gabe, David Kelleher, and Gareth Williams, 118–39. London: Routledge.

HISTORY AND PHILOSOPHY OF SCIENCE

Heresy, Crossroads, and Intersections

Paolo Palmieri, *General Editor*

This series invites book proposals that include innovative strategies for pursuing history and philosophy of science. Especially welcome are scholarly works using non-analytic philosophical perspectives to successfully bring to bear on our understanding of how scientific practices are related to the humanities and the social sciences. The series also welcomes exploration of the sciences in relation to gender, culture, society, and the intellectual and social contexts that illuminate the places, the structures of origination, and the patterns of development over generations. Approaches may include focused analyses of thinkers from unorthodox perspectives that can shed new light on the history and philosophy of science, such as Montaigne, Bruno, Galileo, Newton, Pascal, Emerson, Thoreau, Nietzsche, Jung, Freud. Proposals aimed at probing the philosophical intersections between the sciences and other societal practices that can be configured as heretic are also encouraged. These might include the emergence of the psychoanalytic movements in the twentieth century, how the fine arts have impinged on the historical processes that gave rise to the sciences over the last few centuries, how in turn the intellectual frameworks inaugurated by the sciences have been imported into the avant-garde movements that paralleled the advent of industrialized societies, and finally how contemporary scientific domains of knowledge reverberate in 'deviant' social and artistic practices.

For additional information about this series or for the submission of manuscripts, please contact:

Peter Lang Publishing
Acquisitions Department
29 Broadway, 18th floor
New York, NY 10006

To order other books in this series, please contact our Customer Service Department:

800-770-LANG (within the U.S.)
212-647-7706 (outside the U.S.)
212-647-7707 FAX

Or browse online by series at:

www.peterlang.com

www.ingramcontent.com/pod-product-compliance
Ingram Content Group UK Ltd.
Pitfield, Milton Keynes, MK11 3LW, UK
UKHW020217290926
15470UKWH00001B/250

9 781433 143281